# RADIOISOTOPE ENGINEERING

# RADIOISOTOPE ENGINEERING

*Edited by GEOFFREY G. EICHHOLZ*

*School of Nuclear Engineering*
*Georgia Institute of Technology*
*Atlanta, Georgia 30332*

MARCEL DEKKER, INC., New York 1972

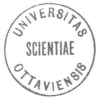

TK
9400
. E5
1972

MARCEL DEKKER, INC.
*95 Madison Avenue, New York, New York 10016*

LIBRARY OF CONGRESS CATALOG CARD NUMBER: 77–142891
ISBN: 0–8247–1156–4


PRINTED IN THE UNITED STATES OF AMERICA

# PREFACE

The use of radioactive materials, substances that emit nuclear radiations spontaneously, has grown enormously during the past decade. This is largely due to the increased production and availability of such materials and to the great volume of research and development performed in many countries all over the world to apply the unique properties of radioisotopes to a wide range of medical and industrial problems. This process of expansion and development has converted many uses that previously were considered only scientific curiosities into commercially important processes that have promise of ever-widening utility. These include such varied applications as radiation sterilization of medical supplies, radiation gauging of material thicknesses, location of oil-bearing horizons far underground, and neutron or gamma-ray radiography of cancerous tumors and metal castings.

In this process, there has been a gradual lessening in many countries of the initially tight government monopoly over all uses of radioisotopes, with commercial interests entering many aspects of the field. Also, there has developed a greater public awareness of the many potential benefits of this area of nuclear engineering, replacing, albeit slowly, the almost superstitious fear associated with all aspects of nuclear energy, engendered by the memory of the birth of large-scale nuclear development under the aegis of the atomic bomb. A great deal of effort is still necessary to inform the public and to accustom it to the increasingly widespread use of radioactive materials, primarily in the industrial radiation field.

This growing use of radioisotopes, both in terms of numbers and in the level of source activity utilized, imposes an obligation on the scientists and engineers involved to design and predict the performance of such nuclear application systems to an ever-increasing degree of reliability and efficiency. Gone are the days when every new application could justify a major research and development effort before a system could be designed. As the number and size of radiation application systems grow, nuclear engineers will be called upon to apply their knowledge and experience to an increasing extent to produce system designs based on *engineering* principles. It is the purpose of this book to discuss many of the engineering aspects of the use of high-level radioisotope sources in medicine and industry and to present in convenient form much information and data material that until now were accessible only through the report literature.

*Geoffrey G. Eichholz*

*Atlanta, Georgia*

# CONTRIBUTORS TO THIS VOLUME

JOHN C. BRADBURNE, JR., Lockheed-Georgia Co., Dawsonville, Georgia

E. ALFRED BURRILL, Consultant, 506 Cuesta Drive, Aptos, California

J. D. CLEMENT, Georgia Institute of Technology, Atlanta, Georgia

KIRK DRUMHELLER, Pacific Northwest Laboratories, Battelle Memorial Institute, Richland, Washington

GEOFFREY G. EICHHOLZ, Georgia Institute of Technology, School of Nuclear Engineering, Atlanta, Georgia

L. GALANTER, Brookhaven National Laboratory, Upton, Long Island, New York

E. J. HENNELLY, Theoretical Physics Division, Savannah River Laboratory, E. I. du Pont de Nemours & Co., Aiken, South Carolina

B. MANOWITZ, Brookhaven National Laboratory, Upton, Long Island, New York

F. X. RIZZO, Brookhaven National Laboratory, Upton, Long Island, New York

ALEXANDER SHEWCHENKO, Atomic Energy of Canada Limited, Ottawa, Ontario, Canada

# CONTENTS

# CONTENTS

# RADIOISOTOPE ENGINEERING

# 1 INTRODUCTION

## GEOFFREY G. EICHHOLZ

GEORGIA INSTITUTE OF TECHNOLOGY
ATLANTA, GEORGIA

## I. GENERAL CONCEPTS

Radioisotope engineering is that branch of nuclear engineering that concerns itself with the production, application, and installation of intense radioisotope sources in a variety of fields of science and industry. It differs from reactor engineering in that the production of large quantities of power is not of primary concern and from the uses of (low-level) radioisotopes as tracers in that the nature of the radioactive materials places a major responsibility on the design engineer in providing for their safe handling, installation, and use. In dealing with such materials, which often possess a combination of unusual chemical properties as well as requiring great care in handling because of the associated radiation levels, many new considerations are encountered by the engineer who is faced

*1*

with the responsibility of planning the production or use of high-intensity radioactive sources. Until recently, this field has been overshadowed by the apparent urgency of solving the many outstanding problems in reactor technology; now, the increasing demand and widespread application of radioisotopes as sources of penetrating radiations are creating a need for the training of engineers capable of dealing with the requirements of this rapidly growing field. Since the major use of such radioisotopes is as sources of radiation, whatever the nature of the nuclear radiation emitted in each case, it is convenient to refer to such a localized and encapsulated radioisotope material simply as a "source."

Radioactivity was discovered by H. A. Becquerel in 1896 when he observed the spontaneous emission of penetrating radiations from uranium ore. Subsequent research at many centers, notably by Pierre and Marie Curie and their associates in Paris and by E. Rutherford and his students in Montreal, Manchester, and Cambridge, helped to elucidate the nature of the radiations emitted and the genetic relationships among the decay products of natural uranium, thorium, and actinium. It was found that radioactive emission was associated with the successive conversion from one daughter substance to another, until the material finally reached a stable substance identifiable as lead or bismuth. F. W. Aston coined the term "isotope" when he showed by means of his mass spectrograph that most elements are made up of various proportions of nuclides with the identical number of electrons determining their place in the periodic table but possessing different atomic masses.

An isotope of mass $A$ of an element of atomic number $Z$ is now defined in terms of the number of protons $Z$ and the number of neutrons $A - Z$ contained in its nucleus. Odd-$Z$ elements possess as a rule only one or two stable isotopes, whereas even-$Z$ elements may have from one (beryllium) to ten (tin) stable isotopes. These stable isotopes tend to be clustered along a line of maximum stability in a nuclide chart that starts with a ratio of neutrons to protons of 1:1 for the light elements and rises slowly with atomic number, to a value of 126 : 83 (1.52 : 1) for bismuth-209 ($^{209}$Bi), the heaviest stable nuclide. Unstable isotopes with neutron–proton ratios in excess of the most stable isotope of any element tend to decay by the emission of one or more negative electrons (beta particles) to reach a stable nuclide. Isotopes with a neutron–proton ratio lower than their most stable isotope tend to decay by positive electron (positron, $\beta^+$) emission toward a stable nuclide. Such decays, involving only the emission of nuclear electrons, do not change the mass of the nucleus but only its charge and the decay product is called an "isobar" of its parent nuclide.

All the unstable, radiation-emitting isotopes are referred to as "radio-active isotopes" or, more briefly, as "radioisotopes."

Apart from the naturally occurring radioisotopes, most of which belong to the elements with atomic number $Z > 83$, it is possible to produce a large number of radioisotopes of the other elements by particle bombardment in accelerators or nuclear reactors. Over 1300 of these artificial radioisotopes have been identified, but only a small number have properties that make them useful for medical or industrial purposes.

Since radioisotopes have the same number of electrons and hence the same chemical properties as their stable brethren of equal $Z$, they have long been used to follow and identify the path of a given element through a chemical or biological process. This use of radioisotopes as "tracers" was first introduced by G. von Hevesy in 1915 when he determined the uptake of lead by plants by means of the radioisotope $^{210}$Pb ("radium-D"). Since then, a vast variety of experiments has been done by means of radioisotope tracers and this class of work accounts for the widest range of demand for radioisotopes of almost all the elements (1–7). The amount of radioactivity involved in any tracer test is of necessity limited, both because the dispersion of the tracers makes it essential to restrict the affected volume and the quantity of radioactive material to the minimum amount required for detection, and because the control of contamination and ultimate disposal of an unencapsulated radioactive material becomes a problem as the total quantity becomes large. Hence such test work is usually restricted to specific research or development applications and the tests must be conducted by persons trained in radioisotope techniques.

The use of encapsulated radioisotopes has also shown a steady growth not only in number of applications but also in the strength of the sources employed (8). It is customary to express the strength of radioactive sources in multiples of "curies," where 1 *curie* (Ci) is equivalent to the quantity of any radioisotope that undergoes $3.70 \times 10^{10}$ disintegrations per second. On this scale, radiotracer tests may involve quantities of radioisotopes ranging in strength from $10^{-7}$ to $10^{-1}$ Ci, rarely more (with the exception of tests involving tritium); encapsulated sources, on the other hand, have been prepared and are being planned with strengths up to $10^8$ Ci. It is this range in source strengths of encapsulated materials that makes it convenient to distinguish between low-level, medium-level, and high-level radioisotope sources. Much of the subsequent discussion will center on the preparation and handling of high-level sources.

The distinctive value of radioactive sources is the fact that they provide a compact, uninterruptible, and uniform source of energy which is emitted

TABLE

CHARACTERISTICS OF ISOTOPES

| Isotope | Half-life, years | Principal chemical form | Density (compound) (g/cm³) | Principal radiation | MPC, ($\mu$Ci/cm³)[a] | Watts/gram (pure isotope) |
|---|---|---|---|---|---|---|
| $^{60}$Co | 5.3 | Co metal | 8.7 | $\gamma$ | $3 \times 10^{-9}$ | 17.4 |
| $^{192}$Ir | 0.21 | Ir metal | 22.4 | $\gamma$ | $4 \times 10^{-8}$ | — |
| $^{90}$Sr | 28 | SrTiO$_3$ | 3.7 | $\beta, X$ | $3 \times 10^{-10}$ | 0.95 |
| $^{137}$Cs | 30 | CsCl | 3.6 | $\beta, \gamma$ | $5 \times 10^{-9}$ | 0.42 |
| $^{144}$Ce | 0.78 | Ce$_2$O$_3$ | 6.6 | $\beta, \gamma$ | $2 \times 10^{-9}$ | 25.6 |
| $^{147}$Pm | 2.6 | Pm$_2$O$_3$ | 6.6 | $\beta$ | $2 \times 10^{-8}$ | 0.33 |
| $^{170}$Tm | 0.35 | Tm$_2$O$_3$ | 7.7 | $\beta$ | $1 \times 10^{-8}$ | 12.1 |
| $^{210}$Po | 0.38 | GdPo | 10 | $\alpha$ | $2 \times 10^{-9}$ | 141 |
| $^{238}$Pu | 87.4 | PuO$_2$ | 10 | $\alpha$ | $7 \times 10^{-13}$ | 0.50 |
| $^{242}$Cm | 0.45 | Cm$_2$O$_3$ | 9 | $\alpha, n$ | $4 \times 10^{-11}$ | 120 |
| $^{244}$Cm | 18 | Cm$_2$O$_3$ | 9 | $\alpha, n$ | $3 \times 10^{-12}$ | 2.8 |

[a]MPC = maximum permissible concentration in air.

[b]For transfers to other U.S. federal agencies only, based on estimated costs in the late 1970s.

[c]Value in parentheses is inches of lead shielding required for a 1-kW source to reduce radiation to 10 mR/hr at 1 m. Does *not* include neutron shielding for curium.

in the form of nuclear radiations: alpha or beta particles, gamma radiation, or neutrons. The absorption or conversion of this energy into heat or other chemical energy has been studied extensively and has led to a large number of actual or potential applications. Of these the most important are the uses of radioisotope sources in medical or industrial radiography, radiation gauges, radiation therapy, radiation processing, preservation, deinfestation, and sterilization of foodstuffs and medical supplies, and various radiation process uses in the chemical and plastics industries. In addition, there are many specialized developments such as the use of radioisotopes as power sources for marine and space applications, radioactive luminescence sources, and deionizing devices. These

1.1

| Watts/gram (compound) | Power density (compound) (watts/cm³) | Curies per watt | Cost range, ($/thermal watt)[b] | Shielding required[c] | Remarks |
|---|---|---|---|---|---|
| 1.7 | 15.2 | 65 | 7–25 | Heavy(9.5) | Currently in large-scale use principally as radiation source |
| — | — | — | — | Heavy (7) | |
| 0.22 | 0.82 | 148 | 25–35 | Heavy(6) | Terrestrial power fuel |
| 0.12 | 0.42 | 207 | 20–30 | Heavy(4.6) | Alternative to $^{60}$Co |
| 3.8 | 25.3 | 126 | 1 | Heavy(10.2) | Being considered for short-lived terrestrial heat sources |
| 0.27 | 1.8 | 2788 | 200–600 | Minor(1) | Being used in thermal conditioning applications |
| 1.07 | 8.2 | 445 | 10–25 | Moderate (2.5) | Being considered as alternative to $^{210}$Po |
| 82.4 | 824 | 32 | 10–25 | Minor(1) | Space: short-lived fuel |
| 0.36 | 3.6 | 30 | 500–700 | Minor(0.1) | Space: long-lived fuel |
| 98 | 882 | 28 | — | Minor(0.4) | |
| 2.5 | 22.5 | 29 | 100–500 | Moderate (2) | Being considered to supplement $^{238}$Pu |

applications have been reviewed in great detail elsewhere (*1, 2, 7, 9–13*) and it is not proposed to dwell on them all in any detail. However, it will be necessary to discuss some of their common features to establish a logical departure point for any treatment of high-level sources.

Before World War II, the only radioisotope source that was readily available for radiographic or therapy purposes, though at considerable expense, was radium-226 or its daughter radon-222, usually dispensed in the form of glass or steel needles that might hold 1–100 $\mu$Ci. The total amount of $^{226}$Ra available world-wide before 1939 was of the order of 100 Ci, most of it supplied by the mines in the Katanga region of the Belgian Congo. The gamma radiation that is the main emission of these sources is actually due to one of the daughter elements, $^{214}$Bi ("radium-C") emitting gamma rays of energy 0.609 MeV* and others of lesser intensity but higher energy, resulting in a spectrum centering on about 0.86 MeV.

The situation changed drastically when it was found, as a result of the atomic energy research effort since 1942, that nuclear reactors were capable of producing many radioisotopes in copious amounts at a fraction of the cost involved in radium production. Most of the reactor-produced sources are made by neutron capture in the target material which results in an isotope one unit heavier than the original atom. Many of these product isotopes will be radioactive and some have properties that make them useful as sources. However, it is also possible to produce radioisotopes by charged particle bombardment in accelerators and by neutron-induced reactions other than the radiative capture process. Because of the large number of neutrons available for nuclear reactions in a nuclear reactor, most high-level sources are made by utilizing either the neutron capture (n, $\gamma$) reaction or the fission (n, f) reaction. The latter occurs when a fissile nuclide, such as $^{235}$U, $^{238}$U, or $^{241}$Pu, is bombarded with neutrons and breaks up into two "fission fragments" of much lower mass that are initially highly radioactive. In addition, by a process of successive neutron captures, production of high-level sources of the transuranium elements occurs, which is of interest because of the high energy density that some of these sources possess.

Apart from the latter group of sources, it is found in practice that the number of radioisotopes that combine a desirable conjunction of radiation characteristics, ease of production, and acceptable life time is exceedingly limited. Since the cost of production, transportation, and installation of high-level sources is large, it is essential that their usable life, the period before they lose a significant part of their strength, should be commensurate with the replacement cost. The source strength of all radioisotopes decreases exponentially with time and it is customary to express the decay characteristic of a radioisotope in terms of its half-life, i.e., the time it takes its activity to decrease to half its initial value. It is found that there are few of the more readily prepared radioisotopes that have half-lives exceeding 3 months, let alone a year. Table 1.1 lists the main characteristics of the radioisotopes most commonly employed in medium-level and high-level sources (*14*). Table 1.2 lists the properties of the potentially most useful products which can be recovered from reactor fuel reprocessing.

---

*See Appendix A for definitions of units.

## II.  RADIOISOTOPES AS ENERGY SOURCES

It is seen that these radioisotopes fall into two groups, those produced by a neutron capture reaction with a high reaction cross section and adequate half-life to justify the cost of production, and those produced by nuclear fission in reactor fuel from which they can be extracted by subsequent processing and separation. The first group includes notably cobalt-60, iridium-192, and, with reservations, thulium-170; the second group comprises cesium-137, strontium–yttrium-90, krypton-85, and promethium-147. Other methods of isotope production, such as accelerator production or fast neutron induced (n, p), (n, $\alpha$), (n, 2n) reactions, are of less significance in this connection because of their low yield and relatively high cost.

Of the sources listed in Table 1.1, cobalt-60 and cesium-137 occupy a special place. This is because at the present time they are the only two materials that can be seriously considered in terms of availability and low cost for the manufacture of kilocurie and megacurie sources. Since cobalt-60 can be made with a pure cobalt metal target by the $^{59}$Co (n, $\gamma$) $^{60}$Co reaction in any reactor with adequate neutron flux, its production, especially for beam therapy units, has received widespread attention and it is now commercially available from many agencies. The quantity made is determined by the activation equation

$$A = N_0 \sigma \phi (1 - e^{-0.69t/\tau_{1/2}}) \tag{1.1}$$

where $A$ = activity of the product at the end of irradiation for time $t$, $N_0$ = number of atoms in the target material, $\phi$ = thermal neutron flux, $\sigma$ = thermal neutron cross section,* and $\tau_{1/2}$ = half-life of product atoms. The number of atoms $N$ of the radioisotope produced by the neutron bombardment is give by the relation

$$A = -dN/dt = \lambda N = (0.693/\tau_{1/2})N$$

or $$\tag{1.2}$$

$$N = \frac{N_0 \sigma \phi \tau_{1/2}}{0.693} (1 - e^{-0.693t/\tau_{1/2}})$$

where $\lambda = 0.693/\tau_{1/2}$ is the decay constant. At any later time $t'$, the activity will have decayed to

---

*See Appendix B for a definition of terms.

TABLE 1.2

PRODUCTS FROM REACTOR FUEL PROCESSING THAT APPEAR MOST REASONABLE AS USEFUL MATERIALS

| Element or isotope | Half-life (years) | Isotopic purity (%) | Current price ($) | Potential uses |
|---|---|---|---|---|
| **A. Fission Products** | | | | |
| $^{85}$Kr | 10.76 | 5 | $22.00/Ci[a] | Special light source, radiation source (phosphors) |
| $^{90}$Sr | 28 | 50 | 0.20/Ci[a] | Heat source, beta source |
| $^{99}$Tc | $2.1 \times 10^5$ | 100 | 55.00/g[a] | Corrosion inhibitor, alloying agent, semiconductor |
| Rhodium | Essentially stable mixture[c] | 100 | 8.00/g[b] | Industrial, electrical, decorative |
| Ruthenium | Stable mixture + 1-year $^{106}$Ru | 3.3% $^{106}$Ru | 1.85/g[b] | Heat and beta source |
| Palladium | Essentially stable mixture[c] | — | 1.45/g[b] | Industrial, electrical, decorative |
| Xenon | Stable mixture | — | 35.00/liter (STP)[d] | Special light sources |
| $^{137}$Cs | 30 | 35 | 0.125/Ci[a] | Heat and gamma sources |
| $^{144}$Ce | 0.78 | 18[e] | 0.15/Ci[a] | Heat and beta sources |
| $^{147}$Pm | 2.7 | 100 | 0.20/Ci[a] | Heat, beta, and X-ray sources |
| **B. Plutonium Isotopes** | | | | |
| $^{238}$Pu | 87.4 | 80 | $1,000/g[f] | Heat and alpha sources |
| $^{239}$Pu | 24,000 | Depends on exposure; can be very high (>95), but likely 40 to 70 | 10/g[g] | Fissionable material and source of heavier isotopes |
| $^{240}$Pu | 6,800 | Depends on exposure; 5 to >40 | 0 | Fertile material and source of heavier isotopes |
| $^{241}$Pu | 13 | Depends on exposure; 1 to >20 | 10/g[g] | Fissionable material and source of heavier isotopes |

| | | | | |
|---|---|---|---|---|
| $^{242}$Pu | $3.8 \times 10^5$ | Depends on exposure; 0.5 to near 100 | 0 | Target for $^{243}$Am formation and source of other heavier isotopes |
| | | **C. Heavier Isotopes** | | |
| $^{236}$U | $2.4 \times 10^7$ | A few tenths | —[h] | Target for $^{237}$Np formation in normal fuel |
| $^{237}$Np | $2.1 \times 10^6$ | Essentially 100 | \$ 225/g[f] | Target for $^{238}$Pu formation |
| $^{241}$Am | 458 | May be 100, but depends on source[i] | 1,000/g[f] | Heat source and target for $^{242}$Cm ($^{238}$Pu) |
| $^{243}$Am | 7,650 | May be 100, but depends on source[i] | — | Target for $^{244}$Cm and other heavier isotopes |
| $^{242}$Cm | 0.45 | May be 100, but depends on source[i] | 20,000/g[j] | Heat source and precursor of $^{238}$Pu |
| $^{244}$Cm | 18.1 | Fairly pure; may contain some $^{245}$Cm | 1,000/g[j] | Heat sources and target for other heavier isotopes |

[a] *Radioisotopes, Stable Isotopes, Research Materials*, Isotopes Development Center, Oak Ridge National Laboratory, Oak Ridge, Tenn.

[b] Current prices (calculated from prices per troy ounce), *Eng. Mining J.* 169, 2 (1968).

[c] Palladium includes very-long-lived, very-low-beta-energy $^{107}$Pd, assumed to be completely nonhazardous and nonobjectionable in all uses. Rhodium will include slight but significant amounts of active $^{102}$Rh. The concentrations in power-reactor fuels have not yet been established.

[d] Price of by-product material from liquid-air manufacturing.

[e] For low exposures; for long exposures (25,000 MWd/T) and a 1-year decay time before processing, composition is about 4.5%.

[f] *Nucleonics Week*, 9 (17), 4 (Apr. 25, 1968).

[g] The estimated fuel value of $^{239}$Pu and $^{241}$Pu is $10/g

[h] Not separated; stays with $^{238}$U or enriched uranium.

[i] Pure $^{241}$Am may be recovered from aged plutonium (from $^{241}$Pu decay); however, from reactor fuel processing it will be mixed with $^{243}$Am and even some $^{242}$Am (152 years); the composition of such mixtures depends on the exposure. At 25,000 MWd/T exposure, the americium is essentially 50:50 $^{241}$Am and $^{243}$Am. Such mixtures also assure that separated curium will also consist of both $^{242}$Cm and $^{244}$Cm, but on aging, fairly pure $^{244}$Cm should result along with pure $^{238}$Pu from the decayed $^{242}$Cm.

[j] H. L. Davis, Radionuclide Power for Space—Part 1, Isotope Cost and Availability, *Nucleonics*, 21 (3) 61–65 (1963).

TABLE   1.3

UNITED STATES AEC PRICES FOR METALLIC COBALT-60 (1968)

Capsules designed with various dimensions for radiography, teletherapy, and heat sources have been fabricated at the Laboratory.[a] Teletherapy and other sources containing more than 1400 Ci are available from the Laboratory. Encapsulated sources containing less than 1400 Ci are commercially available; however, the Laboratory can supply these smaller sources if they are for resale.

| Specific activity (Ci/g) | Quantity in single order (Ci) | Price per curie |
|---|---|---|
| to 15 | 100,000 or more | $0.40 |
| 15 and to 30 | 100,000 or more | 0.50 |
| 30 and to 45[b] | 100,000 to 250,000 | 0.65 |
| | 250,001 to 500,000 | 0.60 |
| | > 500,000 | 0.55 |

Metallic $^{60}Co$ is available with specific activity not to exceed 45 Ci/g provided it is ordered in 100,000-Ci lots. Requests for higher specific activity and/or smaller amounts can be filled only if it has been determined that the material is not available commercially. Price schedules and applicable discounts for these materials are as follows:

| Specific activity (Ci/g) | Price per curie | Quantity ordered (Ci) | Discount (%) |
|---|---|---|---|
| to   30 | $2.00 | to   5,000 | List price |
| 30 and to   40 | 3.00 | 5,000 and to   25,000 | 15 |
| 40 and to   55 | 4.00 | 25,000 and to 100,000 | 30 |
| 55 and to   70 | 5.25 | | |
| 70 and to   85 | 5.65 | | |
| 85 and to 100 | 5.85 | | |
| 100 and to 115 | 6.05 | | |
| 115 and to 130 | 6.20 | | |
| 130 and to 145 | 6.40 | | |
| 145 and to 160 | 6.60 | | |
| 160 and to 175 | 6.80 | | |
| 175 and to 190 | 7.00 | | |
| 190 and to 205 | 7.20 | | |

[a]Refers to Oak Ridge National Laboratory.
[b]Can be supplied only as BNL strips.

TABLE   1.4

UNITED STATES AEC PRICES FOR CESIUM-137

| Order size (Ci) | Unit price ($/Ci) |
|---|---|
| 0   –   10,000 | 0.50 |
| 10,001   –   50,000 | 0.45 |
| 50,001   –   200,000 | 0.35 |
| Over   200,000 | 0.125 |

$$A' = A\,e^{-0.693\,(t' - t)/\tau_{1/2}} \tag{1.3}$$

The "specific activity" $A/N_0$ is of interest because it determines the source volume for a given source strength; this is important whenever a high-intensity point source is desired, such as in beam therapy units. From Eq. (1.1) it is evident that the production of a high specific activity for a given material is ultimately dependent on the available neutron flux $\phi$ and to a lesser extent on the irradiation time $t$. To make high specific-activity material, e.g., $^{60}$Co, high neutron fluxes in excess of $10^{14}$ n/cm$^2$-sec are required. Only a few reactors are available for this purpose at present so that high specific-activity material is more expensive. To illustrate this point, Table 1.3 presents the 1968 U.S. AEC price list of $^{60}$Co. These prices are for the active material only; it will be seen in Chapter 3 that the cost of processing and encapsulation may exceed this cost manifold.

For comparison it should be noted that 1 mCi of $^{60}$Co purchased as $CoCl_2$ in HCl solution costs \$25 commercially (1969).

Cesium-137 is a fission product produced as a byproduct of $^{235}$U fission burnup in nuclear fuel. It is produced by the reaction $^{235}$U(n,f) $^{137}$Cs $+ 3.5$n with a cross section of (585 barns $\times$ 6% yield) $= 35.5$ barns effectively. Its present price and availability depend on the reprocessing rate of burnt-up

TABLE 1.5

UNITED STATES MANUFACTURING COST GOAL RANGES FOR RADIOISOTOPES (REF. *15*)

| Isotope source | 1968 Fission product prices | | |
|---|---|---|---|
| | MCi/yr | Cents/curie | \$/thermal watt |
| $^{90}$Sr | 5–10 | 20 | 30 |
| $^{137}$Cs | 2 | 12.5 | 26 |
| $^{147}$Pm | 6 | 20 | 560 |

| Isotope source | Long-term goal prices |
|---|---|
| | Manufacturing cost, goal range (\$/thermal watt) |
| $^{90}$Sr | 25 – 35 |
| $^{137}$Cs | 20 – 30 |
| $^{147}$Pm | 200 – 600 |
| $^{60}$Co | 7 – 25 |
| $^{170}$Tm | 10 – 25 |
| $^{210}$Po | 10 – 25 |
| $^{238}$Pu | 500 – 700 |
| $^{244}$Cm | 100 – 500 |

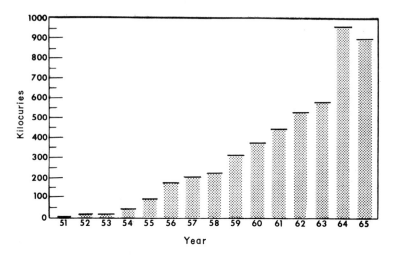

FIG. 1.1   Commercial consumption of cobalt-60 in the United States.

fuel, done usually for plutonium recovery and for easier waste disposal, and the set price can only be regarded as artificial, depending as it does on the plutonium value, the set-off against waste disposal cost and the competitive pressure of cobalt-60. Table 1.4 lists the current (1969) U.S. AEC prices for cesium-137 in quantity to illustrate the price range. Table 1.5 tabulates cost goal ranges for bulk, unencapsulated products, not including depreciation and profit which must be included in commercial prices. They do assume that the isotopes are produced, processed, and converted to a fuel form and sealed in a primary containment capsule at a government-operated facility. In the case of radioisotopes derived from fuel reprocessing, high specific activity is readily achieved by successively separating off all the fission products. Since the installation of nuclear power stations is growing at a very rapid rate, used fuel elements may be plentiful by 1973 and could become a glut on the market. This will certainly boost the availability of cesium-137 as well as the other fission products and will tend to lower their prices regardless of the value of the plutonium content. On the other hand, an increasing demand for high-level sources for industrial uses and food preservation may also be anticipated and it is by no means certain that supply and demand will remain balanced over the next few years. Figure 1.1 presents some data for $^{60}$Co consumption in the United States (16). Figure 1.2 shows some comparative figures for the anticipated production of major radioisotopes (17).

Figure 1.3 is a graph of the increase in number of radiotherapy units

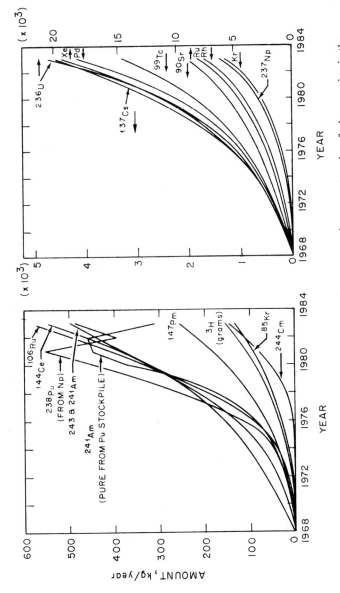

FIG. 1.2  Production of fission products and byproduct isotopes from spent nuclear fuel processing in the United States to 1984.

G. G. EICHHOLZ

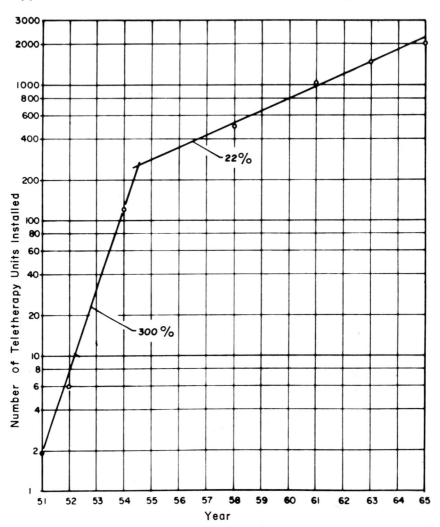

FIG. 1.3  Growth of teletherapy installations throughout the world.

using ⁶⁰Co and, to a lesser extent, ¹³⁷Cs sources in the world as reported by Errington (*16*). In fact, there seems to have occurred a slowdown in new installations of such units, while fresh radioisotope sources were installed in earlier operating machines requiring replacement sources, thus preempting much of the available supply. It is becoming increasingly obvious that it may be necessary to design and operate some reactors pri-

# NUCLEAR ELECTRIC PLANTS

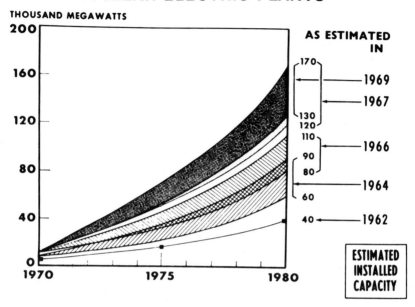

FIG. 1.4 Growth estimates for the U.S. nuclear power industry (18).

marily as radioisotope producers, instead of treating such production as a sideline operation ancillary to power production or heat generation.

The other aspect closely affecting the cost and availability of radioactive sources is the enormous upsurge in the construction of high power nuclear reactors in recent years, as illustrated in Fig. 1.4 which presents American projections only. It has been predicted that the growth in nuclear power capacity in the rest of the Western world will roughly equal the U.S. figures. Most of these reactors will go into operation in the early 1970s and are predominantly of the water-cooled, $^{235}$U-enriched, thermal neutron type. The reprocessing of the fuel elements and the extraction of the longer-lived fission products will entail major capital investment in most industrialized countries and may well build up a large, and largely undesired, stockpile of long-lived fission products. As a rough rule, each megawatt of operation produces one megacurie of fission product activity at the moment of shutdown. Even after several months' storage, the quantity of long-lived fission products in each reactor core that has been taken to its economical burnup value represents a large source of radioactivity.

It has been proposed to utilize used fuel elements as radiation sources without further treatment for maximum economic return. However, economic analysis on the shipment, handling, and replacement cost of such sources, necessitated by the short effective half-life, which is that of $^{95}$Zr–Nb, the dominant medium-life fission product, makes such applications much less attractive.

The use of the long-lived cesium-137, as extracted from the fuel elements, is governed by the cost of extraction and the alternative costs of storage and ultimate disposal, or encapsulation and utilization in radiation sources. At first sight, the latter way seems to be the logical alternative until it is realized that supply is likely to outweigh demand for radiation sources even under the most sanguine expectations for many years to come.

### III.  PHYSICAL AND CHEMICAL PROPERTIES

Although the most obvious and discerning characteristic of radioisotopes is the emission of radiation, their full utilization for industrial applications depends on a combination of physical and chemical properties. Nevertheless, it is customary to specify the quantity of any radioisotope by its activity, in curies, rather than its mass or volume. These can be deduced by the use of Eq. (1.2) for any isotope whose half-life is known.

If the product material can be separated chemically from the target material or dissolved fuel solution without the addition of "carrier" atoms, which might facilitate the separation by providing a macrochemical separation condition, the isotope is referred to as *carrier-free* and has the highest specific activity $A/N$ possible under the circumstances. If carrier-free production is not possible or if the isotope is contained in target material of the same element, which is therefore chemically identical, then the specific activity is given by $A/(N_0+N) \doteqdot A/N_0$ in most cases, where $N_0$ is the number of inert, nonradioactive atoms. A high specific activity is desirable whenever the highest activity is required from a source of minimum dimensions, e.g., for point sources in teletherapy machines or for space power units.

Since radioisotopes are physically and chemically similar to the stable isotopes of the particular element involved, they undergo the same chemical reactions, form the same compounds, and have the same bulk properties in the solid, liquid, or gaseous states. In fact, until the moment of their decay, when they emit radiation and change their chemical "name and address," they are indistinguishable from their stable isotopes, ex-

TABLE 1.6

Fission-Product Beta Emitters

| Nuclide | Fission yield (%) | Half-life (years) | β Energy (MeV) | γ Energy (MeV) | Min. Wt./Ci (mg) | mW/mg | Power/ kCi (W) | MCi/kW | Activity produced/MW-yr of reactor operation (Ci) |
|---|---|---|---|---|---|---|---|---|---|
| 85Kr | 0.293 | 10.3 | 0.67 | 0.54(0.5%) | 2.45 | 0.49 | 1.2 | 0.83 | 190 |
| 90Sr–Y | 5.77 | 28 | 0.55,2.26 | — | 7.10 | 0.85 | 6.0 | 0.17 | 1200 |
| 106Ru–Rh | 0.38 | 1.0 | 3.53(68%) 3.1 (11%) 2.44(10%) | 0.51(21%) 0.62(10%) | 0.28 | 21.4 | ~6.0 | 0.17 | 1600 |
| 144Ce–Pr | 6.0 | 0.78 | 2.98 0.31(76%) 0.18(24%) | 0.13(24%) | 0.31 | 19.3 | ~6.4 | 0.16 | 30,000 |
| 147Pm | 2.7 | 2.64 | 0.223 | — | 1.09 | 0.35 | 0.36 | 2.8 | 5200 |
| 151Sm | 0.45 | 93 | 0.076 | 0.02(I.C.) | 39.3 | 0.001 | 0.04 | 20 | 28 |

cept in matters of atomic mass as determinable by mass spectroscopy of requisite sensitivity. ($N/N_0$ is usually exceedingly small.) This chemical identity underlies the use of radioisotopes as "tracers," a powerful technique widely used in biological, medical, chemical, and metallurgical studies. It is used to establish pathways, flow times, retention times, recovery yields, flow rates, and dispersion volumes of many systems where such information would be difficult to establish by alternative techniques. Since these tracer applications usually involve unencapsulated, low-level radioisotopes, this field lies outside the scope of this book. The reader is referred to the many excellent books on this subject, some of which are listed at the end of this chapter (2, 4, 6, 19–22).

The emission of radiation represents the liberation of energy which may be appreciable in the aggregate. This energy may be fully deposited within the source material or its enclosure, or it can be utilized for external use for sterilization or chemical applications. Since the energy of a 1-MeV energy quantum is equivalent to $1.6 \times 10^{-7}$ erg, it requires a fairly intense source to develop appreciable amounts of heat. Table 1.6 lists the energy characteristics of the principal fission product beta emitters [Silverman (13)]. It is evident that for $^{90}$Sr or $^{144}$Ce, kilowatt heat sources can be produced, e.g., for space applications, from megacurie radioisotope sources. Such sources would have the advantage of being self-contained and requiring no maintenance. Actual selection has to be made on the basis of energy density, useful life as related to mission time, stability, and cost.

The deposition of appreciable amounts of energy can easily disrupt molecular bonds and a whole new branch of chemistry, radiation chemistry, has grown up around investigations to study the consequences of bond breakage, often accompanied by recoil effects, new bond formation, such as by cross linkage in polymers, and catalytic effects of radiation. The most important of these effects is that of radiolysis of water, which results in the creation of free gas ions, free radicals, and measurable concentrations of hydrogen peroxide. These processes affect the corrosion resistance of vessels containing the irradiated water, e.g., in the cooling channels of reactors, and influence the chemical reactions of any aqueous solutions subjected to internal or external radiations. They add appreciably to the cost of fission product extraction by shortening the useful life of ion exchange resins and other materials used. It becomes necessary to select "radiation-resistant" materials, such as Kreidl-type borosilicate glass or stainless steel, to serve as encapsulating materials. Alternatively it becomes necessary to prepare the source material in a form that is stable under the conditions of heat deposition and irradiation encountered. A good example of this is the preparation of stable strontium-90 sources in the foi ~ of ceramic strontium titanate or as a fused glassy fluoride.

From the foregoing and a glance at Table 1.1, it is evident that radioisotopes of practical interest vary widely in their chemical and physical properties. Some are gaseous in their elemental state, such as $^{85}$Kr or $^{3}$H, and some of the others can only be prepared and stored in compound form. Cobalt and iridium alone among the materials listed in Table 1.1 are available and prepared in pure metallic form, a feature which greatly simplifies their handling and encapsulation, with a consequent saving in the cost of source preparation. Most of the others are usually handled as oxides, but as the example of strontium showed, in the preceding paragraph, it is often necessary to search for a more stable and mechanically more satisfactory compound. A particular case is that of krypton-85 which is often prepared as a clathrate compound (23, 24), which means that the large krypton atoms are trapped interstitially in the lattice structure of certain metals.

Since the type of radiation emitted and its energy vary greatly from isotope to isotope, each isotope must be contained in a capsule designed for the specific application. In the case of the beta emitters in Table 1.6 and pure alpha sources such as $^{210}$Po or $^{238}$Pu, the radiation is absorbed almost entirely internally and the capsule has to be capable of dissipating the heat generated and withstanding the constant radiation bombardment without cracking or leaking. In the case of the gamma-ray sources in Table 1.1, the main function of the capsule is the safe containment of the source material, without leakage and without appreciable absorption of the radiation.

For both beta and gamma radiation, the primary absorption in a material is given by a relation of the form

$$I/I_0 = e^{-\mu x} \tag{1.4}$$

where $I_0$ is the incident intensity of radiation of a given energy, $I$ is the intensity after passage through a material thickness $x$. $\mu$ is called the "linear absorption coefficient" and is characteristic of the material and the radiation energy.

The amount of energy deposited in a given volume external to the source per unit volume is called the "dose." It clearly represents the energy lost according to Eq. (1.4) in passing through the material, supplemented by any secondary effects that may have been caused by the passage of the incident particle or photon (25–27). The calculation of

TABLE
TOTAL MASS ATTENUATION
*Data from*

| Mate-rial | Gamma-ray | | | | | | | | |
|---|---|---|---|---|---|---|---|---|---|
| | 0.1 | 0.15 | 0.2 | 0.3 | 0.4 | 0.5 | 0.6 | 0.8 | 1.0 |
| H | 0.295 | 0.265 | 0.243 | 0.212 | 0.189 | 0.173 | 0.160 | 0.140 | 0.126 |
| Be | 0.132 | 0.119 | 0.109 | 0.0945 | 0.0847 | 0.0773 | 0.715 | 0.0628 | 0.0565 |
| C | 0.149 | 0.134 | 0.122 | 0.106 | 0.0953 | 0.0870 | 0.0805 | 0.0707 | 0.0636 |
| N | 0.150 | 0.134 | 0.123 | 0.106 | 0.0955 | 0.869 | 0.0805 | 0.0707 | 0.0636 |
| O | 0.151 | 0.134 | 0.123 | 0.107 | 0.0953 | 0.0870 | 0.0806 | 0.0708 | 0.0636 |
| Na | 0.151 | 0.130 | 0.118 | 0.102 | 0.0912 | 0.0833 | 0.0770 | 0.0676 | 0.0608 |
| Mg | 0.160 | 0.135 | 0.122 | 0.106 | 0.0944 | 0.0860 | 0.0795 | 0.0699 | 0.0627 |
| Al | 0.161 | 0.134 | 0.120 | 0.103 | 0.0922 | 0.0840 | 0.0777 | 0.0683 | 0.0614 |
| Si | 0.172 | 0.139 | 0.125 | 0.107 | 0.0954 | 0.0869 | 0.0802 | 0.0706 | 0.0635 |
| P | 0.174 | 0.137 | 0.122 | 0.104 | 0.0928 | 0.0846 | 0.0780 | 0.0685 | 0.0617 |
| S | 0.188 | 0.144 | 0.127 | 0.108 | 0.0958 | 0.0874 | 0.0806 | 0.0707 | 0.0635 |
| Ar | 0.188 | 0.135 | 0.117 | 0.0977 | 0.0867 | 0.0790 | 0.0730 | 0.0638 | 0.0573 |
| K | 0.215 | 0.149 | 0.127 | 0.106 | 0.0938 | 0.0852 | 0.0786 | 0.0689 | 0.0618 |
| Ca | 0.238 | 0.158 | 0.132 | 0.109 | 0.0965 | 0.0876 | 0.0809 | 0.0708 | 0.0634 |
| Fe | 0.344 | 0.183 | 0.138 | 0.106 | 0.0919 | 0.0828 | 0.0762 | 0.0664 | 0.0595 |
| Cu | 0.427 | 0.206 | 0.147 | 0.108 | 0.0916 | 0.0820 | 0.0751 | 0.0654 | 0.0585 |
| Mo | 1.03 | 0.389 | 0.225 | 0.130 | 0.0998 | 0.0851 | 0.0761 | 0.0648 | 0.0575 |
| Sn | 1.58 | 0.563 | 0.303 | 0.153 | 0.109 | 0.0886 | 0.0776 | 0.0647 | 0.0568 |
| I | 1.83 | 0.648 | 0.339 | 0.165 | 0.114 | 0.0913 | 0.0792 | 0.0653 | 0.0571 |
| W | 4.21 | 1.44 | 0.708 | 0.293 | 0.174 | 0.125 | 0.101 | 0.0763 | 0.0640 |
| Pt | 4.75 | 1.64 | 0.795 | 0.324 | 0.191 | 0.135 | 0.107 | 0.0800 | 0.0659 |
| Tl | 5.16 | 1.80 | 0.866 | 0.346 | 0.204 | 0.143 | 0.112 | 0.0824 | 0.0675 |
| Pb | 5.29 | 1.84 | 0.896 | 0.356 | 0.208 | 0.145 | 0.114 | 0.0836 | 0.0684 |
| U | 1.06 | 2.42 | 1.17 | 0.452 | 0.259 | 0.176 | 0.136 | 0.0952 | 0.0757 |
| Air | 0.151 | 0.134 | 0.123 | 0.106 | 0.0953 | 0.0868 | 0.0804 | 0.0706 | 0.0655 |
| NaI | 1.57 | 0.568 | 0.305 | 0.155 | 0.111 | 0.0901 | 0.0789 | 0.0657 | 0.0577 |
| H$_2$O | 0.167 | 0.149 | 0.136 | 0.118 | 0.106 | 0.0966 | 0.0896 | 0.0786 | 0.0706 |
| Con-crete[a] | 0.169 | 0.139 | 0.124 | 0.107 | 0.0954 | 0.0870 | 0.0804 | 0.0706 | 0.0635 |
| Tissue | 0.163 | 0.144 | 0.132 | 0.115 | 0.100 | 0.0936 | 0.0867 | 0.0761 | 0.1683 |

[a]Type 04.

dose in irradiators, beam therapy units, and radiographic units will be discussed in detail in subsequent chapters. It should be remembered that the optimization of this energy transfer from the source to the object, at minimum cost or risk, is the primary purpose of any engineering design of a radioisotope facility.

Since a radioisotope source will emit radiation uniformly in all directions, not only toward the desired target, and since it is impossible or impractical to scatter back or reflect more than a small fraction of that radiation toward the target, it becomes necessary to absorb and remove

1.7A
COEFFICIENTS ($\mu/\rho$) (cm²/g)
*Ref. 31*

energy (MeV)

| 1.25 | 1.5 | 2 | 3 | 4 | 5 | 6 | 8 | 10.0 |
|---|---|---|---|---|---|---|---|---|
| 0.113 | 0.103 | 0.0876 | 0.0691 | 0.0579 | 0.0502 | 0.0446 | 0.0371 | 0.0321 |
| 0.0504 | 0.0459 | 0.0394 | 0.0313 | 0.0266 | 0.0234 | 0.0211 | 0.0180 | 0.0161 |
| 0.0568 | 0.0518 | 0.0444 | 0.0356 | 0.0304 | 0.0270 | 0.0245 | 0.0213 | 0.0194 |
| 0.0568 | 0.0517 | 0.0445 | 0.0357 | 0.0306 | 0.0273 | 0.0249 | 0.0218 | 0.0200 |
| 0.0568 | 0.0518 | 0.0445 | 0.0359 | 0.0309 | 0.0276 | 0.0254 | 0.0224 | 0.0206 |
| 0.0546 | 0.0496 | 0.0427 | 0.0348 | 0.0303 | 0.0274 | 0.0254 | 0.0229 | 0.0215 |
| 0.0560 | 0.0512 | 0.0442 | 0.0360 | 0.0315 | 0.0286 | 0.0266 | 0.0242 | 0.0228 |
| 0.0548 | 0.0500 | 0.0432 | 0.0353 | 0.0310 | 0.0282 | 0.0264 | 0.0241 | 0.0229 |
| 0.0567 | 0.0517 | 0.0447 | 0.0367 | 0.0323 | 0.0296 | 0.0277 | 0.0254 | 0.0243 |
| 0.0551 | 0.0502 | 0.0436 | 0.0358 | 0.0316 | 0.0290 | 0.0273 | 0.0252 | 0.0242 |
| 0.0568 | 0.0519 | 0.0448 | 0.0371 | 0.0328 | 0.0302 | 0.0284 | 0.0266 | 0.0255 |
| 0.0512 | 0.0468 | 0.0407 | 0.0338 | 0.0301 | 0.0279 | 0.0266 | 0.0248 | 0.0241 |
| 0.0552 | 0.0505 | 0.0438 | 0.0365 | 0.0327 | 0.0305 | 0.0289 | 0.0274 | 0.0267 |
| 0.0566 | 0.0518 | 0.0451 | 0.0376 | 0.0338 | 0.0316 | 0.0302 | 0.0285 | 0.0280 |
| 0.0531 | 0.0485 | 0.0424 | 0.0316 | 0.0330 | 0.0313 | 0.0304 | 0.0295 | 0.0294 |
| 0.0521 | 0.0476 | 0.0418 | 0.0357 | 0.0330 | 0.0316 | 0.0309 | 0.0303 | 0.0305 |
| 0.0510 | 0.0467 | 0.0414 | 0.0365 | 0.0349 | 0.0344 | 0.0344 | 0.0349 | 0.0359 |
| 0.0501 | 0.0459 | 0.0408 | 0.0367 | 0.0355 | 0.0355 | 0.0358 | 0.0368 | 0.0383 |
| 0.0502 | 0.0460 | 0.0409 | 0.0370 | 0.0360 | 0.0361 | 0.0365 | 0.0377 | 0.0394 |
| 0.0544 | 0.0492 | 0.0437 | 0.0405 | 0.0402 | 0.0409 | 0.0418 | 0.0438 | 0.0465 |
| 0.0554 | 0.0501 | 0.0445 | 0.0414 | 0.0411 | 0.0418 | 0.0427 | 0.0448 | 0.0477 |
| 0.0563 | 0.0508 | 0.0452 | 0.0420 | 0.0416 | 0.0423 | 0.0433 | 0.0454 | 0.0484 |
| 0.0569 | 0.0512 | 0.0457 | 0.0421 | 0.0420 | 0.0426 | 0.0436 | 0.0459 | 0.0489 |
| 0.0615 | 0.0548 | 0.0484 | 0.0445 | 0.0440 | 0.0446 | 0.0455 | 0.0479 | 0.0511 |
| 0.0567 | 0.0517 | 0.0445 | 0.0357 | 0.0307 | 0.0274 | 0.0250 | 0.0220 | 0.0202 |
| 0.0508 | 0.0465 | 0.0412 | 0.0367 | 0.0351 | 0.0347 | 0.0347 | 0.0354 | 0.0366 |
| 0.0630 | 0.0575 | 0.0493 | 0.0396 | 0.0339 | 0.0301 | 0.0275 | 0.0240 | 0.0219 |
| 0.0567 | 0.0517 | 0.0445 | 0.0363 | 0.0317 | 0.0287 | 0.0268 | 0.0243 | 0.0229 |
| 0.0600 | 0.0556 | 0.0478 | 0.0384 | 0.0329 | 0.0292 | 0.0267 | 0.0233 | 0.0212 |

all radiation traveling in all other directions. This is important because of the effect of radiation on body tissues and other organs that makes unnecessary exposure to ionizing radiation undesirable and potentially hazardous. As guidelines and target figures, maximum permissible levels of external radiation have been set by international agreement (*28, 29*) and by national law (e. g., *30*) to avoid dangerous exposure both of personnel associated with the operation of the radioisotope facility ("radiation workers") and of the general public. Since radiation workers are expected to be aware of the radiation field and to carry suitable monitoring

TABLE

TOTAL GAMMA-RAY ATTENUATION

| Ma-terial | Density (g/cm³) | Gamma-ray | | | | | | | |
|---|---|---|---|---|---|---|---|---|---|
| | | 0.1 | 0.15 | 0.2 | 0.3 | 0.4 | 0.5 | 0.6 | 0.8 |
| Be | 1.85 | 0.244 | 0.220 | 0.202 | 0.1748 | 0.1567 | 0.1430 | 0.1323 | 0.1162 |
| C | 2.25 | 0.335 | 0.302 | 0.275 | 0.239 | 0.2144 | 0.1958 | 0.1811 | 0.1591 |
| Na | 0.9712 | 0.147 | 0.126 | 0.115 | 0.099 | 0.0886 | 0.0809 | 0.0748 | 0.0657 |
| Mg | 1.741 | 0.279 | 0.235 | 0.212 | 0.185 | 0.1643 | 0.1497 | 0.1384 | 0.1217 |
| Al | 2.70 | 0.435 | 0.362 | 0.324 | 0.278 | 0.2489 | 0.2268 | 0.2098 | 0.1844 |
| Si | 2.42 | 0.416 | 0.336 | 0.303 | 0.259 | 0.2309 | 0.2103 | 0.1941 | 0.1709 |
| P | 1.83 | 0.318 | 0.251 | 0.223 | 0.190 | 0.1698 | 0.1548 | 0.1427 | 0.1254 |
| S | 2.07 | 0.389 | 0.298 | 0.263 | 0.224 | 0.1983 | 0.1809 | 0.1668 | 0.1463 |
| K | 0.87 | 0.187 | 0.130 | 0.110 | 0.092 | 0.0816 | 0.0741 | 0.0684 | 0.0599 |
| Ca | 1.55 | 0.369 | 0.245 | 0.205 | 0.169 | 0.1496 | 0.1358 | 0.1254 | 0.1097 |
| Fe | 7.86 | 2.704 | 1.438 | 1.085 | 0.833 | 0.7223 | 0.6508 | 0.5989 | 0.5219 |
| Cu | 8.933 | 3.814 | 1.840 | 1.313 | 0.965 | 0.8183 | 0.7325 | 0.6709 | 0.5842 |
| Mo | 9.01 | 9.280 | 3.505 | 2.027 | 1.171 | 0.8991 | 0.7668 | 0.6857 | 0.5838 |
| Sn | 7.298 | 11.53 | 4.109 | 2.211 | 1.117 | 0.795 | 0.6466 | 0.5663 | 0.4722 |
| I | 4.94 | 9.040 | 3.201 | 1.675 | 0.815 | 0.563 | 0.4510 | 0.3912 | 0.3226 |
| W | 19.3 | 81.25 | 27.79 | 13.66 | 5.655 | 3.358 | 2.413 | 1.949 | 1.473 |
| Pt | 21.37 | 101.51 | 35.05 | 16.99 | 6.924 | 4.082 | 2.885 | 2.287 | 1.710 |
| Tl | 11.86 | 61.20 | 21.35 | 10.27 | 4.104 | 2.419 | 1.696 | 1.328 | 0.9773 |
| Pb | 11.34 | 59.99 | 20.87 | 10.16 | 4.037 | 2.359 | 1.644 | 1.293 | 0.9480 |
| U | 18.7 | 19.82 | 45.25 | 21.88 | 8.452 | 4.843 | 3.291 | 2.543 | 1.780 |
| NaI | 3.667 | 5.757 | 2.083 | 1.118 | 0.568 | 0.407 | 0.3304 | 0.2893 | 0.2409 |
| H₂O | 1.00 | 0.167 | 0.149 | 0.136 | 0.118 | 0.106 | 0.0966 | 0.0896 | 0.0786 |
| Con-crete$^a$ | 2.35 | 0.397 | 0.327 | 0.291 | 0.251 | 0.2242 | 0.2045 | 0.1889 | 0.1659 |

$^a$Type 04.

equipment, they are permitted to work and operate in higher potential radiation fields than the general public. The ultimate cumulative dose that is considered "safe" or acceptable is, of course, the same in all cases though there are some statistical arguments on population dynamics that attempt to differentiate. More details on this subject are given in Section VI. The main effect of this need for protection against unwanted radiation exposure is to introduce the design of collimators and shielding arrangements into the overall consideration of any radiation facility at an early stage.

Shielding or collimation of gamma radiation depend on the attenuation equation, Eq. (1.4), as a first approximation. For thicker shields, secondary effects become increasingly more significant, giving rise to "build-up," i.e., an increased radiation field without clear directional correlation

## 1.7B

CROSS SECTIONS ($\mu_t$) (in cm$^{-1}$)

| energy (MeV) | | | | | | | | | |
|---|---|---|---|---|---|---|---|---|---|
| 1.0 | 1.25 | 1.5 | 2 | 3 | 4 | 5 | 6 | 8 | 10.0 |
| 0.1045 | 0.0932 | 0.0849 | 0.0729 | 0.0579 | 0.0492 | 0.0433 | 0.0390 | 0.0333 | 0.0298 |
| 0.1431 | 0.1278 | 0.1166 | 0.0999 | 0.0801 | 0.0684 | 0.0608 | 0.0551 | 0.0479 | 0.0437 |
| 0.0590 | 0.0530 | 0.0482 | 0.0415 | 0.0338 | 0.0294 | 0.0266 | 0.0247 | 0.0222 | 0.0209 |
| 0.1092 | 0.1975 | 0.0891 | 0.0770 | 0.0627 | 0.0548 | 0.0498 | 0.0463 | 0.0421 | 0.0397 |
| 0.1658 | 0.1480 | 0.1350 | 0.1166 | 0.0953 | 0.0837 | 0.0761 | 0.0713 | 0.0651 | 0.0618 |
| 0.1537 | 0.1372 | 0.1251 | 0.1082 | 0.0888 | 0.0782 | 0.0716 | 0.0670 | 0.0615 | 0.0588 |
| 0.1129 | 0.1008 | 0.0919 | 0.0798 | 0.0655 | 0.0578 | 0.0531 | 0.0500 | 0.0461 | 0.0443 |
| 0.1314 | 0.1176 | 0.1074 | 0.0927 | 0.0768 | 0.0679 | 0.0625 | 0.0588 | 0.0551 | 0.0328 |
| 0.0538 | 0.0480 | 0.0439 | 0.0381 | 0.0318 | 0.0284 | 0.0265 | 0.0251 | 0.0238 | 0.0232 |
| 0.0983 | 0.0877 | 0.0803 | 0.0699 | 0.0583 | 0.0524 | 0.0490 | 0.0468 | 0.0442 | 0.0434 |
| 0.4677 | 0.4174 | 0.3812 | 0.3333 | 0.2837 | 0.2594 | 0.2460 | 0.2389 | 0.2319 | 0.2311 |
| 0.5226 | 0.4654 | 0.4252 | 0.3734 | 0.3189 | 0.2948 | 0.2823 | 0.2760 | 0.2707 | 0.2725 |
| 0.5181 | 0.4595 | 0.4208 | 0.3730 | 0.3289 | 0.3144 | 0.3099 | 0.3099 | 0.3144 | 0.3190 |
| 0.4145 | 0.3656 | 0.3350 | 0.2978 | 0.2678 | 0.2591 | 0.2591 | 0.2613 | 0.2686 | 0.2795 |
| 0.2821 | 0.2480 | 0.2272 | 0.2020 | 0.1828 | 0.1778 | 0.1783 | 0.1803 | 0.1862 | 0.1946 |
| 1.235 | 1.050 | 0.9496 | 0.8434 | 0.7817 | 0.7759 | 0.7894 | 0.8067 | 0.8453 | 0.8975 |
| 1.408 | 1.184 | 1.071 | 0.9510 | 0.8847 | 0.8783 | 0.8933 | 0.9125 | 0.9574 | 1.019 |
| 0.8005 | 0.6677 | 0.6025 | 0.5361 | 0.4981 | 0.4934 | 0.5017 | 0.5135 | 0.5384 | 0.5740 |
| 0.7757 | 0.6452 | 0.5806 | 0.5182 | 0.4774 | 0.4763 | 0.4831 | 0.4944 | 0.5205 | 0.5545 |
| 1.416 | 1.150 | 1.025 | 0.9051 | 0.8322 | 0.8228 | 0.8340 | 0.8509 | 0.8957 | 0.9556 |
| 0.2116 | 0.1863 | 0.1705 | 0.1511 | 0.1346 | 0.1287 | 0.1272 | 0.1272 | 0.1298 | 0.1342 |
| 0.0706 | 0.0630 | 0.0575 | 0.0493 | 0.0396 | 0.0339 | 0.0301 | 0.0275 | 0.0240 | 0.0219 |
| 0.1492 | 0.1332 | 0.1215 | 0.1046 | 0.0853 | 0.0745 | 0.0674 | 0.0630 | 0.0571 | 0.0538 |

based on the scattering properties of the shield, primarily as a result of the Compton effect. Table 1.7 collects the main characteristics of the more important shielding materials for $^{170}$Tm, $^{192}$Ir, $^{137}$Cs, and $^{60}$Co gamma rays (31).

For a detailed discussion of shielding theory, the reader is referred to the books of Goldstein (27), Rockwell (32), and Jaeger (26). The design effects of shielding considerations in specific applications are discussed in subsequent chapters.

## IV. APPLICATIONS OF SEALED RADIOISOTOPE SOURCES

There are four well-established areas of applications where medium-level encapsulated radioisotope sources are used in industry. These are in radiography, radiogauging, well-logging, and as portable power sources. Apart from radiotherapy they constitute the largest number and the most widespread utilization of radioisotope sources. The source strengths typically are in the millicurie and curie range depending on whether portability or high radiation dose is the dominant design criterion. The design of these devices has been fairly well established, is almost entirely in commercial hands, at least in the United States and Western Europe, and will be discussed here only briefly. The use of radioisotope power sources has so far been largely confined to space applications and cannot yet be considered to have reached commercial maturity (*33, 34*). In all cases one is dealing with radioisotope sources that are permanently encapsulated and usually designed to perform a single specific function. As a rule, licensing requirements specify a periodic leak test of the source to ensure continued integrity of the containment. Since the radiation level surrounding these sources is quite high, they are usually installed in a shield assembly to which they are attached mechanically; only in the case of radiographic systems is provision made for automatic movement of the source from the shield into the camera assembly for limited and preset periods.

## A.  Radiography

The field of radiography for the inspection of cast and machined metal objects and other manufactured items has been flourishing since the early days of X-ray technology. Radium sources and X-ray machines have been in use for many years and are an established part of quality inspection procedures (*35–37*). With the increased requirements of industrial quality control, the use of radioisotopes, principally $^{60}$Co, $^{192}$Ir, $^{137}$Cs, and $^{170}$Tm, has become more popular both on account of the lower cost and greater portability of radioisotope sources and because of greater ease in matching the gamma-ray spectrum of the source with the type and thickness of material to be inspected. For optimum sensitivity and contrast, the thickness of the work to be radiographed should be of the order of the half-value thickness of the effective X- or gamma radiation from the source. Table 1.8 lists the characteristics of the most widely used radiographic sources (*38*). Where a wide range of material thicknesses is to be inspected, no single source can be expected to meet all requirements.

To achieve economic utilization of the sources, it is obviously important to obtain as many exposures per day as possible, so that the source

TABLE 1.8

CHARACTERISTICS OF RADIOGRAPHIC SOURCES

| Isotope | Half-life | Typical source strength (Ci) | Output (R/hr m) | Useful range (in.) | | Approximate cost (encapsulated) ($) |
|---------|-----------|------------------------------|-----------------|--------------------|--|-------------------------------------|
| $^{226}$Ra | 1600 yr | 0.5 | 0.42 | 0.5 – 2 | (steel) | 10,000 |
| $^{60}$Co | 5.3 yr | 0.5 – 50 | 0.7 – 70 | 0.5 – 6 | (steel) | 200–2000 |
| | | | | 1 – 12 | (Al) | |
| $^{192}$Ir | 74 days | 10 – 50 | 5.5 – 28 | 0.2 – 3 | (steel) | 150–400 |
| | | | | 0.5 – 6 | (Al) | |
| $^{137}$Cs | 30 yr | 10 – 50 | 3.6 – 18 | 0.3 – 4 | (steel) | 500–1000 |
| $^{70}$Tm | 127 days | 5 – 20 | 0.015 – 0.05 | 0.02 – 0.25 | (steel) | 1000–2200 |
| $^{75}$Se | 120 days | 5 – 10 | 0.06 – 0.12 | 0.02 – 0.3 | (steel) | n.a. |
| $(^{90}$Sr):Pb | 28 yr | 1 – 5 | | 0.2 – 0.3 | (Al) | 500–1000 |
| | | | | 0.075 – 0.5 | (steel) | |

strength selected is based on the competitive factors of individual exposure time and number of exposures per working day versus the amortized cost of the encapsulated source and its shield-camera assembly. Figures 1.5 and 1.6, taken from Clarke's paper (38), show the relation between exposure time and steel thickness for various sources. A great deal of engineering ingenuity has been devoted to the design of various radiographic cameras which are really portable source holders with a mechanical or pneumatic transfer system or shutter, bringing the source close to the work to be inspected. Similar considerations apply to the diagnostic use of X rays or gamma rays in medicine, but here radioisotope sources have found less ready acceptance than X-ray machines whose technology has been familiar for many years.

A more recent entry into this field is neutron radiography. Medical, diagnostic applications of neutron sources are still at the research stage and whether the use of machine sources or radioisotope sources, like antimony–beryllium or californium-252, will be preferred ultimately cannot be predicted at this time. On the other hand, for industrial purposes neutron radiography is becoming well established wherever reactor or accelerator neutrons are readily available (39). Its application with portable sources may depend largely on the rate at which $^{252}$Cf sources are becoming available (40).

The production and encapsulation of sources for radiographic purposes presents no particular problem and will be included in the description of encapsulation procedures in Chapter 3.

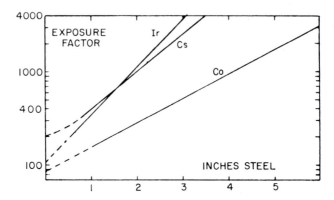

Fig. 1.5 Exposures required to yield density 2.0 on medium speed film for three isotopes:

$$\left[ \text{exposure time} = \frac{\text{exposure factor} \times (\text{source to film in inches})^2}{\text{millicuries}} \right]$$

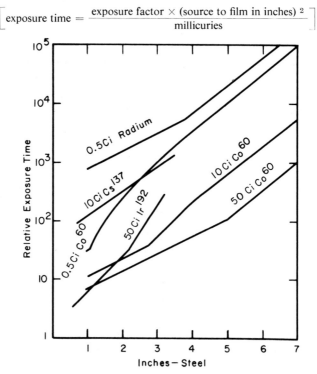

Fig. 1.6 Relative exposure times for several sources on steel, maintaining source-film distance greater than 100 × source diameter and greater than 6 × specimen thickness.

## B. *Radiation Gauges*

The field of radiogauging, i.e., the measurement and control of thickness, density, mass, or water content by means of measurement of the absorption or back-scattering of nuclear radiations, has reached commercial maturity many years ago (*41–45*). Radiation gauges are well established in such industries as paper-making, metal-foil rolling, soil and cement moisture measurements, and cigaret making, but their full industrial potential is far from being reached at this time, particularly in North America. Basically, the material to be measured is interposed between source and radiation detector and for optimum response and sensitivity the material thickness should be of the order of the half-value thickness for the radiation from the source selected. The gauge response depends on the change in count rate with change in thickness or density during the passage of the scanned material volume through the space seen by the detector. The gauge sensitivity depends on the minimum statistical change in counts required to indicate minimum tolerable changes in the parameter under observation, obtainable for a given source strength and source-detector geometry. These relations have been discussed in detail by Gardner and Ely (*19*), who present an excellent review of the relevant theory and its application to the design of gauges for different purposes.

For beta-ray gauges the most widely used sources include $^{90}$Sr–Y, $^{147}$Pm, $^{63}$Ni, $^{204}$Tl, and $^{144}$Ce, for gamma-ray gauges $^{85}$Kr, $^{60}$Co, $^{137}$Cs, and $^{75}$Se. Related to these is the use of high-energy beta sources as generators of bremsstrahlung X rays for thickness gauges and X-ray fluorescence analyzers (*8, 46*); recently K-capture sources like $^{109}$Cd and $^{55}$Fe have appeared on the market for applications of this kind. Neutron gauges tend to employ Pu–Be, Am–Be, and Ra–Be sources; however, the impending availability of $^{252}$Cf spontaneous fission sources may change this situation. For extensive targets, like paper sheets, foils, or ore on a conveyor belt, the use of several sources or several long detectors may be equally feasible, but considerations of cost and containment tend to favor the use of only one or two sources with a number of long detectors in appropriate positions. For safety, the source should be integrally mounted in a shield that reduces all radiations to the immediate environment to acceptable levels at a distance of closest approach and contains provisions for a shutter that cuts off the radiation beam whenever the gauge is not in use.

The optimization procedure for the overall design of a gauge starts with the choice of a source material that emits radiation of energy appropriate to the target thickness and desired sensitivity. Next, a suitable detector is chosen, bearing in mind the requirements of reliability, ease of replacement, low cost, and environmental conditions inherent in the industrial application. The detector sensitivity and the detector-source geometry, in turn, determine the source strength for a specified count rate and counting statistics needed for requisite accuracy of measurement. If the detector is unduly insensitive or inefficient, this will increase the source strength needed and, hence, the size of the shield surrounding the source and in this way force up the overall cost of the device. In many applications the design details are constrained by problems of fluctuation in line voltage, serious electrical interference, climatic factors, e.g., high humidity or extreme temperatures, or by dust or vibration conditions (8, 43).

## C.  Well-Logging Devices

These problems are accentuated in well-logging devices as used in geophysical prospecting. In these devices small accelerators or gamma-ray or neutron sources are lowered down drill holes to determine continuously the composition of the surrounding material by measuring the intensity of backscattered gamma-rays or neutrons (8, 47, 48). The radio-isotope sources employed are sealed sources of the order of a few curies with a collimated shield assembly adapted to bore-hole use. Some work is under way to extend such well-logging gauges to borehole analysis by means of X-ray fluorescence or neutron activation (8, 49). Both of these methods are also likely to find increasing use for field prospecting and on-line analysis in the mining industry.

## D.  Radiation Therapy

By far the largest contribution to the growth in demand for high-level radioactive sources shown in Fig. 1.3 has been provided by the rapid increase in radiation therapy units, using mainly cobalt-60 sources, all over the world. The advantages of being able to employ a fairly compact source, capable of being rotated around the patient to focus the beam on the tumor site without burning the intervening tissue, and of lower cost compared with conventional X-ray equipment, combined with improved health services in all countries, boosted the demand for such high-level sources to unprecedented levels. In order to obtain a well-collimated beam, it is important to have as near a point source as possible. This implies using cobalt-60 sources with as high a specific activity as is available

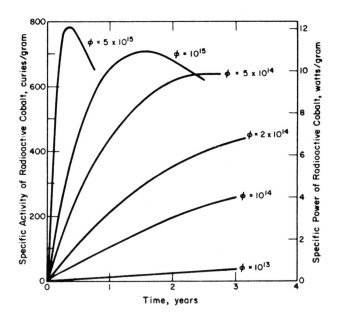

FIG. 1.7   Production conditions of cobalt-60.

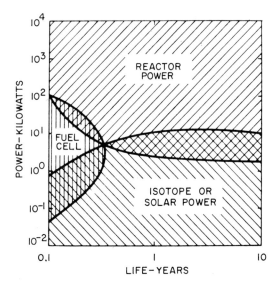

FIG. 1.8   Application chart for power sources.

TABLE

CHARACTERISTICS OF ATTRACTIVE

| | Cobalt–60 | Strontium–90 | Cesium–137 | Promethium–147 |
|---|---|---|---|---|
| Specific power (W/g) | 17.4 | 0.95 | 0.42 | 0.33 |
| Half-life (yr) | 5.3 | 28 | 30 | 2.7 |
| Isotopic purity (%) | 10 | 50 | 35 | 95 |
| Compound form | Metal | $SrTiO_3$ | Glass | $Pm_2O_3$ |
| Density of compound (g/cc) | 8.9 | 4.6 | 3.2 | 6.6 |
| Active isotope in compound (%) | 10 | 24 | 16 | 82 |
| Specific power of compound (W/g) | 1.7 | 0.23 | 0.067 | 0.27 |
| Power density (W/cc of compound) | 15.5 | 1.16 | 0.215 | 2.22 |
| Volume for 2 kW heat (cc) | 129 | 1840 | 9300 | 1120 |
| Availability annual $kW_t$ (1967- )[a] | Available | Available (67 kW) | Available (48 kW) | Available (11 kW) |
| Shielding requirement | Heavy | Heavy | Heavy | Minor |
| Biological hazard (MPC)[a] | $3 \times 10^{-9}$ | $3 \times 10^{-10}$ | $5 \times 10^{-9}$ | $2 \times 10^{-8}$ |
| Estimated cost ($/W)[a] | 33 | 19[a] | 21[a] | 91[a] |
| Estimated cost ($/g) | 570 | 18[a] | 9[a] | 30[a] |
| Curies per gram | 1130 | 142 | 87 | 914 |
| Curies per watt | 65 | 150 | 207 | 2770 |
| Spontaneous fission half-life (yr) | | | | |

[a] From proposed Hanford Isotope Plant, HW-77770 ($kW_t$ = thermal kilowatts).
[b] Except for shielding against neutrons.
[c] From AEC data; also *Nucleonics* **21** (3), 63, (1963); ("projected" costs).

and economically feasible (*50, 51*). Since [60]Co has a 5.3-year half-life, it is essential to activate the target material at a much higher rate than its rate of decay; as Fig. 1.7 shows, this necessitates a neutron flux in excess of $10^{14}$ n/cm$^2$ sec and limits the maximum specific activity attainable even in the highest available neutron fluxes. For many years the majority of cobalt therapy sources were supplied from Canada and only in recent years have other sources of supply become available in adequate numbers.

The sources used in therapy units are typically in the range of 10,000–60,000 Ci. This imposes safety problems in shipping and installation, as well as design problems in attempting to obtain a well-collimated beam with optimum source-to-patient geometry. These aspects will be discussed fully in Chapter 4. It is encouraging to see how an important radioisotope application can in fact be developed to full public acceptance once the benefits are fully realized and the proper degree of salesmanship is brought to bear on the subject.

1.9

RADIOISOTOPIC HEAT SOURCES

| Polonium–210 | Plutonium–238 | Americium–241 | Curium–242 | Curium–244 |
|---|---|---|---|---|
| 141 | 0.56 | 0.11 | 120 | 2.8 |
| 0.38 | 89 | 458 | 0.45 | 18 |
| 95 | 80 | 90 | 90 | 90 |
| Metal | $PuO_2$ | Metal | $Cm_2O_3$ | $Cm_2O_3$ |
| 9.3 | 10 | 11.7 | 11.75 | 11.75 |
| 95 | 70 | 90 | 82 | 82 |
| 134 | 0.39 | 0.1 | 98 | 2.3 |
| 1210 | 3.9 | 1.17 | 1150 | 27 |
| 1.65 | 513 | 1710 | 1.74 | 74 |
| Available | Limited | Limited | Potentially | Potentially |
|  | Available | Production | Available | Available |
| Minor | Minor | Minor | Minor[b] | Minor[b] |
| $2 \times 10^{-9}$ | $7 \times 10^{-13}$ | $2 \times 10^{-12}$ | $4 \times 10^{-11}$ | $3 \times 10^{-12}$ |
| 26,500[c] | 894 | 200 | 17 | 357 |
| 188 | 500[c] | 1820 | 2000 | 1000[c] |
| 4500 | 17 | 3.25 | 3310 | 84 |
| 32 | 30 | 30 | 28 | 30 |
|  | $4.9 \times 10^{10}$ | $1.4 \times 10^{13}$ | $7.2 \times 10^{6}$ | $1.4 \times 10^{7}$ |

## E. Power Sources

Their relative compactness and lack of moving parts make radio-isotopes ideal energy sources where maintenance problems or geographic isolation override problems of cost or low efficiency. Such conditions may exist for unattended beacons at sea or in the Antarctic and for low-power applications in space satellites (*10, 16*). Figure 1.8, taken from a paper by English (*16*), shows the regions of applicability for different energy sources. Table 1.9 compares a number of radioisotope heat sources; the cost information represents 1966 figures and can be readily compared with the more recent figures in Table 1.1. Cobalt-60, which looks attractive on the basis of power density and cost per watt (*52*), becomes considerably less so when it is realized that heavy shielding will be required for any handling and preflight launching. The highest power density is obtained for the shorter-lived alpha emitters $^{210}Po$ and $^{242}Cm$. Clearly the expected

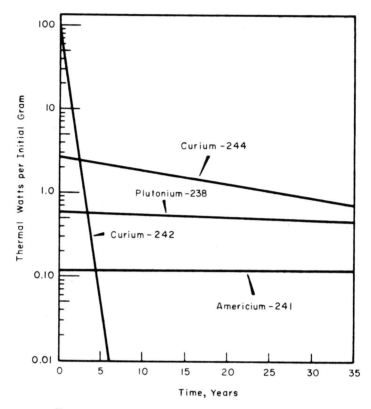

FIG. 1.9   Heat production of four transuranium sources.

life and intended mission of the device play an important part in the selection of the source material. Figure 1.9 compares the heat production of four transuranium isotopes as a function of time (*16*); the production of such material is discussed in detail in Chapter 2. In the United States, work on isotopic power sources has been carried on under the "SNAP" program. Table 1.10 summarizes the current status of this program (*14*). Of particular interest are the activity levels employed, ranging from a few kilocuries to nearly a megacurie of polonium or plutonium. These, obviously, are not energy sources that are likely to be economically competitive with conventional power sources employing electrochemical or combustion processes for terrestrial applications for a long time yet. In Europe sufficient interest in isotopic generators has developed in recent years that an Isotopic Generator Information Centre has been set up by

TABLE 1.10

Radioisotope-Thermoelectric Generators [U.S. Program (14)]

| | SNAP-3A | SNAP-9A | SNAP-11 | SNAP-17 | SNAP-19 | SNAP-27 | SNAP-29 | AMSA Unit |
|---|---|---|---|---|---|---|---|---|
| Environment | Earth orbit | Earth orbit | Lunar surface | Earth orbit | Earth orbit | Lunar surface | Earth orbit | Earth orbit |
| Reference space mission | Navigation satellite | Navigation satellite | 90-day surveyor | Small military communications satellite | Nimbus-"B" | ALSEP | Various | Various |
| Isotope | $^{238}Pu$ | $^{238}Pu$ | $^{242}Cm$ | $^{90}Sr$ | $^{238}Pu$ | $^{238}Pu$ | $^{210}Po$ | $^{147}Pm$ |
| Approximate activity (kCi) | 18 | 15 | | | 18 | 45 | 800 | 200 |
| Capsule operating surface temperature (°C) | 510 | 510 | | | 760 | 760 | 980 | 320 |
| Thermal power (kW$_t$) | 0.060 | 0.5 | | | 0.6 | 1.5 | 25 | 0.060 |
| Power level W$_e$ | 2.7 | 25 | 21-25 | 25 | 25 | 50 | 500 | 3 |
| Specific power (watts/pound) | 0.59 | 0.93 | 0.83 | 1.0 | 1.0 | 1.5 | 1.0 | — |
| Fuel[a] | Pu metal | Pu metal | $^{242}Cm$ | $^{90}SrTiO_3$ | $PuO_2$(microspheres) | $PuO_2$(microspheres) | GdPo | $Pm_2O_3$ |
| Conversion material | PbTe | PbTe | PbTe | PbTe and SiGe | PbTe | PbTe | PbTe | |
| Safety criteria[b] | Burnup | Burnup | Intact | Burnup | Intact | Intact | Intact | |
| Flight readiness | 1961 | 1963 | Ground demonstration 1966 | Not being developed | 1967 | 1968 | Early 1970s | |

[a] Useful lifetimes for the $^{238}Pu$ systems are from 1 to 6 years; for the $^{242}Cm$ and $^{210}Po$ systems, about 3 to 5 months.
[b] Design criteria for atmospheric re-entry after orbit decay or launch failure.

the European Nuclear Energy Agency of the Organization for Economic Cooperation and Development (OECD) in Paris (*34*).

The isotopic power generators as a rule consist of two parts: the radio-isotope source and, surrounding it or embedded in it, the converter-generator. For low-power systems, the converter usually is a thermopile consisting of a large number of lead telluride thermocouples connected in parallel. For high-power systems, thermionic converters and closed Ran-kine or Brayton cycle generators have been studied. One of the limitations on the efficiency of the system is imposed by the maximum heat source temperatures that can be employed at present. Additional limitations, particularly for space systems, are presented by reentry problems in case of failure or abort of the mission. Few health physicists are prepared to face calmly the possibility of having half a megacurie of plutonium dis-tributed as a fine vapor over any part of the countryside; hence, the cap-sule must be designed to sustain reentry temperatures safely and to permit ready identification and recovery.

## V.  HIGH-LEVEL IRRADIATORS

The level of engineering design involved in the medium-level isotope source applications described in the preceding section can be considered as largely conventional in the sense that the source capsule can be handled, transported, and shielded by readily predicted means and the source assembly itself does not necessarily constitute the most complex component of the system. This situation changes when radiation sources in the kilocurie and megacurie range are employed in facilities designed for the large-scale irradiation of food, industrial products, or other goods. The interplay of radiation physics, mechanical design, and optimization of economic factors required by the large capital investment involved in these cases constitutes the major portion and main objective of this book. Although details of design and design approach still vary considerably from project to project, the general principles involved are readily dis-cerned and will be discussed in subsequent chapters.

### A.  *Sterilization Plants*

Since bacteria are relatively radiation-resistant, the radiation dose for sterilization is relatively high, of the order of 1.5–4 Mrad, depending on the organisms involved. This implies that all parts of a target package must receive at least the minimum sterilization dose, either in a single ex-posure or as an integrated dose received during repeated passes past the radiation source. To ensure adequate plant capacity, each passage of the

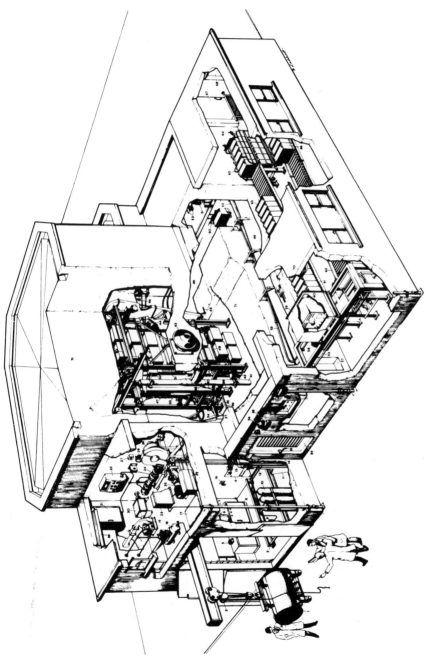

FIG. 1.10  View of automatic continuous irradiation plant.

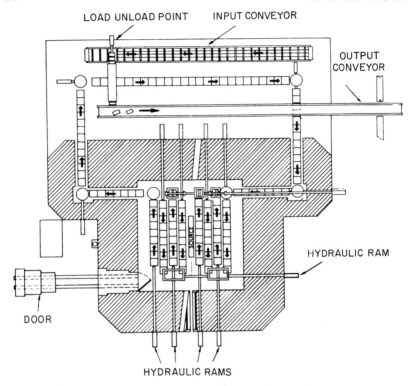

FIG. 1.11   Simplified plan of irradiator cell.

target material should be as rapid as possible, dictating a source strength capable of imparting the requisite dose to the target material during the time of exposure. As will be seen in Chapters 5 and 6, these requirements have to be optimized for minimum cost of operation, and a number of satisfactory plants have in fact been operating for some years under economically competitive conditions.

As an example of the type of plant involved, Fig. 1.10 shows a sketch of a plant for the irradiation and sterilization of medical sutures (*53*). The overall design is dominated by the source handling and storage facilities and by conveyor systems for the suture packages designed to utilize the radiation from the source to the fullest extent. Figure 1.11 shows in more detail the arrangement of the actual irradiation cell and the conveyor system within it. Other plants for sterilization of medical supplies along similar lines have been constructed in many countries around the world. Several plants have also been built for the radiation sterilization of hospital mattresses by a batch process (*54*).

## B. *Radiation Processing*

Ionizing radiation is capable of catalyzing and initiating chemical re-actions in a wide variety of materials, particularly organic substances, and a whole new branch of chemistry, radiation chemistry, has grown up a-round these effects. In spite of very intensive research around the world during the past 20 years, the number of commercially useful and industrially competitive processes that have emerged has been fairly limited. It has been estimated that one new process per year has been developed. In the United States, the dollar volume of sales for such products has been estimated to be about $100 million annually at present, with a growth rate of 20–25 % for radiation processing of chemicals and plastics (*55*), or even higher (*56*).

The major processes in operation include the following:

(1) Cross linking of polyethylene in films and coatings.
(2) Preparation of specialty copolymers for battery separators.
(3) Synthesis of ethyl bromide.
(4) Synthesis of new graft copolymer fibers.
(5) Production of wood-plastic compounds in monomer-injected wood panels.
(6) Controlled degradation of certain polymers.
(7) Curing of surface coatings by machine irradiation.

The radiation source for these processes may be a machine or radioisotope source (*9, 13, 16, 57*) depending on the scale of operations and plant capacity. Dose levels range from $10^5$ to $2 \times 10^7$ rads and target size may vary considerably with the nature of the product. As a rule, the irradiation step is just one stage in a more complex manufacturing process and the irradiator must be designed as an integral part of the plant system. Due to the steady growth of this field, new irradiators will have to be designed for a variety of specific applications (*12, 58*).

## C. *Food Irradiation*

In view of the increased pressure put on the world's food resources by the rapidly growing population, considerable importance attaches to any method that reduces food losses by spoilage in transit or storage. Radiation methods have been shown to be effective in doing this for a variety of food stuffs either by killing insect pests or by retarding sprouting (*59–61*). The marketing of wheat flour and rice that have been irradiated for deinfestation and of potatoes, where irradiation inhibits sprouting, has been cleared by licensing in several countries. Onions, bacon, and leguminous and root crops have been irradiated with promising results and may appear on the world market soon. High-cost fruit, like strawberries, papaya, mango, and bananas, have been preserved for commercially significant periods. Various types of marine products have been studied with a view to extending their shelf life; if commercially feasible, this would extend market areas accessible to sea food and greatly increase available food reserves (60).

The dose requirements for sprout inhibition and delayed ripening of fruit are of the order of 20–40 krad. Pasteurization and sterilization processes require doses one or two orders of magnitude higher with a consequent increase in unit cost and a greater risk of affecting the taste of the food product. Though at this stage irradiation tests have proceeded in many countries on a laboratory or pilot plant scale only, it seems reasonable to expect the erection of full-scale plants in many places as soon as regulatory problems are overcome and the demand for food and its preservation force a realistic look at the benefits of irradiation in relation to the costs involved.

Plant designs have been proposed (59, 62) that will permit irradiation of more than one food crop, as each comes into season, to improve utilization of irradiation facilities. In Canada, a demonstration potato irradiator has been built, which can be moved to different areas wherever potato harvesting is in progress. To avoid reinfestation, many food stuffs will have to be prepackaged before irradiation and some plant designs incorporate packaging assemblies. To be commercially feasible each proposed irradiator will have to be assessed in terms of its capacity, throughput, market capacity for the added food, transportation and storage facilities, and the capital investment (see Chapter 6). This field offers a great challenge to the economist, the nuclear engineer—and the politician.

## VI.  SAFETY ASPECTS

The ionizing radiations emitted by medium and high-level radioisotope sources can be extremely hazardous and some safety precautions in handling and installation must invariably be provided. Although ingestion of such sources may be considered extremely unlikely, the external radiation exposure from an unshielded source may cause serious harm through both genetic and somatic effects. The latter may involve burns of varying intensity, radiation sickness, and leukemia, in some cases appearing after a long interval since the original exposure. Table 1.11 lists the levels of ex-

TABLE 1.11

SUMMARY OF EFFECTS RESULTING FROM ACUTE WHOLE BODY EXTERNAL EXPOSURE OF RADIATION TO MAN[a]

| 0–25 R | 25–100 R | 100–200 R | 200–300 R | 300–600 R | 600 R or more |
|---|---|---|---|---|---|
| No detectable clinical effects. | Slight transient reductions in lymphocytes and neutrophils. | Nausea and fatigue, with possible vomiting above 125 R. | Nausea and vomiting on first day. | Nausea, vomiting and diarrhea in first few hours. | Nausea, vomiting and diarrhea in first few hours. |
| Delayed effects may occur. | Disabling sickness not common, exposed individuals should be able to proceed with usual duties. | Reduction in lymphocytes and neutrophils with delayed recovery. | Latent period up to two weeks or perhaps longer. | Latent period with no definite symptoms, perhaps as long as one week. | Short latent period with no definite symptoms in some cases during first week. |
|  | Delayed effects possible, but serious effects on average individual very improbable. | Delayed effects may shorten life expectancy in the order of one per cent. | Following latent period symptoms appear but are not severe: loss of appetite, and general malaise, sore throat, pallor, petecheae, diarrhea, moderate emaciation. | Epilation, loss of appetite, general malaise, and fever during second week, followed by hemorrhage, purpura, petecheae, inflammation of mouth and throat, diarrhea, and emaciation in the third week. | Diarrhea, hemorrhage, purpura, inflammation of mouth and throat, fever toward end of first week. |
|  |  |  | Recovery likely in about 3 months unless complicated by poor previous health, superimposed injuries or infections. | Some deaths in 2 to 6 weeks. Possible eventual death to 50% of the exposed individuals for about 450 R. | Rapid emaciation and death as early as the second week with possible eventual death of up to 100% of exposed individuals. |

[a] Adapted from "The Effects of Nuclear Weapons," U.S. Government Printing Office, Washington, D.C., 1957.

posure and the nature of effects to be expected for whole-body exposures to high doses of radiation.

In no other field of scientific and technical development has so much attention been paid to the supposed or potential hazards of operations as in the field of nuclear development. While most of this is part of the heritage of the violent beginnings of the field, it is essential to realize that, outside the field of medical radiology which is not normally included in these considerations, the use and applications of radiation and nuclear energy actually have an unexcelled safety record (63). It is appropriate, therefore, to establish the need and desirability of a project first, before considering routinely the protective features required for its feasible development, so that an unemotional assessment of the benefit factors as against any reasonable risks can be made.

It goes without saying that any source installation must include adequate shielding and other safeguards to obviate any danger of excessive radiation exposure to the operator or the general public, both when the source is in its storage position or when the system is operated normally. To this end it is necessary to make the shielding an integral part of the overall system design, to incorporate fail-safe and interlock devices to prevent accidental exposure to anybody, and to guard against the effects of any accidental malfunctions of the electric or mechanical components of the installation.

While no system can ever be designed practically and economically that protects against willful disregard of regulations, deliberate tampering with safety devices, or sabotage, it is incumbent on the design engineer to design a system that is as safe and "fool-proof" as any industrial system can reasonably be made without sacrificing effectiveness and without intolerable cost. The shielding and engineered safeguards then form one of the most distinctive features in the design of high-level radiation sources and irradiators.

Most countries have a system of licensing the possession of radioisotopes and their use. However, as the use of irradiators and radiographic sources grows more widespread, a more effective and uniform system of testing and licensing of the operators of such units must probably be devised than is customary at present. In the United States there have been a number of cases where isotope licenses had to be cancelled because of deliberate or careless disregard of regulations by some users, especially of radiographic sources. However, it would not be practical nor should it be necessary to employ a full-fledged nuclear engineer or health physicist merely to utilize a radiation gauge or irradiator unit for routine operations.

An additional safeguard customarily included in U.S. source licenses is the requirement for leak tests on sources to be carried out at specified intervals to check if the encapsulation is intact and to prevent contamination.

There has been, in the past, perhaps an overemphasis on radiation hazards and safety requirements, which has contributed to the psychological barriers and cost of installations, preventing a more widespread utilization of radiation gauges and other radiation equipment by industry and slowing down public and legal acceptance of irradiated materials. It behooves the nuclear engineer to be aware of this problem, to incorporate the necessary safety features in any radiation system as a matter of course, and to assure the users of this fact just as much, but no more, than the electrical or chemical industries assure their customers that they are protected against any inherent and foreseeable hazards in those cases. (In the case of medical therapy units and other radiological devices, the father figure of the doctor in charge already performs this function.)

Table 8.2 (Appendix A) lists the maximum permissible exposure levels to radiation workers or members of the general public for varying periods of exposure under normal conditions (28, 29, 64). It does not take into account any deliberate exposure of specific organs carried out under doctor's orders as part of a therapeutic treatment or for diagnostic purposes. The figures in Table 8.2 serve as a general guide to the design of shielding assemblies surrounding radiation sources, both mobile or stationary, and to the total exposure permissible during the handling and exposure of radiography sources. Whenever possible, of course, the system should be designed to keep possible exposures well below the levels listed.

These safety aspects of radioisotope systems are responsible for the large body of legal requirements that have come into being in most countries, covering the packing, labeling, and transportation of radioactive sources (65), as well as the siting of plants where high-level radiation sources are handled. Up to now, preparation of radioisotope sources has usually been handled by government-owned facilities in most countries, but as more source preparation facilities are set up by private industry, considerations of plant hygiene and of environmental conditions are receiving more attention, particularly with respect to potential hazards of air or water pollution or in waste disposal.

With regard to the shipment of radioiostopes, the shipping of low-level, millicurie amounts, for medical or tracer uses, by air or rail, is common and conditions of labeling and packing are prescribed to ensure low external radiation levels (65–68). Medium- and high-level sources cannot normally be shipped in this fashion since the quantity may exceed that permitted by regulations. Stronger sources will require specially designed shipping casks and special arrangements must be made to transport such heavy and bulky containers by road, flat car, or ship. As will be seen later, the cost of the cask and the transportation of the source may form a significant item in the economic analysis of an irradiator system and its competitiveness compared with accelerator installations.

Another area of concern is the ultimate fate of unwanted sources that may have decayed below a level that is considered usable in a given application and yet contain enough activity to make their handling potentially hazardous. In some cases a second-hand use may be found, e.g., some decayed therapy sources may be split up for use as radiography sources, but in general the hot-cell facilities required for reprocessing or loading may add appreciably to the cost of such a secondary source. In that case, some long term storage or underground disposal site may need to be utilized, all of which entail expenses which together with the cost of safe transportation to the disposal site have to be taken into consideration in any estimate of the operational costs of the radiation facility. Very rarely would it be possible or legal to dispose of a fully or partially decayed source through local, municipal services.

## REFERENCES

1. J. Kohl, R. Zentner, and H. R. Lukens, *Radioisotope Applications Engineering,* Van Nostrand, Princeton, New Jersey, 1961.
2. L. G. Erwall, H.G. Forsberg, and K. Ljunggren, *Industrial Isotope Techniques,* Wiley, New York, 1964.
3. E. Broda and T. Schönfeld, *The Technical Applications of Radioactivity,* Vol., 1, Pergamon Press, New York, 1966.
4. C. Leymonie, *Radioactive Tracers in Physical Metallurgy,* Wiley, New York, 1963.
5. H. Piraux, *Les Radioisotopes et Leurs Applications Industrielles,* Philips Tech. Library, 1962.
6. P. Daudel. *Radioactive Tracers in Chemistry and Industry,* Charles Griffin, London, 1960.
7. "Radioisotope Applications in Industry" (Bibliography), International Atomic Energy Agency, Vienna, 1963.
8. "Radioisotope Instruments in Industry and Geophysics," Proc. Warsaw Conf., 1965, 2 vols., International Atomic Energy Agency, Vienna, 1966.
9. A. Charlesby, *Atomic Radiation and Polymers,* Pergamon Press, New York 1960.
10. W. R. Corliss and D.G. Harvey, *Radioisotopic Power Generation,* Prentice-Hall, Englewood Cliffs, New Jersey, 1964.
11. "Food Irradiation," *Isotopes Radiation Technol.* **3,** 30 (1965).
12. "Industrial Radioisotope Economics, "*IAEA Tech. Report Series No. 40.,* International Atomic Energy Agency, Vienna, 1965.
13. "Large Radiation Sources in Industry," Proc. Warsaw Conf. 1959. International Atomic Energy Agency, Vienna, 1960.

*14.* "Radioisotopes: Production and Development of Large-Scale Uses. II. Applications," *Isotopes Radiation Technol.* **6,** 238 (1969).

*15.* P. S. Baker (ed.) "Radioisotopes: Production and Development of Large-Scale Uses.," *Isotopes Radiation Technol.* **6,** 131 (1968).

*16.* "Large Scale Production and Applications of Radioisotopes," (Proc. ANS Augusta Meeting), SRL Rept. DP-1066, Savannah River Lab., E.I. DuPont de Nemours, Aiken, South Carolina 1966.

*17.* C. A. Rohrmann,. "Values in Spent Fuel from Power Reactors," *Isotopes Radiation Technol.* **6,** 19 (1968).

*18.* "The Nuclear Industry – 1969," U.S. Atomic Energy Commission, Washington, D. C., 1970.

*19.* R. P. Gardner and R.L. Ely, *Radioisotope Measurement Applications in Engineering,* Reinhold, New York, 1967.

*20.* C. W. Sheppard, *Basic Principles of the Tracer Method,* Wiley, New York, 1962.

*21.* "Radioisotopes in Hydrology," Proc. Tokyo Conf. 1963, International Atomic Energy Agency, Vienna, 1963.

*22.* C. H. Wang and D. L. Willis, *Radiotracer Methodology in Biological Science,* Prentice-Hall, Englewood Cliffs, New Jersey, 1965.

*23.* D. Chleck, R. Maehl, and O. Cucchiara. "Kryptonates: $Kr^{85}$ becomes a universal tracer," *Nucleonics* **21,** No. 7, 53 (1963). Also, D. Chleck, R. Maehl, O. Cucchiara, and E. Carnevale, "Radioactive Kryptonates. I. Preparation; II. Properties," *Int. J. Appl. Radiation Isotopes* **14,** 581, 593 (1963).

*24.* J. E. Carden. "Radio-Release in Review," *Isotopes Radiation Technol.* **5,** 104 (1967).

*25.* S. V. Starodubtsev and A. M. Romanov, *The Passage of Charged Particles Through Matter,* Izdatelstvo A. N. Uzbek. SSR Tashkent, 1962. (English transl., Israel Program for Scientific Translations, Jerusalem, 1965, issued as U.S. AEC Rept. AEC-tr-6468, Washington, D. C., 1965.

*26.* R.G. Jaeger (ed.), *Engineering Compendium on Radiation Shielding,* Vol. 1, Springer, Berlin, 1968.

*27.* H. Goldstein, *Fundamental Aspects of Reactor Shielding,* Addison-Wesley, Reading, Massachusetts, 1959.

*28.* "Radiation Protection," Recommendations of the International Commission on Radiological Protection (revised), ICRP Publication 6, MacMillan, New York, 1964.

*29.* "Basic Safety Standards for Radiation Protection," 1967 ed, IAEA Safety Series No. 9, International Atomic Energy Agency, Vienna, 1967.

*30.* "Standards for Protection against Radiation," U.S. AEC Rules and Regulations (as amended) Title 10, Code of Federal Regulations, Part 20.

*31.* G. W. Grodstein, *X-ray attenuation coefficients from 10 keV to 100 MeV,* NBS Circular 583, National Bureau of Standards, Washington, D. C., 1957.

*32.* T. Rockwell (ed.), *Reactor Shielding - Design Manual,* Van Nostrand, Princeton, New Jersey, 1956.

*33.* "An Evaluation of Systems for Nuclear Auxiliary Power—January 1964," U.S. AEC Rept. TID-20079, 1964.

*34.* J. G. Morse. "Isotopic Power in Europe II," *Isotopes Radiation Technol.* **6,** 100 (1968).

*35.* R. Halmshaw, *Physics of Industrial Radiology,* Elsevier, Amsterdam, 1966.

*36.* H. R. Clauser, *Practical Radiography for Industry,* Reinhold, New York, 1952.

*37.* M. H. Qureshi, *Industrial Radiography Course,* 2nd ed., Rept. PAECL/N19, Pakistan Atomic Energy Centre, Lahore, 1968.

*38.* E. T. Clarke, "Industrial Inspection with Reactor Isotopes." *Proc. Intern. Conf. Peaceful Uses At. Energy, Geneva, 1955,* **15,** 188 (1956).

39.  H. Berger, *Neutron Radiography*, Elsevier, Amsterdam, 1965.
40.  "Californium-252; its Use and Market Potential," U.S. AEC, Washington, D. C., 1969.
41.  H. Hart and E. Karstens, *Radioaktive Isotope in der Dickenmessung,* VEB Verlag, Berlin, 1958.
42.  N. N. Shumilovskii, I. M. Taksar, G. D. Latyshev, V. I. Verkhovskii, V. I. Sinitsyn, and V. A. Yanushkovskii (eds.), "Radioactive Control and Regulation Methods of Industrial Processes." (*Conf. Trans. Riga,* 1959),. U. S. AEC Rept. AEC-tr-4139, Washington, D.C., 1960.
43.  N. N. Shumilovskii, L. V. Melttser, *Radioactive Isotopes in Instrumentation and Control,* Pergamon Press, New York, 1964.
44.  "Symposium on Applied Radiation and Radioisotope Test Methods, " ASTM Special Technical Publication No. 268, 1959.
45.  R. S. Rochlin and W. W. Schultz, *Radioisotopes for Industry,* Reinhold, New York, 1959.
46.  L. Reiffel and R. F. Humphreys, "Beta-ray-Excited X-Ray Sources," *Proc. Intern. Conf. Peaceful Uses At. Energy, Geneva, 1955*, **15,** 291, 1956.
47.  H. Faul (ed.), *Nuclear Geology,* Wiley, New York, 1954.
48.  H. Israel and A. Krebs, *Nuclear Radiation in Geophysics,* Academic Press, New York, 1963.
49.  "Nuclear Techniques and Mineral Resources," *Proc. Buenos Aires Symposium, 1968*, International Atomic Energy Agency, Vienna, 1969.
50.  "Use of Radioisotopes and Supervoltage Radiation in Radioteletherapy," International Atomic Energy Agency, Vienna, 1960.
51.  T. J. Deeley and Constance A. P. Wood (eds.), *Modern Trends in Radiotherapy,*. Appleton, New York, 1967.
52.  J. W. Joseph, H. F. Allen, C. L. Angerman, and A. H. Dexter, "Radioactive Cobalt for Heat Sources." U. S. AEC Rept. DP-1012, 1965.
53.  B. D. Baines, "Irradiation Plant Economics," *Industrial Uses of Large Radiation Sources* **2,** 243 (1963), International Atomic Energy Agency, Vienna, 1963.
54.  A. V. Bibergal, V. I. Sinitsyn, and N. I. Leshchinskii, *Gamma Irradiation Facilities,*. Atomizdat, Moskow, 1960. (English transl., Israel Program for Scientific Translations, Jerusalem, 1965. Issued as US AEC Rept. AEC-tr-6469, Washington, D. C., 1965.)
55.  D. S. Ballantine, "Study of Radiation Processing," *Isotopes Radiation Technol.* **6,** 164 (1968).
56.  Nuclear Industry - 1968. *Nucl. News* **12,** No. 1, 19–51 (1969).
57.  A. Charlesby (ed.), *Radiation Sources,* Macmillan, New York, 1964.
58.  "Industrial Uses of Large Radiation Sources," Proc. Salzburg Conf. 1963 (2 vols.), International Atomic Energy Agency, Vienna, 1963.
59.  "Food Irradiation," Proc. Karlsruhe Symp., 1966. International Atomic Energy Agency, Vienna, 1966.
60.  D. M. Yates, G. W. Collings, J. L. Kline, J. R. Kircher, J. H. Litchfield, and O. Wilhelmy, "The Commercial Prospects for Selected Irradiated Foods," U.S. AEC Rept. TID-24058; *Isotopes Radiation Technol.* **6,** 77, (1968).
61.  K. G. MacQueen, "Potential Role of Radiation in Alleviating Some World Food Problems," *Isotopes Radiation Technol.* **5,** 126 (1967).
62.  J. B. Huff. "Designing for Lower Food Irradiation Costs," *Isotopes Radiation Technol.* **6,** 154 (1968).
63.  "Radiation in Perspective," (C. R. McCullough, J. H. Sterner, M. Eisenbud, C. Starr, F. J. Jankowski, contribs.) *Nucl. Safety* **5,** 226 (1964); **5,** 325, (1964); **6,** 31 (1964); **6,** 143 (1964); **6,** 380 (1965); **7,** 11 (1965).

*64.* "Standards for Protection Against Radiation." Title 10, U.S. Code of Federal Regulations, Part 20, as amended.

*65.* "Regulations for the Safe Transport of Radioactive Materials (1967)," IAEA Safety Series No. 6, International Atomic Energy Agency, Vienna, 1967.

*66.* U. S. Dept. of Transportation Regulations—Hazardous Materials Regulations Board, Title 49, U. S. Code of Federal Regulations Parts 171-177, as amended.

*67.* "Packaging of Radioactive Materials for Transport." Title 10, U.S. Code of Federal Regulations, Part 51, as amended, 1966.

*68.* F. E. Mackinney, S.A. Reynolds and P. S. Baker, "Isotope User's Guide," U. S. AEC Rept. ORNL-IIC-19, 1969.

# 2   LARGE-SCALE PRODUCTION OF RADIOISOTOPES*

## E. J. HENNELLY

SAVANNAH RIVER LABORATORY
E. I. DU PONT DE NEMOURS AND CO.
AIKEN, SOUTH CAROLINA

---

*The information contained in this article was developed during the course of work under Contract AT(07-2)-1 with the U.S. Atomic Energy Commission.

47

## I. INTRODUCTION

Since the birth of the nuclear age in the early 1940s, the production of radioisotopes has evolved from small-scale laboratory operations using charged-particle accelerators or natural Ra–Be neutron sources to large-scale operations involving nuclear reactors and hundreds of millions of dollars. Production of $^{239}$Pu for weapons was the first large-scale radioisotope production operation and was initiated in 1944 at the AEC Hanford Plant near Richland, Washington. Approximately ten years later the Savannah River Plant near Aiken, South Carolina, began production operations for the AEC. The combined productive capacity of these two plants provided the United States with a large capability for producing radioisotopes (1). The spectacular growth of the nuclear electrical power industry has added a new dimension to the nation's and the world's isotope production potential (1a). The combined potential of production and power reactors to produce radioisotopes forms the basis for this chapter.

The application of reactor-produced radioisotopes has grown from the initial use of $^{239}$Pu for nuclear weapons to many fields ranging in scope from tracer use in medicine to large-scale food irradiation and power supplies in space exploration. A multitude of potential applications arises from specific advantages of radionuclides as unique, compact, and portable sources of alpha and beta particles, gamma and X rays, and neutrons. Radioisotope production rates are sometimes governed by the availability of starting materials. Growth of applications is governed principally by the ability of radioisotopes to compete economically with alternative means of achieving a given technical mission.

The attractive long-range potential of large-scale low-cost production, coupled with many unique applications, more than justifies a look at how radioisotopes are made and what these facts portend for the future. For some time to come, matching production with specific requirements will be difficult because radioisotope production requires extensive advanced planning. As a further complication in long-range planning, if a desired radioisotope is not available in sufficient quantity for a particular application, a less attractive alternative isotope or another type of energy source may be used. Even so, application of radioisotopes continues to grow at a very rapid rate, and acceptance of only a few of the many potentially large-scale uses will require that a supply be made available.

The methods of production to be described are limited to cases of radioisotopes produced by neutron absorption or nuclear fission in reactors designed to produce electrical power or designed specifically for production of isotopes. In addition to radioisotope production methods employing reactors, there are two other promising methods which will not be covered in detail. These are the intense neutron generator (ING), which has been under consideration in Canada (2), that could be used as a source of neutrons for isotope production, and the use of underground nuclear explosions in which recoverable quantities of radioisotopes may be produced as a byproduct (3). Both of these methods provide high neutron flux or neutron density. The ING, which appears to be postponed indefinitely, would have been useful for radioisotope production where neutron fluxes $>10^{15}$ n/cm²-sec are required. Underground nuclear explosions, such as Par and Barbel in the U.S. AEC Plowshare program, have already produced detectable quantities of high mass nuclides. Up to 19 neutrons have been added to $^{238}$U to produce a nuclide with a mass of 257, which is well beyond the mass of reactor-produced $^{252}$Cf discussed in later sections. The expense of building and operating substantial chemical processing equipment required to recover trace quantities of such products from vast amounts of bomb debris limits the utility of the method. Both methods are potentially useful, but are rather speculative at this time (1970). The experimental evidence currently available indicates that they would have eventual application only in special cases.

## II.  RADIOISOTOPES OF INTEREST

### A.  *Nuclides Produced by Neutron Absorption*

Nuclides that can be produced by neutron absorption and which have potential large-scale use as heat or radiation sources are summarized in

TABLE 2.1

Neutron-Produced Radionuclides of Interest for Large-Scale Production

| Product | Target | Principal emission | Product half-life | Specific power of pure isotope (W/g) | Applications |
|---------|--------|--------------------|-------------------|--------------------------------------|--------------|
| $^{238}$Pu | $^{237}$Np | $\alpha$ | 87 yr | 0.57 | Heat |
| $^{227}$Ac | $^{226}$Ra | $\alpha\ (\beta)^a$ | 21.8 yr | 14.3 (after 300 days) | Heat |
| $^{244}$Cm | $^{243}$Am | $\alpha$ | 17.6 yr | 2.84 | Heat |
| $^{242}$Cm | $^{241}$Am | $\alpha$ | 163 days | 120 | Heat |
| $^{210}$Po | $^{209}$Bi | $\alpha$ | 138 days | 141 | Heat |
| $^{204}$Tl | $^{203}$Tl | $\beta$ | 3.8 yr | 0.73 | Heat |
| $^{171}$Tm | $^{170}$Er ($^{170}$Tm) | $\beta$ | 1.92 yr | 0.22 | Heat |
| $^{170}$Tm | $^{169}$Tm | $\beta$ | 127 days | 13 | Heat and radiation |
| $^{60}$Co | $^{59}$Co | $\gamma$ | 5.3 yr | 17.3 | Heat and radiation |
| $^{252}$Cf | —$^b$ | $\alpha$,n | 2.65 yr | 40 $2.3 \times 10^{12}$ n/sec g | Heat Neutron source |

$^a$A low-energy $\beta$ emitter with 5 short-lived $\alpha$-active daughters.
$^b$Made by successive neutron additions to uranium, plutonium, americium, curium, berkelium, and/or californium isotopes.

Table 2.1. The five alpha emitters provide a wide range of potential heat source material and usually require chemical separation before use. The three beta-emitting nuclides can normally be produced in a reactor in final form. $^{60}$Co is the only gamma emitter listed and has wide application for use as radiation and heat sources. $^{252}$Cf is unique among all known nuclides as an intense source of neutrons. The actinides are produced from target nuclides formed by reactor irradiation of uranium; the other nuclides by irradiation of naturally occurring target material. A more detailed discussion of the production process of each nuclide follows.

**1. Plutonium-238.** $^{238}$Pu is produced directly by irradiating $^{237}$Np with neutrons. The neptunium target material is obtained as a byproduct from chemical processing of irradiated uranium fuel. $^{237}$Np may be formed by two routes:

$$
\begin{array}{ccc}
\text{Fission} & & ^{237}\text{Np} \\
\uparrow & & \uparrow \\
| & & \beta\ (\tau_{1/2} = 6.7\ \text{days}) \\
| & & | \\
^{235}\text{U} \xrightarrow[\text{n},\gamma]{} & ^{236}\text{U} \xrightarrow[\text{n},\gamma]{} ^{237}\text{U} & \xleftarrow[\text{n, 2n}]{} ^{238}\text{U}
\end{array}
$$

In uranium-fueled reactors containing a large fraction of $^{238}$U, such as most pressurized water (PWR), boiling water (BWR) nuclear power plants, and graphite and $D_2O$ moderated, near-natural, or natural uranium-fueled reactors, the fast neutron $^{238}$U (n, 2n) contribution is the most important production route in fuel that experiences low burnup of $^{235}$U. However, $^{236}$U is formed by neutron capture in $^{235}$U at about 20% the $^{235}$U fission rate. Therefore after long fuel exposures [ $>10^4$ megawatt days per metric ton (MWD/T)], the formation of $^{237}$Np via the $^{236}$U route predominates. Deliberate recycle through reactors of uranium fuel containing previously produced $^{236}$U increases the $^{237}$Np production rate. Thus the $^{237}$Np supply, primarily a reactor byproduct, is limited by the integrated fission power generated in $^{235}$U, the presence of $^{238}$U and the efficiency of $^{236}$U recycle.

After recovery of $^{237}$Np by chemical processing, $^{238}$Pu is then produced by reirradiation in a reactor via the following route:

$$^{238}\text{Pu} \longrightarrow \text{Higher Pu Isotopes}$$
$$\uparrow \beta \, (\tau_{1/2} = 2.1 \text{ days})$$
$$^{237}\text{Np} \xrightarrow{\text{n, } \gamma} {}^{238}\text{Np} \longrightarrow \text{Fission and Capture}$$

Loss from fission and capture in $^{238}$Np ($\tau_{1/2} = 2.1$ days) is a function of the neutron flux.

The present limited supply of $^{237}$Np target material for $^{238}$Pu production should be alleviated late in this decade when the nuclear power industry achieves its projected growth and the $^{237}$Np is available for recovery from residues of chemically processed power reactor fuel (Fig. 2.1) (3a). Pure $^{238}$Pu can also be produced via alpha decay of chemically separated $^{242}$Cm, made by neutron absorption in $^{241}$Am. However, $^{241}$Am is projected to be available in substantially less quantity than $^{237}$Np (Fig. 2.1).

$^{238}$Pu is also formed directly in the fuel of nuclear power reactors from neutron absorption in $^{237}$Np and by $^{242}$Cm alpha decay. However the product is isotopically mixed, as a minor constituent ($\sim$1%) in plutonium fuel containing predominantly $^{239}$Pu. $^{239}$Pu is the major isotope produced in power reactors and is formed by neutron capture in $^{238}$U to form $^{239}$U followed by double beta decay. The $^{238}$Pu is regarded as an isotopic contaminant and is not available for heat source application because it remains with the fuel when plutonium is recycled for further power production. The $^{238}$Pu would burn up by neutron capture to form $^{239}$Pu.

Efficient application of $^{238}$Pu as a source of heat will probably require high temperatures and hence the use of oxide (mp$\sim$2240°C).

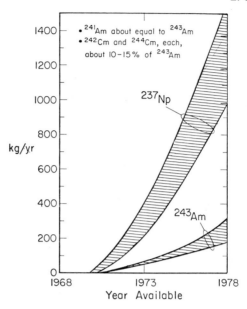

FIG. 2.1. Predicted U.S. availability of actinide targets for radioisotope production.

Microspheres of plutonium oxide have been developed for this purpose. Plutonium metal can be used for lower temperature application, i.e., $<600\,°C$.

**2. Actinium-227.** $^{227}$Ac is made by neutron irradiation of radioactive but naturally occurring $^{226}$Ra. Although principally (98.3%) a low-energy beta emitter, it is a potentially attractive candidate heat source because of the high power density caused by the decay cascade that includes five short-lived alpha-active daughters: $^{227}$Th, $^{223}$Ra, $^{219}$Rn, $^{215}$Po, and $^{211}$Bi. After a buildup of about a year, the equilibrium decay follows the $^{227}$Ac half-life. Formation is by the following route:

$$^{227}\text{Ac}$$
$$\bigg\uparrow \beta \,(\tau_{1/2} = 41 \text{ min})$$
$$^{226}\text{Ra} \xrightarrow{\text{n, } \gamma} {}^{227}\text{Ra}$$

In-reactor burnup, loss of $^{227}$Ac ($\sigma_{\text{th}} \sim 800$ b) to form $^{228}$Ac ($\tau_{1/2} = 6.1$ hr), which leads rapidly by beta decay to unwanted $^{228}$Th, can be kept to a minimum by short target irradiation times ($\sim$3 weeks). To keep expensive target inventories small, the irradiation is followed rapidly by chemical removal of $^{227}$Ac and immediate recycle of the radium target to the reactor (4). Thus inventory of rare radium is kept to a minimum. The $^{228}$Th, which is unavoidably formed, contributes undesirable $\gamma$-rays from $\beta, \gamma$ disintegrations in the decay chain, particularly $^{208}$Tl, so that even trace quantities of thorium should be removed in the chemical processing used to purify $^{227}$Ac after separation from the $^{226}$Ra target. Unshielded residual gamma emission would then amount to about 7 R/hr-g at 1 m.

**3. Curium-244.** $^{244}$Cm is produced directly by irradiating $^{243}$Am target that is chemically recovered from residues of fuel in which plutonium was produced and/or irradiated. It is also possible, with intermediate beta decay, to add five successive neutrons to a $^{239}$Pu target until $^{244}$Cm is produced. Irradiation of target mixtures of the intermediate plutonium isotopes, $^{240}$Pu, $^{241}$Pu, and $^{242}$Pu, provides other alternatives. The complete path to $^{244}$Cm is shown below:

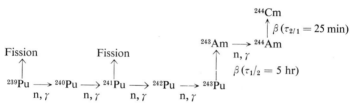

In reactors in which the plutonium formed contributes substantial power, such as in most nuclear power plants, and in reactors especially designed to burn plutonium (5), $^{243}$Am and $^{244}$Cm are produced in recoverable amounts. If plutonium produced in nuclear power fuel is reirradiated, availability of higher plutonium isotopes as well as of $^{243}$Am and $^{244}$Cm is enhanced further (6). These conditions are becoming increasingly probable indicating the prospect of having large-scale availability of $^{244}$Cm and target material from which it can be produced. High-temperature ($\sim$2000°C) applications of $^{244}$Cm will probably require use of curium oxide (mp > 2200°C).

**4. Curium-242.** $^{242}$Cm ($\tau_{1/2} = 163$ days) has a relatively short half-life and hence high power density. It is formed by irradiation of $^{241}$Am, which in turn is a decay product of $^{241}$Pu ($\tau_{1/2} = 13$ yr). A heat source containing $^{242}$Cm was used in a demonstration of the "SNAP 2" thermoelectric generator in 1966. This device had been planned to power scientific experiments on the moon. $^{242}$Cm was also a source of alpha particles in Surveyor V equipment, which made the first direct chemical analysis of lunar surface by measuring alpha-particle interactions. $^{242}$Cm is formed via the following route:

$$^{242}\text{Cm}$$
$$\uparrow \quad \beta\,(\tau_{1/2} = 16\text{ hr}),\ 82\%$$

$$\overset{n,\gamma}{^{241}\text{Am} \longrightarrow}\ ^{242}\text{Am} \longrightarrow \text{Fission}$$

Fission $\quad\uparrow\quad \searrow\ ^{242\text{m}}\text{Am}\,(\tau_{1/2} = 150\text{ yr})$

$$\uparrow \quad n,\gamma$$

$$\uparrow \quad \beta\,(\tau_{1/2} = 13\text{ yr})$$

$$^{239}\text{Pu} \longrightarrow {}^{240}\text{Pu} \longrightarrow {}^{241}\text{Pu} \dashrightarrow {}^{242}\text{Pu}$$
$$n,\gamma \qquad n,\gamma$$

Product is lost by $^{242\text{m}}$Am formation (about 17%), by $^{242}$Am fission, which is a function of the neutron flux, by electron capture of $^{242}$Am to form $^{242}$Pu (18%) and by $^{242}$Cm alpha decay, depending on delivery time, giving an optimum yield of about 0.65 g/g of $^{241}$Am burned up. The availability of target $^{241}$Am is limited by the $\beta$-decay rate of $^{241}$Pu formed in the irradiation of plutonium. Storage of chemically separated plutonium to allow $^{241}$Pu to decay would give pure $^{241}$Am; however, separation of americium from irradiated power reactor fuel would provide a mixture of $^{241}$Am and $^{243}$Am in varying ratios. Rather than using the $^{242}$Cm as product, it has been proposed (7) to let it decay to $^{238}$Pu. Because the respective neutron cross sections are about 9:1, $^{241}$Am:$^{243}$Am, the americium isotope mixtures could be irradiated initially in reactors to burn up $^{241}$Am preferentially to produce predominantly $^{242}$Cm. The separated curium isotope mixture, rich in $^{242}$Cm, would supply $^{238}$Pu from $^{242}$Cm alpha decay. After chemical separation of the americium, the $^{243}$Am richer target mixture could be irradiated to produce $^{244}$Cm, with smaller $^{242}$Cm content (7a), or by continued irradiation, $^{252}$Cf.

Generally speaking, for future large-scale production, $^{244}$Cm and $^{238}$Pu produced from their respective targets, $^{243}$Am and $^{237}$Np, probably will provide the major sources of actinide isotopic power. The production and application of $^{242}$Cm have some merit as an alternative to short-lived $^{210}$Po or $^{170}$Tm. However if not needed when produced, $^{242}$Cm $\alpha$-decays to produce $^{238}$Pu product with delivery delayed by the $^{242}$Cm decay rate and quantities limited by $^{241}$Am availability.

**5. Polonium-210.** $^{210}$Po is produced by irradiating naturally occurring bismuth (100% $^{209}$Bi). $^{210}$Po was used in 1959 to demonstrate the "SNAP 3" a prototype electrical generating device. The route to $^{210}$Po is as follows:

$$^{210}\text{Po}\,(\tau_{1/2} = 138\text{ days})$$
$$\uparrow \beta\,(\tau_{1/2} = 5\text{ days})$$
$$^{209}\text{Bi} \longrightarrow {}^{210}\text{Bi}$$
$$n,\gamma$$

Two obstacles to making $^{210}$Po are (a) the low neutron absorption cross section of $^{209}$Bi ($\sigma_{th}$ ~15 mb) which limits $^{210}$Po production in any reactor by the amount of bismuth that can be packed into a reactor volume, and (b) the short half-life of $^{210}$Po ($\tau_{1/2}$ = 138 days) that results in substantial product loss before use. Pure $^{210}$Po has the advantage of a high power density and does not require the long lead time for buildup of target material necessary for making $^{238}$Pu, $^{242}$Cm, and $^{244}$Cm. However, source fabrication is completely dependent on availability of chemical processing facilities for separating $^{210}$Po from bismuth targets. $^{210}$Po would have application where its short half-life can be tolerated and its high power density is desirable. Because of the low melting point of $^{210}$Po (mp = 254°C), its use as a heat source requires fabrication of rare-earth polonides with higher melting points, ~2000°C.

6.  **Thallium-204.**  $^{204}$Tl has a desirable half-life and convenient $\beta$ decay properties for an isotopic power source. $^{204}$Tl is made directly by irradiating $^{203}$Tl (29.5% abundant in natural thallium). Most of the shielding required is to absorb the effect of the bremsstrahlung accompanying the 0.76-MeV $\beta$ decay. The inherently low specific power of irradiated natural thallium, ~0.06 W/g after 1 yr at a neutron flux of $10^{15}$ n/cm$^2$ sec, and the relatively low melting point of the thallium metal (mp = 300°C) and oxide (mp = 760°C) are undesirable properties for heat source application. Isotopic separation of $^{203}$Tl target material from natural thallium prior to irradiation or isotopic separation of $^{204}$Tl after irradiation would improve product power density substantially, but would not alter the unfavorable physical properties.

7.  **Thulium-171.**  $^{171}$Tm has attractive properties from the user point of view. Thulium oxide is physically and chemically quite stable at high operating temperatures, and the pure $^{171}$Tm isotope requires very little shielding because it has high self-absorption for its soft 0.067-MeV gamma ray. $^{171}$Tm is produced by irradiation of $^{170}$Er or by double neutron capture in $^{169}$Tm.

$$^{171}\text{Tm} \qquad\qquad\qquad\qquad ^{170}\text{Yb}$$

$$\uparrow \beta\ (\tau_{1/2} = 7.5\ \text{hr}) \qquad\qquad \uparrow \beta\ (\tau_{1/2} = 130\ \text{days})$$

$$^{170}\text{Er} \longrightarrow {}^{171}\text{Er} \qquad\qquad ^{169}\text{Tm} \longrightarrow {}^{170}\text{Tm} \longrightarrow {}^{171}\text{Tm}$$

$$\text{n, }\gamma \qquad\qquad\qquad\qquad \text{n, }\gamma \qquad\quad \text{n, }\gamma$$

$$(a) \qquad\qquad\qquad\qquad (b)$$

Route (a) requires complete separation of the $^{170}$Er isotope (14.9% abundant), before irradiation, to be efficient and to yield an isotopically pure, chemically separable product; route (b) requires a high neutron flux to minimize product loss by beta decay of the intermediate [170]Tm target, but inherently leaves significant residual [170]Tm contamination that requires extra shielding. Processes for chemical separation of [171]Tm from erbium target and ytterbium decay products have been developed (8). The principal deterrent to large-scale production of isotopic power using [171]Tm is the low specific energy per disintegration. What proves to be an advantage for shielding purposes imposes a serious limitation on reactor capacity for producing enough [171]Tm to create significant total power in comparison with other radioisotopes.

**8.   Thulium-170.**   [170]Tm can be used as a heat source where the very high melting thulium oxide (mp $= 2400\,°C$) fuel form and the ability to preform the final product prior to irradiation are advantages that could outweigh the relatively short half-life. [170]Tm has a higher specific power than [171]Tm but requires heavier shielding. [170]Tm also has application as an X-ray radiography source by virtue of its photoemission resulting from the dominant 84-keV $\gamma$ transition and X rays from internal conversion. [170]Tm is made directly by irradiating natural [169]Tm, an isotopically pure, naturally occurring element. The power density of [170]Tm in the resultant product has a practical limit of about 25% of pure [170]Tm because of burnup and decay of [170]Tm during irradiation. The favorable neutron absorption cross section (Table 2.11) of [169]Tm permits rapid and efficient production of [170]Tm in reactors.

**9.   Cobalt-60.**   Of all radioisotopes that can be produced directly in reactors, [60]Co offers the greatest potential for immediate large-scale heat generation and use in radiation source applications. It is perhaps for this reason that [60]Co applications have been studied in such wide diversity and great detail. [60]Co is produced directly from natural isotopically pure [59]Co by neutron absorption; about half passes through [60m]Co (10.4 min) by isomeric transition. To demonstrate a record high level of activity, a small pellet of cobalt was irradiated in a Savannah River reactor (9) to about 700 Ci/g of cobalt, which represents about 65% of the specific activity of pure [60]Co. [60]Co up to 400 Ci/g can be produced routinely on a large scale.

[60]Co has many attractive properties as an isotopic power source such as the comparatively long half-life, the good metallurgical properties of cobalt and its compatible decay product nickel, and the potential for preforming the final product prior to irradiation. For heat generation, its principal disadvantage is the substantial shielding required. However, when [60]Co is used as a heat source for large installations, the calculated tungsten shield weights range from only 1000 to 2000 pounds for 2–20

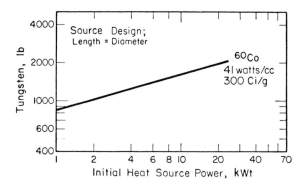

FIG. 2.2.   Shielding $^{60}$Co heat sources.

thermal kilowatts (kW$_t$) (Fig. 2.2), showing a factor of 5 advantage in the shield-weight per unit power for the larger source (10).

The use of $^{60}$Co as a radiation source is widespread and is discussed in more detail in Chapters 4 and 6. Efficient utilization involves the following considerations. Shielding a radiation source facility is an expected cost and weight penalty because efficient irradiation of materials depends on gamma rays escaping from $^{60}$Co sources. In fact, for use in radiation sources, gamma-ray self-shielding of the cobalt and the resultant heating within the source are undesirable and reduce radiation efficiency, with a consequent increase in cost. This is emphasized by the fact that $^{60}$Co source costs are projected to be the major fraction of the capital requirements of a large-scale radiation processing plant, i.e., a plant with about a megacurie of $^{60}$Co. For this reason, cobalt radiation sources should be thin, with sufficiently high specific activity to provide the proper source strength per unit source area.

**10.   Californium-252.**   Of all the nuclides of interest, $^{252}$Cf is currently the least available, but it offers the greatest challenge for both large-scale production and application. Primarily an alpha emitter with an effective half-life of 2.65 yr and as such a potential heat source, $^{252}$Cf undergoes spontaneous fission at about 3.2% of the alpha decay rate and has great possibilities as an absolutely unique intense source of neutrons with an emission rate of 2.3 × 10$^{12}$ n/sec-g. However, its production requires successive addition of 14 neutrons to $^{238}$U, the naturally occurring starting material. Intermediate plutonium, americium, curium, and californium isotopes, if available, could also be used as starting targets to shorten the required irradiation time and to increase the yield of $^{252}$Cf. Uncertainty still exists about some neutron absorption cross section data in the buildup chain so that forecasts of $^{252}$Cf availability contain unavoidable uncertainties. Predictions of kilogram quantities of $^{252}$Cf are long-term projections (*10a*) over 10–15 years, and the assumption is made that suitable target material will be available as residue byproducts in the fuel of operating nuclear power plants (Fig. 2.1).

### B.  Fission Products

Fission products are not "produced" in the usual sense that neutrons are absorbed intentionally in a target nuclide to make a desired product radioisotope, but are made as inevitable byproducts of the fission process. Fission product yields vary widely according to the now-classical two-humped distribution in Fig. 2.3, but for those fission products of primary interest as radiation and heat sources, i.e., $^{90}$Sr, $^{137}$Cs, $^{144}$Ce, and $^{147}$Pm, the initial yields per fission are between 2.1 and 6.2%.

The potential availability and cost of the fission products are functions of their concentrations in irradiated fuel, which in turn depend on the fission yield, the accumulated fuel exposure, the fission product half-life, and neutron cross section for burnup. These parameters account for the variations in average yield as functions of fuel exposure listed in Table 2.2.

For example, with its half-life of only 2.62 yr, $^{147}$Pm availability in fuel exposed to $\sim$25,000 MWD/T (3–4 yr exposure) drops well below the initial fission yield of $\sim$2.5% to an average net yield of less than 1%. However, $^{147}$Pm concentration still increases significantly in the first 10,000 MWD/T ($\sim$1.5 yr exposure), thus reducing incremental recovery plant costs per gram of product, which are roughly inversely proportional to concentration (*12*). $^{147}$Pm decay and burnup account for the losses. Greater "losses" occur for shorter-lived $^{144}$Ce ($\tau_{1/2} = 285$ days) and lesser "losses" for longer-lived $^{90}$Sr ($\tau_{1/2} = 30$ yr), but the unit recovery costs for these products are projected to differ by only a factor of about two because of the substantial concentration of each in the fission product residues in irradiated power reactor fuel.

**1.  Cesium-137.**   $^{137}$Cs is produced with an initial fission yield of about 6.2% in $^{235}$U fuel and slightly higher, $\sim$6.6%, in $^{239}$Pu, but the final separated cesium product contains only about one-third $^{137}$Cs because of dilution by stable $^{133}$Cs and relatively stable $^{135}$Cs ($\tau_{1/2} \sim 2.3 \times 10^6$ yr); the latter two are produced in a ratio of fission yields of about two. Average $^{137}$Cs yields are nearly constant with power reactor fuel exposure because its half-life is long compared with fuel cycle time; $^{137}$Cs burnup

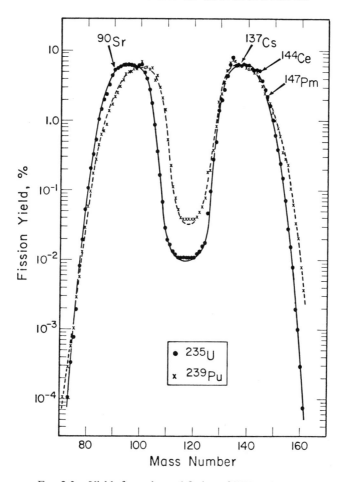

FIG. 2.3.   Yields from thermal fission of $^{235}$U and $^{239}$Pu.

losses are relatively small ($\sigma_{th} \sim$0.1 b) and the yields in plutonium and $^{238}$U fast fissions are comparable to $^{235}$U fissions. $^{137}$Cs is primarily a beta emitter, but its 2.6-min daughter, $^{137m}$Ba, is a source of 0.66-MeV gamma activity. Thus, although possibly useful as a heat source, the unfavorable physical properties of cesium compounds, low power density, and poor high temperature properties, tend to limit application to gamma-emitting radiation sources where $^{60}$Co is the primary isotope competitor. The small quantity (of the order of 1–2%) of gamma-emitting $^{134}$Cs ($\tau_{1/2} =$ 2.1 yr), formed by neutron absorption in the stable fission product $^{133}$Cs, does

TABLE 2.2

RADIOFISSION PRODUCTS OF INTEREST FOR LARGE-SCALE USE[a]

| Product | Principal emission | Half-life | Energy pure isotope (W/g) | Isotopic purity (%) | Average yield from power fuel at discharge[a] (mg/MWD) | | | Principal application |
|---|---|---|---|---|---|---|---|---|
| | | | | | Initial | 14,000 MWD/T | 25,000 MWD/T | |
| $^{137}$Cs | $\beta,\gamma$ | 30 yr | 0.42 | 35 | 39 | 33.5 | 32 | Radiation |
| $^{90}$Sr | $\beta$ | 28 yr | 0.96 | 55 | 24 | 19 | 15 | Heat |
| $^{147}$Pm | $\beta$ | 2.62 yr | 0.33 | 100 | 17 | 10 | 7 | Heat |
| $^{144}$Ce | $\beta$ | 285 days | 25.2 | <15 | 35 | 17 | 10 | Heat |

[a] Based on generally accepted fission yields for initial yield with low exposure and on measurements of Yankee fuel for exposed fuel (11).

not provide operational problems when fission product cesium is used as a radiation source.

The long half-life, the relative abundance, the ease of chemical separation and the desirability to find useful means for its disposal have stimulated development of $^{137}$Cs as a radiation source.

**2. Strontium-90.**   $^{90}$Sr results from a fission yield of 5.6% in $^{235}$U but only 2.1% in $^{239}$Pu. This lower yield from plutonium accounts for the drop in the yield of $^{90}$Sr observed in power reactor fuel with long exposure where plutonium fissions become a major contribution to reactor power (Table 2.2). Other strontium isotopes are also produced so that, of the total strontium present, only about half is $^{90}$Sr and most of the remainder is stable $^{88}$Sr. In chemical processing, care must be taken not to add chemicals that contain trace amounts of naturally occurring strontium that would further dilute the final product. The intense, high-energy $\beta$ activity of $^{90}$Y ($\tau_{1/2} = 62$ hr), the decay daughter of $^{90}$Sr in secular equilibrium, results in high-energy bremsstrahlung for which heavy shielding is required in heat source application. Aging to reduce short-lived $^{89}$Sr ($\tau_{1/2} = 51$ days), normally present in trace quantity at the time of reactor discharge, improves product quality by minimizing this other high-energy radiation source. Strontium is often prepared as the oxide (mp $= 2460\,°C$) or titanate (mp $= 1910\,°C$) in final source fabrication. $^{90}$Sr is frequently considered for heat source application in thermoelectric generators and use has been demonstrated in the SNAP-7 series in ocean buoys.

**3. Promethium-147.**   $^{147}$Pm has desirable properties as a heat source, e.g., the high melting point of $Pm_2O_3$, $\sim 2100\,°C$. The major source of supply will be from power reactor fuel residues. Final yield is substantially reduced from the initial fission yield of 2.5% by decay and burnup during projected exposures and by the additional 2- to 3-year decay required prior to source preparation to permit decay to a negligible level of the energetic gamma-emitting contaminant $^{148m}$Pm ($\tau_{1/2} = 42$ days). $^{148}$Pm is formed in small amounts by neutron absorption in $^{147}$Pm. Trace quantities ($\sim 4$ ppm) of gamma-emitting $^{146}$Pm ($\tau_{1/2} = 5.5$ yr) prevent use of $^{147}$Pm as a pure low energy beta emitter and prolonged decay or aging increases the $^{146}$Pm/$^{147}$Pm ratio. $^{146}$Pm results primarily from the $^{147}$Pm (n,2n) reaction.

The technology of $^{147}$Pm heat sources is well developed and fuel-form materials have good physical properties. Large-scale application awaits adequate availability, which will continue, however, to be limited by the decay and yield penalties cited above.

**4.   Cerium-144.**   $^{144}$Ce will abound as a heat source as seen in Fig. 2.4. The major energy generation comes from decay of its daughter $^{144}$Pr ($\tau_{1/2} = 17.3$ min). High fission yields of ~5.6% from $^{235}$U and 4.1% from $^{239}$Pu, and high specific power are advantages for special short-term application. The melting point of $Ce_2O_3$ is also desirably high, ~2150°C.

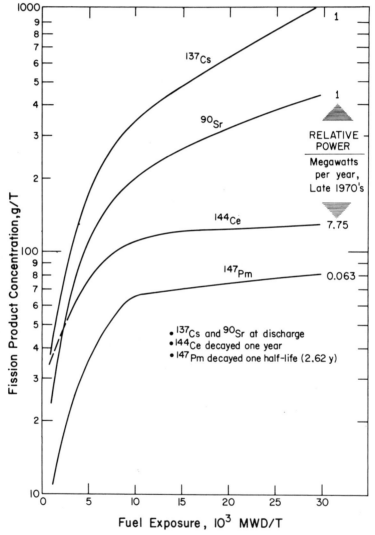

FIG. 2.4.   Fission product buildup in nuclear power fuel.

However, being available only as an incidental fission product, the use of short-lived $^{144}$Ce cannot be scheduled as effectively as longer-lived fission products. The total amount of product available and its specific power are therefore necessarily uncontrollable.

$^{144}$Ce is diluted by two stable cerium fission product isotopes, $^{140}$Ce and $^{142}$Ce, that are nearly equally abundant and limit $^{144}$Ce in power reactor residues to $<15\%$ isotopic abundance. The power density of the resultant isotopic mixture, therefore, is reduced from a theoretical 25 W/g to a practical value of less than 3.7 W/g depending on fuel exposure in the reactor and time elapsed after fuel discharge and chemical separation. This reduction in isotopic purity and the variability that is dependent on product history are drawbacks to any large-scale application. In addition the extremely energetic activity of the daughter product, $^{144}$Pr, provides a further disadvantage when shielding is considered. $^{141}$Ce ($\tau_{1/2} = 32.5$ days) is a radioisotope impurity that is reduced to manageable proportions by decay during the normal delay period required prior to chemical processing.

On the credit side, $^{144}$Ce will always be a major source of immediate fission product power, and this factor alone may stimulate solutions that would compensate for any disadvantages from its physical properties and may bring about large-scale applications. The inherent difficulties in matching the predictable supply with a varying demand may not be serious because the supply is potentially very large in relation to foreseeable demands.

## III. LARGE-SCALE PRODUCTION CONSIDERATIONS

### A. An Equivalent Neutron Absorption Comparison

For the present purpose, "large-scale production" will be understood as requiring reactor-years of operation and/or millions of dollars of expenditure.

Most people would agree that kilogram quantities of plutonium are large amounts and that a gram of californium is relatively small. What is probably not generally recognized is that both quantities may be classified as requiring "large-scale production." To make kilograms of plutonium, reactor irradiation of tons of uranium would be required. To make gram quantities of californium, additional years of time-consuming reactor exposure of the plutonium and its reaction products must occur.

Thus from the production point of view, "large scale" for products between plutonium and californium includes quantities covering a range of at least $10^3$.

Potential users of radioisotopes are interested in the same general quantity range because, although single large uses of radioisotopes as heat or radiation sources draw attention and capture the imagination, supplying sources for multiple small applications may in the long run equal or surpass requirements for a few larger applications.

Table 2.3 gives approximate relative ultimate yields of the neutron-produced radionuclides of interest if sufficient target material were available, and provides comparison of production potential for equivalent "large-scale" efforts. Simply stated, the ultimate yield is the amount of product produced for each gram atom of target consumed. For a single neutron capture, this is readily seen to be the yield. For products where multiple neutron capture in a sequence of nuclides must occur to make the product, the ultimate yield is the amount of product produced for each gram atom of target consumed after all of the intermediates have been converted to the final product. The word ultimate is used to indicate that substantial time may pass before that yield is achieved.

The reader should use Table 2.3 only for approximate projections. Too many factors not yet discussed are implicit in estimating relative yields, particularly the assumptions that target material is always available and

TABLE 2.3

ULTIMATE YIELD FOR ONE GRAM OF NEUTRON
ABSORPTION IN A GRAM ATOM OF TARGET

| Target nuclide | Radionuclide of interest | Specific power (W/g) | Ultimate yield (g) | Ultimate yield (W) | Ultimate yield (W/yr) |
|---|---|---|---|---|---|
| $^{237}$Np | $^{238}$Pu | 0.57 | 167 | 95 | 12,000 |
| $^{226}$Ra | $^{227}$Ac | 14.3 | 170 | 2430 | 77,000 |
| $^{243}$Am | $^{244}$Cm | 2.84 | 220 | 625 | 16,000 |
| $^{241}$Am | $^{242}$Cm | 120 | 157 | 18,800 | 12,100 |
| $^{241}$Am | $^{238}$Pu from $^{242}$Cm $\alpha$-decay | 0.57 | 154 | 88 | 11,100 |
| $^{209}$Bi | $^{210}$Po | 141 | 7 | 987 | 540 |
| $^{203}$Tl | $^{204}$Tl | 0.73 | 190 | 139 | 765 |
| $^{170}$Er | $^{171}$Tm | 0.22 | 144 | 32 | 89 |
| $^{169}$Tm | $^{170}$Tm | 13 | 85 | 1105 | 570 |
| $^{59}$Co | $^{60}$Co | 17.3 | 55 | 950 | 7300 |
| $^{244}$Cm | $^{252}$Cf | $\alpha$-source 40 | $\sim$0.25 | $\sim$1 | $\sim$4 |
| | | 2.3 $\times$ $10^{12}$ n/sec-g | $\sim$0.6 $\times$ $10^{12}$ n/sec | | |

that target can be converted rapidly to product. However, the wide range of grams, watts and watt-years for equivalent neutron absorption emphasizes the potential range covered in the term "large-scale production."

## B. Comparison of Availability and Time

Another means of defining "large-scale production" involves consideration of target availability. The relative yield calculations in Table 2.3 assumed that target availability matched requirements. However, at the present time target material is lacking for the heavy actinides: $^{237}Np$, $^{243}Am$, $^{241}Am$, and $^{242}Cm$–$^{244}Cm$ mixtures that are needed to make $^{238}Pu$, $^{244}Cm$, $^{242}Cm$, and $^{252}Cf$, respectively. Targets for the other products occur naturally and, in principle, are available in abundant quantity; however availability of $^{226}Ra$ is limited because it occurs naturally in uranium ore in concentrations of only 0.3 ppm of uranium and as a minor byproduct is not always recovered in typical uranium mining operations. Tailings from high grade uranium ore provide a rich source that has supplied most of the current limited demand.

Availability of actinide target nuclides in the United States is a function of past reactor power generation with $^{235}U$ and $^{239}Pu$ fuel, which up to now has taken place primarily in AEC production reactors. Looking to this decade, however, the availability of target material from chemically processing fuel irradiated by the nuclear power industry is potentially very large. Latest estimates given in Fig. 2.1 show the range of target availability (3a) predicted for some of the target nuclides; availability according to these figures would influence potential production predicted from Table 2.3 yield comparisons. Growth projections, such as these, are under constant upward revision as the future of nuclear electrical power brightens. Nuclide availability, from the chemical processing of fuel irradiated in power reactors outside the United States, is estimated to be at least 50% as large over the same period of time. The range of uncertainty in current estimates is shown by the shaded areas in Fig. 2.1. It is evident that the definition of "large scale" for $^{237}Np$ can vary by a factor of 10 or more as a function of time over the 1970s. At a given time it may also vary considerably for the two different isotopes, $^{237}Np$ and $^{243}Am$, simply because target availability of the two nuclides will increase rapidly but at different rates. 100% utilization of the quantities projected during the 1970s would be truly "large scale" by any standard.

Recycle of plutonium as fuel in nuclear power plants in the early 1970s would have a marked effect on annual availability of americium and curium isotope mixtures by increasing the expected quantities of these nuclides, industry-wide, by a factor of two or more in the late 1970s (*6*).

### C.  Scope of Potential Production

The potential for $^{60}$Co production in the United States of hundreds of megacuries per year was announced at the Geneva Conference (*1*) in 1964. This shows an acknowledged capability for radioisotope production far in excess of current $^{60}$Co demand and near-term projected needs. Thus in terms of total quantity, "large-scale production" means quantities from the current megacurie level to a potential of hundreds of megacuries (1 MCi = 15.5 kW for $^{60}$Co). Similar large-scale projections apply to fission products for the late 1970s when hundreds of megacuries will have been accumulated.

## IV.  LARGE-SCALE PRODUCTION METHODS

### A.  Introduction

Radioisotopes can be produced as primary products in production reactors or as byproducts in research and power reactors. Since production reactors are designed to use a substantial portion of available neutrons for radioisotope production, they are as a rule likely to be more efficient producers. On the other hand, byproduct generation of radioisotopes in power reactors, where the cost of reactor operation is borne largely by the sale of generated electricity, may result in more economical production of some radioisotopes. The growth of nuclear power will result in the production of larger quantities of target and product nuclides in this decade and beyond. These factors will be discussed in the remaining sections of this chapter.

Regardless of the type of reactor employed, certain basic facts apply in estimating production of radioisotopes:

(1)  An average of about 2.5 neutrons are emitted per fission.

(2)  Of these neutrons, one must be reserved to continue the chain reaction to keep the reactor operating at power.

(3)  Of the remaining, at least 0.5 neutron is lost by leakage from the reactor, capture in structural and coolant materials, and parasitic capture in the fuel.

(4)  Approximately one neutron per fission is thus available to make the desired product.

(5)   About $3.1 \times 10^{16}$ fissions per second equal one megawatt (energy release is $\sim$200 MeV per fission).

The primary problem of reactor physics, as applied to radioisotope production, involves the determination of how efficiently a particular reactor utilizes the excess neutrons not needed to maintain the chain reaction. The principal factors for estimating potential radioisotope production are the efficiency of excess neutron utilization in producing the desired product and the total number of fissions or the integrated power, usually expressed in megawatt-days.

The simple procedure of using neutron flux, neutron absorption cross section, and time of reactor exposure, and multiplying these factors by the amount of target material in the reactor, so useful in estimating activation in small sample irradiations, should generally be avoided in making large-scale estimates unless detailed reactor physics considerations are taken into account to determine valid operating values of neutron flux, neutron cross section, and permissible amount of target material.

## B.   Reactor Types

The types of reactors capable of producing radioisotopes may be separated into five general categories:

(1)   Heavy water moderated production (Savannah River) and power reactors (Canadian).
(2)   Graphite moderated production (Hanford) and gas-cooled power reactors (HTGR and Great Britain).
(3)   Light water moderated boiling water (BWR) and pressurized water (PWR) reactors for generating electrical power.
(4)   Fast breeders and resonance or intermediate spectrum reactors (projected).
(5)   Research and test reactors, such as the General Electric Test Reactor (GETR) and the High Flux Isotope Reactor (HFIR).

The following discussion on production includes appropriate reference to these reactor types and their characteristics.

## C.   Full-Scale Production

Three factors that determine the full-scale production rate in a reactor are: reactor power, reactor operating efficiency, and efficiency of neutron utilization. Neutron flux considerations enter into overall production efficiency if the product decays substantially during irradiation, e.g., $^{210}$Po or $^{170}$Tm, or if an intermediate target decays, e.g., $^{170}$Tm in the two-stage formation of $^{171}$Tm from $^{169}$Tm irradiation, or if an intermediate is destroyed, e.g., by neutron capture in $^{238}$Np during formation of $^{238}$Pu, or if high specific activity of product is desired, e.g., for $^{60}$Co and $^{170}$Tm sources.

In principle, any of the reactor types could be devoted to full-scale production of any of the radionuclides of interest. However, those reactors designed for radioisotope production have advantages for the following reasons:

### (a)  Higher Power

Production reactors generally do not produce usable thermal power so that the coolant temperature rise across a reactor and hence the power removal capability of the circulating coolant can be larger than in an equivalent reactor designed for efficient electrical power generation, where for thermodynamic efficiency of associated turbines the temperature *rise* is smaller.

Compared with test reactors in the 10–100 MW range, production and power reactors operate at sizable power levels as judged for example by the announced capability of about 800 $MW_e$ or about 4000 $MW_t$ of the Hanford NPR.

### (b)  Better Efficiency

At the lower average operating temperature of production reactors, aluminum with its low neutron absorption and substantially lower cost can be used as a structural and cladding material instead of either stainless steel, which has high neutron absorption, or costly zirconium alloy, both of which are used in nuclear power plants.

Production, research, and test reactors are designed for rapid and frequent removal of target material, so important for the shorter half-life products, in contrast to year-long fuel replacement cycles and comparatively lengthy refueling periods typical of nuclear power reactors.

Intermediate or fast spectrum reactors have specialized potential for radioisotope production, not the broad capability of thermal neutron production reactors. As an example of the limitations of these reactors, the higher atomic weight actinides have sizable fission cross sections in fast reactors and might be destroyed rather than produced (*12a*).

Finally, another factor which is sometimes overlooked and which affects the efficiency of product delivery, is the speed with which the product can be chemically separated, especially if the half-life is short. Similarly, if the target supply is limited, efficiency depends upon how rapidly the target material can be recycled back into the reactor for further irradiation. Production reactor sites usually have associated separation facilities to expedite target turnaround; such facilities may not be readily available to other types of large-scale reactor operations. These considerations apply equally to actinide production and to fuel reprocessing plants where long-lived fission products must be extracted. However, in the case of $^{60}$Co or $^{170}$Tm, postirradiation chemical processing is not required and the material is available for use soon after reactor discharge.

   **1. Fuel and Target Selection.** First-principle reactor physics determines how fuel and targets are selected. For a reactor to achieve criticality the net neutron multiplication factor $k$ must equal unity. To operate at power this factor must initially be greater than unity to allow for such negative reactivity effects as fuel burnup, negative temperature coefficients required for stable operation, and parasitic neutron absorptions in fission products formed. The extra reactivity is compensated initially by neutron absorbers (control rods) at appropriate positions within the reactor. As the need arises, control rods are moved out of the reactor core to compensate for the negative reactivity effects at power.

   To illustrate the relationship between fuel and target neutron absorption, the case of $^{235}$U fuel is chosen first. The maximum multiplication constant, or neutrons emitted per neutron absorbed in fuel, is 2.07 for an infinitely large thermal reactor, i.e., one with no neutron leakage and with no nonfission neutron absorptions except in $^{235}$U to form $^{236}$U. Then $k = \eta = 2.07$, where $\eta$ = neutrons emitted per neutron absorbed in fuel.

   When a neutron absorber is added as the irradiation target, the resultant neutron utilization to make the desired product is given by $(1 - f)$, and the multiplication constant is reduced to $k = \eta f$, i.e., neutrons emitted per *total* number absorbed. The factor $f$ applies to thermal neutron absorptions. However, if neutrons are absorbed with energies intermediate between the average energy of fission, $\sim2$ MeV and thermal energies, $\sim0.02$ to 0.05 eV, another factor $p$, the resonance escape probability, which accounts for epithermal absorptions, reduces $k$ further and $k = \eta f p$.

   Finally, if materials such as $^{238}$U or $D_2O$ are present, extra neutrons from fast fission and $(\gamma,n)$ events, respectively, can add neutrons and hence reactivity. The fast fission effect $\varepsilon$ is the larger effect, but is usually only a few percent greater than 1.

   Therefore $k$ is often expressed by the "four-factor formula" $k = \eta f p \varepsilon$. To achieve a measure of the required excess reactivity, $k - 1$, for a particular operating reactor charge, the size of the reactor must also be considered because $(k-1)$ must at least equal the neutron leakage fraction. However, for most reactors of the size required for large-scale production, neutron leakage is small and $k$ is in the range of 1.05 to 1.15. A nominal value of 1.10 will be selected for further discussion.

Assuming for simplicity, but without sacrificing reasonable accuracy, that p and $\varepsilon$ equal unity, e.g., that there is no $^{235}$U present, then

$$k = 2.07 \times \left( \frac{\text{neutrons absorbed in fuel}}{\text{total neutrons absorbed}} \right) = 1.10 \quad \text{and}$$

$$2.07 \times (\text{neutrons absorbed in fuel}) = 1.10 \times (\text{neutrons absorbed in fuel}) + 1.10 \times (\text{neutrons absorbed in target})$$

Rearranging

$$1.10 \times (\text{neutrons absorbed in target}) = 0.97 \times (\text{neutrons absorbed in fuel})$$

and

$$\frac{\text{neutrons absorbed in target}}{\text{neutrons absorbed in fuel}} = 0.88$$

Since the ratio of thermal absorption to fission in $^{235}$U is about 1.18,

$$\frac{\text{neutrons absorbed in target}}{\text{fissions in fuel}} = 0.88 \times 1.18 = 1.04$$

This means that for each fission event approximately one neutron is available for productive absorption in the target. Similar calculations can be made for $^{239}$Pu and $^{233}$U fuel. They are compared in Table 2.4 with the $^{235}$U values.

$^{235}$U is used most commonly as a reactor fuel because it occurs naturally in larger amounts and is cheaper than the other two. However, Table

TABLE 2.4

MAXIMUM TARGET ABSORPTIONS PER FISSION

| Fissionable nuclide | $^{235}$U | $^{239}$Pu | $^{233}$U |
|---|---|---|---|
| $\nu$, neutrons/fission | 2.44 | 2.87 | 2.51 |
| $\eta$, neutrons/fuel absorption | 2.07 | 2.11 | 2.28 |
| Absorption/fission | 1.18 | 1.36 | 1.10 |
| For $k = 1.10$ in a reactor $\dfrac{\text{target absorptions}}{\text{fuel absorptions}}$ | 0.88 | 0.92 | 1.07 |
| $\dfrac{\text{target absorptions}}{\text{fuel fissions}}$ | 1.04 | 1.25 | 1.18 |

2.4 shows that $^{233}$U could be the most efficient reactor fuel from neutron utilization considerations. The high calculated target-to-fuel absorption ratio, $\sim$1.07, indicates why $^{233}$U is a potential thermal breeder fuel, i.e., at thermal energies more than one target absorption can be made per fuel atom destroyed. In contrast, $^{239}$Pu has the largest target absorption-to-fission ratio, indicating the greatest potential production rate per unit of reactor power. Viewed strictly as neutron producers, either $^{233}$U or $^{239}$Pu are superior to $^{235}$U, unless $^{237}$Np, which is formed from byproduct $^{236}$U and leads to $^{238}$Pu product, is desired.

To approach the efficiencies in Table 2.4, the moderator must be non-absorbing. Structural and cladding material must be kept to a minimum and the unavoidable neutron leakage must be compensated by surrounding the reactor with productive neutron absorbing blankets or efficient reflectors. In addition, control rod absorptions must be productive, which would eliminate from consideration often-used nonproductive absorbing materials such as $^{10}$B and natural Cd.

Heavy water with its low absorption cross section makes an ideal moderator for minimizing unwanted parasitic neutron absorptions. Graphite is the next most desirable and natural water the least.

Because the chemistry of water contributes to corrosion and the hydraulic effects to erosion in most thermal neutron reactors, aluminum can be used to support $^{235}$U and to clad and support target material only when maximum coolant temperatures are below 120°C. Coextruded tubes of $^{235}$U–Al alloy clad with aluminum have been used at record high specific power and heat flux (13). However, power reactor water temperatures in the range of 300°C require use of zirconium or stainless steel as cladding and support materials.

For final selection of fuel and target design to achieve optimum isotope production conditions, the following factors must be taken into consideration: reactor power; operating efficiency; product yield; unit cost; and total cost. Interrelations among these factors are discussed in succeeding parts of this Section.

In summary, target material for making the desired product is limited to an amount which will reduce the multiplication constant $k$ to about 1.1. Fuel type and configuration are selected on the basis of neutron flux desired, overall cost, availability, and need for byproduct residues. Cladding and support material are chosen to contain the fuel and target adequately and to reduce neutron absorption losses acceptably.

**2. Nuclides Produced in Targets.** Most of the nuclides of interest, other than fission products, are produced by irradiating the target material in reactor positions physically separated from fuel. These could be in adjacent positions, within the fuel assembly, in reflectors, blankets, or in control rods.

The amount of target needed is set by the quantity required to bring the multiplication constant $k$ of the loaded reactor to the desired value $\sim 1.1$. This in turn depends on the amount of fissionable fuel to be used in a particular reactor loading.

The effectiveness of a target to absorb neutrons in competition with the fuel is proportional to

$$\frac{N_1 \, \sigma_1 \, \phi_1}{N_2 \, \sigma_2 \, \phi_2} = \frac{\text{absorption in target}}{\text{absorption in fuel}}$$

where subscripts 1 and 2 refer to target and fuel, respectively; $N$ = number of atoms; $\sigma$ = effective absorption cross section, $10^{-24}$ cm$^2$/atom or barn; $\phi$ = neutron flux, n/cm$^2$ sec; and $\phi\sigma$ = specific reaction rate, neutrons absorbed/sec atom.

If the cross section is large, i.e., $\sigma > 100$ b, and the target is thick, i.e., $\sim 0.25$ cm, the outer layers of pure target absorb neutrons preferentially while the inner region is exposed to a reduced neutron density. This effect is called self-shielding and results in a depression of the neutron flux. The effectiveness of a target and also the fuel to absorb neutrons is thus dependent on how it is dispersed. Practical considerations usually require that both be concentrated in specific assemblies in the reactor so that product can be removed separately when required and heat can be removed by coolant from the fuel during operation. Targets in limited supply, such as $^{237}$Np, $^{243}$Am, $^{241}$Am, and $^{244}$Cm, should be dispersed so that each atom is exposed to a high neutron flux to permit the most rapid conversion to product. Self-shielding slows the conversion rate, particularly when the target supply is limited.

Such targets as cobalt and thulium have an advantage for subsequent use if they can be preformed to final shape prior to irradiation. Sample thickness acceptable to final applications is usually controlled to nominal values of 0.03–0.10 cm. The self-shielding that occurs (14) reduces the product specific activity but can be tolerated in many cases in the interest of overall economics and improved production efficiency by using preformed targets. The relatively easy availability of most target materials permits full utilization of reactor neutrons and production rates are therefore not affected by self-shielding.

In some cases it is desirable to precoat target material, such as $^{59}$Co with nickel or $^{169}$Tm with molybdenum, to aid in reducing contamination during postirradiation handling and to speed up delivery for final use. These coatings reduce reactor neutron utilization by the fraction of neutrons absorbed in the coating but are justified by overall economic and safety considerations. At the present time actinide irradiation and production would be aided by the use of aluminum to disperse the target because postirradiation aluminum removal by chemical separations processes is a well-developed technique and facilities are available.

Bismuth irradiation for $^{210}$Po production provides an exception to most of the above generalizations. Bismuth has a very small absorption cross section for producing $^{210}$Po, $\sim$0.015 b (total absorption $\sigma = 0.034$ b); this compares with an aluminum absorption cross section of $\sim$0.23 b, about 15 times greater. Thus, *if* aluminum is used to clad bismuth, and the relative productive bismuth-to-parasitic aluminum absorption ratio is to be only unity, *then* the Bi/Al weight ratio in the target must be at least 119 and the required volume ratio per unit length becomes 33. Consequently, for a bismuth slug about 12 in. long with a reasonable 20-mil cladding of aluminum and a net thickness of 1 in. aluminum in the end plugs, the Al-to-Bi absorption ratio is raised to 4.5. In addition, only half the total bismuth absorptions produce $^{210}$Po. This unavoidably low efficiency of $^{210}$Po production per neutron absorption in the target, plus decay of product prior to use, accounts for the relatively low ultimate yield of $^{210}$Po given in Table 2.3.

One other factor must be considered in general target design. Relatively modest amounts of heat, several watts per gram of target-plus-cladding, are generated in the targets by absorption of $\gamma$ rays resulting from fissions in the fuel and neutron capture. Compared with gamma heating, relatively large amounts of additional heat can originate from fissions which occur in the following target irradiations:

(1)  from fission in $^{239}$Pu and $^{241}$Pu formed as unavoidable byproducts in production of $^{238}$Pu from $^{237}$Np;

(2)  from fission in $^{238}$Np, the intermediate in the formation of $^{238}$Pu from $^{237}$Np;

(3)  from fission in $^{239}$Pu and $^{241}$Pu in plutonium isotopic mixtures irradiated to produce $^{243}$Am and $^{244}$Cm;

(4)  from fission in $^{242}$Am, the intermediate in the formation of $^{242}$Cm from $^{241}$Am;

(5)  from fission in $^{245}$Cm and $^{247}$Cm in curium isotopic mixtures irradiated to produce $^{252}$Cf.

Specially designed targets are required to remove fission heat for each

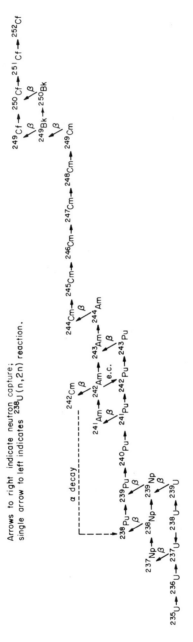

Arrows to right indicate neutron capture;
single arrow to left indicates $^{238}U(n,2n)$ reaction.

FIG. 2.5.    Production chain of radionuclides.

specific reactor selected for the irradiation. The specific fission power generation is a function of the neutron flux, target concentration, and time of irradiation, and must be considered in detail each time targets are irradiated.

**3. Nuclides Produced in Reactor Fuel.** Some of the nuclides of interest and/or target material from which they can be produced must be recovered from irradiated fuel. These include the fission products $^{137}$Cs, $^{90}$Sr, $^{147}$Pm, and $^{144}$Ce as well as the transuranium actinides. A measure of availability of these nuclides can be estimated from experimental data and reactor calculations for nuclear power plants (6, 11, 15).

Estimates of fission product availability from the nuclear power industry are shown in Fig. 2.4. As fuel exposure increases, the concentrations of $^{137}$Cs and $^{90}$Sr continue to increase; whereas the concentrations of the shorter-lived $^{144}$Ce and $^{147}$Pm approach a constant value for the reasons cited in Section II.B. The annual U.S. availability (MW/yr) in the late 1970s, shown at the right, indicates the isotopic power that could be utilized if the currently projected growth rate of the nuclear power industry materializes and the fuel exposure goal of about 30,000 MWD/T is achieved.

Reactors fueled with $^{235}$U produce byproduct $^{237}$Np and $^{238}$Pu. Reactors containing $^{238}$U also produce byproduct $^{237}$Np; in addition they produce plutonium in major quantities. The resultant $^{241}$Pu $\beta$ decays to $^{241}$Am which can be converted to $^{242}$Cm; resultant $^{242}$Pu converts to target $^{243}$Am, which is then available to produce $^{244}$Cm. Resultant curium isotopic mixtures can be converted to $^{252}$Cf. The actinide production chains are shown in Fig. 2.5; for simplicity, fissions are not shown.

The calculated concentrations-at-discharge of actinides, in grams per metric ton of uranium fuel, over the range of fuel exposure, megawatt-days per metric ton of uranium fuel, are plotted in Fig. 2.6 for typical 1000 MW$_e$ nuclear power plants of current construction. Expectations for pressurized water reactors (PWR) and boiling water reactors (BWR) are nearly identical, with the exception that BWR fuel contains about 20% less $^{237}$Np and about 50% more $^{241}$Am at equivalent exposures because of differences in neutron spectrum and power density. Experimental data from Yankee Reactor fuel are shown in Fig. 2.6 for $^{237}$Np; data for the other actinides correspond closely with the PWR calculations. Figure 2.7 provides a comparison of actinide target production when plutonium and uranium from the first fuel exposure cycle, after an exposure of ~24,000 MWD/T, are recycled with $^{235}$U added to achieve the required reactivity. Gains in concentration for all nuclides would result, with the largest for

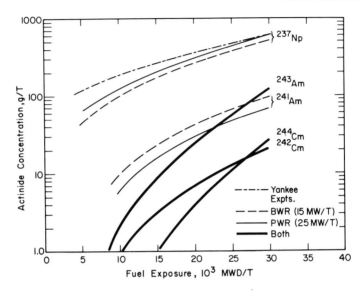

FIG. 2.6.   Actinide buildup in nuclear power reactor fuel at discharge.

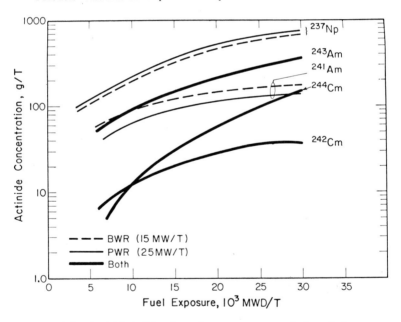

FIG. 2.7.   Actinide buildup in nuclear power reactor fuel at discharge
(first recycle of Pu and U).

$^{244}$Cm, which is the furthest along the production chain from uranium.

In this decade, operating characteristics of nuclear power reactors will change because there are economic incentives and it is feasible for designers to double the specific power (MW/T) and for operators to increase fuel exposure to about 35,000 MWD/T. Increases in specific power reduce some nuclide yields, but extra exposure more than compensates, within the same time span, so that reasonable long-term estimates of nuclide expectations can be made using the data in Figs. 2.6 and 2.7 (where $^{241}$Am about doubles one year after discharge) and the growth data in Fig. 2.1.

The key point is that for the longer fuel exposures, >20,000 MWD/T, which are the goals of the electrical industry for economic electric power production, actinide and fission product concentrations in irradiated fuel are great enough to permit recovery at a reasonable cost if facilities are available at chemical fuel reprocessing plants. Recovery unit costs vary inversely as the concentration in the fuel. A recent study of the technical feasibility (12) showed unit costs of chemical separation over a seven-year period dropping from $102 to $15 per gram of $^{237}$Np and from $234 to $31 per gram of americium. The reduction reflects unit cost savings in processing the increased concentrations and throughput from greater amounts of irradiated fuel with longer reactor exposure that would be available at the end of that time period.

A helpful generalization is that, at similar concentrations in the fuel, all isotope recovery unit costs are comparable, at least to within ±50% of the average.

One final note about fuel-produced nuclides relative to neutron spectrum. Yankee experimental data for $^{237}$Np show an interesting phenomenon; the quantity of $^{237}$Np produced per megawatt-day is nearly constant up to fuel exposure of 30,000 MWD/T. However, calculations of $^{237}$Np for the 1000 MW$_e$ power plants (15) show an increase in the $^{237}$Np production rate as shown in comparison in Table 2.5.

TABLE 2.5

AVERAGE $^{237}$Np PRODUCTION RATE

| Exposure (MWD/T) | $^{237}$Np, mg/MWD | | |
|---|---|---|---|
| | Yankee | 1000 MW$_e$ PWR | 1000 MW$_e$ BWR |
| 10,000 | 18 | 12 | 10 |
| 20,000 | 18 | 15 | 12.5 |
| 30,000 | 20 | 20 | 17 |

The differences between the Yankee and the 1000 MW$_e$ designs apparently arise because the closer packing of fuel rods in the Yankee core provides a proportionally higher $^{238}$U (n,2n) contribution to $^{237}$Np production, at low exposure, than the more open fuel packing in the newer, higher power designs. However, as exposure increases, the early Yankee advantage is lost because the buildup of $^{236}$U from neutron captures in $^{235}$U provides a target for increased production of $^{237}$Np and because the early $^{237}$Np is burned up. $^{237}$Np availability is thus dependent on the fuel-lattice arrangement as well as fuel exposure. As will be shown in Section VI, the production of other actinides is also dependent on the neutron spectrum and the yield predictions should be calculated using specific reactor design data.

Data on fission product and actinide generation presented in this subsection provide material for making reasonably accurate estimates of radioisotope availability in the next decade. More specific and detailed reactor design data, which would help to provide more accurate estimates, are often difficult to obtain or are considered proprietary by the power industry. In any case, uncertainties in predicting nuclide availability are more affected by the timing of reactor construction and by chemical processing factors, because the rapid growth rate of the industry equates uncertainties in quantity estimates of a factor of 2 to uncertainties in time estimates of about two to three years. This is indicated by the shading in Fig. 2.1 for $^{237}$Np and $^{243}$Am–$^{241}$Am mixtures.

4. **Effect of Neutron Flux.** Because pedagogical examples often use neutron flux and cross section values to predict isotope production, comparison of this method with the method outlined in previous sections relating production to fissions requires a basic discussion of the character of neutron flux.

The implication of the units of flux, neutrons/cm$^2$ sec, is that a high flux is desirable generally for a more rapid production rate and specifically for improving the production rate of short-lived products. This is true when

(1) The supply of target material is limited, e.g., in $^{252}$Cf production;

(2) The intermediate precursor in the neutron addition chain decays, e.g., $^{170}$Tm ($\tau_{1/2} = 130$ days) in the production of $^{171}$Tm from $^{169}$Tm;

(3) The cross section of an intermediate decay precursor is less than that of the product, e.g., $\sigma^{239}$Np ($\tau_{1/2} = 2.1$ days) $= 60$ b, is less than $\sigma^{239}$Pu $= 1010$ b;

(4) High specific activity of the product is the main goal, as in the case of $^{60}$Co and $^{170}$Tm source production; and $^{210}$Po in Bi.

(5) Early delivery of product is desirable, e.g., production of $^{244}$Cm from $^{242}$Pu, where the comparatively low cross section ($\sim$20 b) and the limited availability of $^{242}$Pu restricts the production rate of final product $^{244}$Cm.

However, in going to higher flux a price must be paid in lower neutron utilization efficiency and lower reactor power, and this price must be compensated by a higher product value.

The reason for lower neutron utilization at higher neutron flux can be shown by examining the design of a high flux reactor. Neutron flux in a thermal reactor containing fissionable $^{235}$U fuel can be calculated accurately using the following simple relationship:

$$\phi = K\,(P/U)$$

where $P$ = power in megawatts (MW), $U$ = quantity of $^{235}$U (g), and

$$K = \frac{[3.1 \times 10^{16}\ \text{fissions/(sec} \times \text{MW)]}}{[(2.56 \times 10^{21}\ \text{atoms}\ ^{235}\text{U/g}) \times (\sigma_{\text{fiss}}\ ^{235}\text{U})]}$$

The effective fission cross section for $^{235}$U ($\sigma_{\text{fiss}}$) must be calculated for the neutron spectrum in the fuel.* An average value of 450 b was calculated at Savannah River for the world's highest flux of $6 \times 10^{15}$ n/cm$^2$/sec (13). Thus, for that reactor

$$\phi = 2.7 \times 10^{16}\ P/U$$

and the neutron flux is directly proportional to the specific power per gram of $^{235}$U. To increase the specific power in an existing reactor, it is necessary to reapportion the coolant flow to fewer fuel assemblies, so that the power removal rate per assembly can increase, and to reduce the fuel concentration to the minimum required for operation at power. These modifications result in a reduction of total reactor power, but give a net increase in neutron flux. This lowering of reactor power accounts for a large part of the lower production efficiency of high flux operations.

Previously it was shown that for $^{235}$U, the ratio

$$\frac{\text{neutron absorptions in target}}{\text{fissions in fuel}} = 1.04.$$

This holds approximately true for any $^{235}$U–D$_2$O reactor because D$_2$O absorbs few neutrons, and is nearly true for graphite which also has a low

---

*For methods of calculation refer to Section VII.

cross section. The percent "productive" absorptions in the target, compared to nonproductive absorption in structural material, is a function that depends on the unavoidable parasitic absorption in the cladding and support material of both fuel and target. Thus, for a given reactor heat removal and power generating capability, the highest neutron flux requires a minimum $^{235}$U. Consequently *no productive target can be present* and all so-called "target" absorption takes place in the necessary support and cladding material and, therefore, is unavailable for productive use.

In the case of the Savannah River high flux operation, the minimum $^{235}$U was about 8.5 kg (*13*), which occurred at the end of the fuel cycle. Therefore, almost all "target" absorption occurred in structural and cladding aluminum since control rods are withdrawn at end-of-cycle, where $^{235}$U is a minimum, and useful target absorptions were relatively few. At the highest possible neutron flux, the following approximate relationship applied:

$$\frac{\text{absorptions in Al}}{\text{fissions in fuel}} = 1.04.$$

Reactor physics considerations require that the ratio of "absorption" to fission remain nearly constant for the reactor to operate at power and if productive neutron absorber is added, compensating $^{235}$U must also be added. If total "target" doubles, fissionable fuel must also double, thus making productive absorptions equal to aluminum parasitic absorptions; but the flux is halved because $^{235}$U has been doubled. If more fuel and target are added, the neutron flux would continue to drop and the productive to nonproductive absorptions would increase. Figure 2.8 shows this for the example chosen.

If some structural or cladding aluminum could have been traded for productive absorber by replacing it with a less absorbing support material, production would be shifted upward as shown in Fig. 2.8 for the equivalent of a 25% reduction in aluminum. In any case, *there is a maximum flux* where *production is zero* and at lower fluxes the efficiency of neutron utilization is a function of the percent parasitic captures in support, cladding, moderating materials, and fission products. Neutron leakage is large from this type of reactor, but it is assumed in this example that a surrounding blanket in the reflector absorbs neutrons productively.

Because maximum neutron utilization is incompatible with operation at the maximum attainable flux, when neutron flux is used to calculate production, care must be taken to consider how any absorber material might reduce the flux and whether the desired overall production goal is

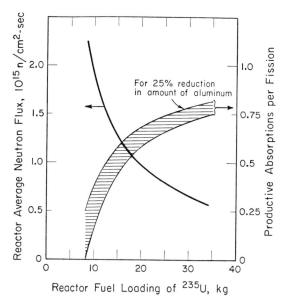

FIG. 2.8.    High flux production and reactor fuel loading.

thereby achieved. Since $D_2O$ is an ideal moderator, with proper design to minimize self-shielding of target nuclei, the actual neutron flux in the target material in a heavy water reactor can be quite close to the fuel flux calculated above.

The high flux reactor at Oak Ridge (HFIR) operates in the thermal neutron flux range in excess of $10^{15}$ n/cm² sec. High flux is achieved in a small central region using the "flux trap" principle (16). Nevertheless, production limitations based on target capacity and power level also apply in this case.

Knowledge of target flux and *effective* cross section is important for calculating radioisotope production mentioned earlier in this section, such as:

(1)   Losses in $^{171}$Tm production from $^{169}$Tm and $^{238}$Pu from $^{237}$Np.
(2)   Specific activity of $^{60}$Co in cobalt and $^{170}$Tm in thulium.
(3)   Production rates of products with limited target quantities, e.g., $^{252}$Cf, $^{244}$Cm.

Section VII describes means for obtaining the required cross sections.

   **5.   Reactor Power and Operating Efficiency**.   To operate a reactor at power, part of the fuel is consumed by fission and an additional fraction

TABLE 2.6

FISSIONABLE NUCLIDES CONSUMED AT POWER[a]

| Nuclide | Fissioned (g/MWD) | Total destroyed (g/MWD) |
|---------|-------------------|-------------------------|
| $^{235}U$ | 1.05 | 1.24 |
| $^{233}U$ | 1.04 | 1.15 |
| $^{239}Pu$ | 1.02 | 1.41 |

[a]200 MeV per fission, $^{235}U$, $^{233}U$; 208 MeV per fission, $^{239}Pu$.

of fuel is destroyed by capture. Fissioning of about one gram of fuel is equivalent to one megawatt day of energy. Comparison of consumption of fissionable nuclides that might be considered as fuel is made in Table 2.6. Thus a reactor, to operate at power, must contain an excess of fuel over that required for initial criticality. To continue to operate for days or months, substantial excess fuel is needed, or fresh fuel must be produced by productive neutron absorption as in converter or breeder reactors. Continuing with the example of the Savannah River high flux operation, the initial $^{235}U$ loading was 14.1 kg and the final 8.5 kg; the actual burnup of 5.6 kg provided the reported accumulated exposure of 4500 MWD (1.24 g $^{235}U$/MWD). At the rated power of 710 MW, the minimum operating time is 6.35 days or about 7 days when a gradual approach to power is included. About 3 days was required for charge–discharge of fuel and general maintenance so that $\sim70\%$ operating efficiency at power is calculated, which was very close to actual performance. However, the burnup of fuel at constant power leads to an increase in the neutron flux.

Thus during high neutron flux operation, the flux is not constant with time and must be interrupted at frequent intervals for recharging fuel to the reactor. If a smaller initial loading had been used, the neutron flux over the operating cycle would have been higher, but the efficiency of operation at a given power would decrease because the time for charge–discharge remains constant. For example, if 9.4 kg were the initial loading, only 0.9 kg would be available for burnup, equivalent to one day's operation. The effective operating period at the higher flux would thus be only one day out of four, resulting in about a 25% efficiency. At fixed power, the productive rate approaches zero at the maximum flux because *both* operating efficiency *and* efficiency of neutron utilization drop to zero.

Improvement in operating efficiency can be achieved by adding fuel and target to the reactor. However, if power remains constant, the neutron flux drops. As shown in the previous subsection, neutron utilization improves at lower flux, as does operating efficiency. Improvements can be achieved in the following ways.

(1) By using a more effective neutron absorbing control system to permit an increased fuel loading, the same percent burnup of fuel is possible and the number of operating days at power between fuel replacement will increase.

(2) By using target material that will burn up along with fuel, thus extending the time an amount of fuel can undergo fission while still maintaining the multiplication constant $k$ at the needed value.

(3) By using fertile target material that will form fresh fuel material by productive neutron absorption in the target.

Thus at a substantially lower flux, nuclear power plants running at higher power (3000 $MW_t$) but at thermal neutron fluxes of only $\sim 3 \times 10^{13}$ n/cm$^2$ sec, will operate for about 9 months before shutdown for partial fuel discharge. Equilibrium fuel exposure of 1000 days ($\sim$24,000 MWD/T) are predicted for $\sim$60% burnup of the initial $^{235}$U. Plutonium buildup in the uranium helps to extend fuel exposure times even though $^{239}$Pu actually replaces less than half the burned-up $^{235}$U.

Thus reactor operating time is functionally related inversely to neutron flux. It was shown previously that productive absorptions are related to fissions in fuel and that, integrated over time, they are functionally inversely proportional to flux.

Knowledge of four factors, reactor power, neutron utilization, operating efficiency, and neutron flux, is required to determine potential productivity. Section VI covers losses due to burnup and decay of actual product. Failure to consider all of the above factors can lead to substantial errors in predicting nuclide availability from full-scale production.

**6. Effect of Neutron Spectrum.** In all nuclear reactors there is a continuum of neutron energies extending from the upper end at fission energies, at about 2 MeV, down to thermal energies (0.025 eV) where neutrons have come to equilibrium with the temperature of the surrounding medium. Neutrons of energies over the entire range are present in all reactors. The characterization of the neutrons as a function of energy describes the spectrum. Whether a reactor is regarded as having a fast, intermediate, or thermal neutron spectrum is one of degree only. Thermal reactors are well-moderated reactors, i.e., there is sufficient moderator space between fuel assemblies for neutrons to slow down from fission energy by nonabsorbing collisions with the moderator. A neutron is regarded as thermal once it has an energy less than 0.6 eV, where it becomes part of the neutron population that follows an approximate thermal Maxwellian energy distribution (Section VII). However there are still substantial numbers of higher-energy neutrons that can be absorbed. For example, even in those nuclear power plants which are regarded as thermal reactors the ratio of thermal to epithermal fissions is only 2 to 1.

The intermediate or resonance energy region extends from above thermal to about 10 keV. However, most of the so-called absorption or fission cross section resonances are in the range 1–100 eV. Fast breeder reactor spectra may vary from 10 keV upward, depending on the fuel density and coolant selected. Breeding-blankets surrounding fast reactors can have a neutron spectrum extending over the entire energy range. A reactor spectrum is identified by the energy region where the majority of neutron absorptions and fissions occur.

In the Savannah River high flux reactor core, the predominant neutron absorption events are thermal. If fuel and compensating neutron absorber were added to this core design, at constant power the ratio of thermal-to-epithermal absorption events in the fuel would decrease. Although the reactor would still be a thermal reactor, the spectrum would be considered "harder." If the moderator could be displaced leaving only $D_2O$ coolant, the ratio of thermal-to-epithermal events would be further reduced, so that the spectrum could then have a majority of neutron absorptions and fissions in the resonance or intermediate energy region. The spectrum would then be considered "intermediate" or "resonance." If $D_2O$ coolant could be then replaced by a nonmoderating coolant material, a fast reactor of sorts would exist. This example is given to show how to proceed conceptually from one end of the neutron spectrum to the other. Actual design would involve substantial and complicated calculations and experiments to define the spectrum and to select materials of construction.

It is unlikely that deliberate spectrum adjustment to higher energies will play much of a role in radioisotope production unless advantages over existing thermal reactors become evident. Advantages that could come from the "harder" resonance spectra are:

(1)  Product is made faster because target nuclei have high resonance absorption cross sections.
(2)  Yield of product is increased because the capture-to-fission ratio in a chain of precursors is increased.
(3)  Product burnup relative to formation is reduced at the harder spectrum.

Some idea of the losses in neutron utilization for intermediate spectrum or resonance reactors in comparison with thermal reactors can be obtained by looking at the increase in parasitic capture that occurs in fuel for a neutron energy of 100 eV, a typical average energy for fission for resonance reactor design (17). The capture-to-fission ratio increases with neutron energy for $^{235}$U and $^{239}$Pu but not for $^{233}$U. The results are compared with the thermal neutron equivalents in Table 2.7.

The calculations show that raising the energy of the neutrons reduces the potential neutron utilization by a substantial amount, with the exception of $^{233}$U-fueled reactors which would be unaffected. $^{233}$U seems to have ideal properties for neutron utilization efficiency from this point of view.

The reduced productivity caused by the increase in capture-to-fission in fuel can be turned to advantage if the same holds true for target chains where the capture product is desired and fission is regarded as a loss. This would be true for $^{252}$Cf production *if* the fissionable precursors $^{245}$Cm and $^{247}$Cm show similar responses to spectrum change as $^{235}$U and $^{239}$Pu. The combined gain in yield for each curium isotope might more than compensate for the loss in reactor productivity in going to the harder spectrum. Theoretical correlations (18) indicate that capture-to-fission ratio will increase; however, cross section measurements at this time (1970) do not.

The resonance integral for $^{238}$Pu is about 30% of the thermal cross section, but for its target $^{237}$Np the resonance integral is about three times the thermal cross section so that the ratio of production rate to burnup rate increases as the spectrum is hardened, thus improving product yield for a given burnup of target.

TABLE 2.7

COMPARISON OF NEUTRON UTILIZATION—THERMAL AND 100 eV NEUTRONS

| Fuel | $^{235}$U | | $^{239}$Pu | | $^{233}$U | |
|---|---|---|---|---|---|---|
| $v$, Neutrons/fission | 2.44 | | 2.89 | | 2.51 | |
| Neutron energy, eV | 0.025 | 100 | 0.025 | 100 | 0.025 | 100 |
| $\eta$, Neutrons/fuel absorption | 2.07 | 1.60 | 2.08 | 1.68 | 2.28 | 2.28 |
| Absorption to fission ratio | 1.18 | 1.52 | 1.39 | 1.72 | 1.10 | 1.10 |
| For $k = 1.1$ in a reactor | | | | | | |
| $\dfrac{\text{Target absorptions}}{\text{Fuel absorptions}}$ | 0.88 | 0.45 | 0.89 | 0.53 | 1.07 | 1.07 |
| $\dfrac{\text{Target absorptions}}{\text{Fuel fission}}$ | 1.04 | 0.69 | 1.24 | 0.91 | 1.18 | 1.18 |

Finally, for a harder resonance spectrum, the resonance integral plays an important role in setting the production rate for targets of limited availability. In some cases a resonance reactor production rate could exceed that of high thermal flux operation with the same amount of target material available. For example $^{242}$Pu, which is a potential target for $^{244}$Cm via $^{243}$Am, and $^{236}$U, which leads to $^{238}$Pu via $^{237}$U and $^{237}$Np have low thermal cross sections of about 20 and 5 b, respectively. Here, there is an advantage in going to high flux to increase the production rate when target availability is limited as in these cases at this time (1970). The resonance integral to thermal cross section ratio is 59 for $^{242}$Pu and 72 for $^{236}$U compared to only 0.48 for $^{235}$U fission. Therefore in studies of possible production acceleration for equal fission powers, the advantages of the hardened neutron spectrum of a resonance reactor must be compared with the advantages of a high flux thermal reactor in selecting the preferred method. If unlimited target material is available, thermal reactors have an advantage because of the potential for superior total neutron utilization. However, even with unlimited amounts of initial target material, resonance reactors would still have a production rate advantage if in the production chain a target in small supply is formed with a large resonance to thermal absorption ratio. For example, in the production of $^{252}$Cf from $^{244}$Cm, $^{246}$Cm ($RI/\sigma \approx 100$), and $^{248}$Cm ($RI/\sigma \approx 170$) are formed in relatively small amounts because of fission losses in $^{245}$Cm and $^{247}$Cm. A proper resonance spectrum could accelerate conversion to the desired higher actinides.

7. **Product Quality.** It is virtually impossible to obtain an isotopically pure product of any radionuclide because radioisotopes are either not pure originally or accumulate decay products. Product quality is defined by the nearness to the desired product purity. Quality definitions can be broken up into four categories: specific activity, isotopic purity, chemical purity, and decay product buildup.

High specific activity of $^{60}$Co in cobalt and $^{170}$Tm in thulium is usually desirable because this often permits design of more efficient power or radiation sources. High specific activity is achieved by irradiation at high neutron flux. Activity as high as about 700 Ci/g (11 W/g) $^{60}$Co has been produced equivalent to $\sim65\%$ $^{60}$Co in cobalt (9). The nickel decay products are metallurgically compatible with the cobalt. However, chemical separation of nickel would increase specific activity still further. At similar neutron flux levels $\sim2.5$ W/g $^{170}$Tm has been produced which is about 20% $^{170}$Tm in thulium, and decay product ytterbium is also similarly compatible. In both cases high quality means high specific activity. In neither case is 100% product purity achieved.

In general high isotopic purity is a good measure of high quality because undesired isotopes dilute power density. For example, $^{238}$Pu produced from $^{237}$Np absorbs neutrons during irradiation which unavoidably produces heavier plutonium isotopes, as high as $^{242}$Pu. Irradiation time can be shortened to reduce this loss of product purity and the resultant product power dilution. However, in practice, concentrations greater than 80% $^{238}$Pu are considered an acceptable quality. Very high purity product, $\sim$100% $^{238}$Pu, can be made by $\alpha$-decay of separated $^{242}$Cm.

Heavier isotopic impurities are also produced in $^{244}$Cm. For this product about 95% $^{244}$Cm is considered high quality. Typical obtainable isotopic purities of these nuclides are shown in Table 2.8.

Low concentrations of some impurities can reduce product quality. $^{236}$Pu ($\tau_{1/2} = 2.9$ yr), although present in only trace amounts in $^{238}$Pu, introduces an extra shielding requirement because it decays by an $\alpha$-cascade to $^{208}$Tl, a hard $\gamma$ emitter. $^{236}$Pu is made by unavoidable $^{237}$Np (n, 2n) or ($\gamma$, n) reactions. $^{236}$Pu is not formed in $^{241}$Am irradiations which lead to $^{238}$Pu via $^{242}$Cm $\alpha$-decay. Low $^{236}$Pu concentrations, <1 ppm, give a high-quality product. $^{236}$Pu is also a potential radiation problem in handling of recycled power reactor plutonium fuel. $^{242}$Cm generates energy at a rate about 43 times $^{244}$Cm so that it can be a nuisance even in small amounts. Low $^{242}$Cm concentration, 0.02%, gives high-quality $^{244}$Cm product. Neutrons from spontaneous fission in $^{244}$Cm ($\sim$10$^7$ neutrons/sec g) are unavoidable and undesirable (19).

High-quality $^{227}$Ac must be chemically pure. $^{228}$Th (an $\alpha$-decay daughter of $^{236}$Pu), which in this case is an irradiation byproduct of $^{226}$Ra irradiation to produce $^{227}$Ac, must be reduced to the ppm concentration range to keep gamma-ray shielding requirements low. The hard gamma emitter, $^{208}$Tl, is again the culprit in the decay chain.

TABLE 2.8

Isotopic Purity of Representative $^{238}$Pu and $^{244}$Cm Products

| $^{238}$Pu product | | $^{244}$Cm product | |
|---|---|---|---|
| Isotope | At. % | Isotope | At. % |
| $^{236}$Pu | $0.9 \times 10^{-4}$ | $^{242}$Cm | 0.02 |
| $^{238}$Pu | 81 | $^{243}$Cm | 0.02 |
| $^{239}$Pu | 15 | $^{244}$Cm | 96 |
| $^{240}$Pu | 2.9 | $^{245}$Cm | 1 |
| $^{241}$Pu | 0.8 | $^{246}$Cm | 3 |
| $^{242}$Pu | 0.1 | $^{247}$Cm | 0.07 |
| | | $^{248}$Cm | 0.05 |

[204]Tl isotopic dilution by natural thallium is also undesirable. Isotopic separation provides the only means to increase power density. Unavoidable [170]Tm contamination of [171]Tm increases shielding requirements significantly. On the other hand, isotopic dilution of [252]Cf in deliverable californium has a negligible effect on the desirability of the product, although trace quantities of [254]Cf ($\tau_{1/2} = 60$ days) could be troublesome in some applications.

Chemical purity is particularly important for the $\alpha$-decay radionuclides because light element impurities create targets for ($\alpha$, n) reactions and the resultant neutron activity requires additional and undesirable neutron shielding of the source. The following example illustrates the extent that ($\alpha$, n) reactions need reduction. [238]PuO$_2$ is a candidate fuel form for an isotopic energy source. If used in biological applications, radiation should be held to a minimum. It was shown experimentally (20) that in oxide prepared with naturally occurring oxygen, the neutrons from [18]O (0.209 at. %) ($\alpha$, n) [21]Ne reactions are the major source ($\sim$90 %) of neutron emission. Oxide prepared with depleted oxygen containing only 0.0016 at. % [18]O had essentially the neutron emission rate per gram of [238]Pu. that results from unavoidable spontaneous fission, i.e., $\sim$2850 neutrons/g sec. The ($\alpha$,n) yield for [18]O has been measured to be $31 \times 10^{-6}$ neutrons/$\alpha$ particle. Other potential ($\alpha$, n) sensitive impurities have to be controlled equally to limit neutron emission to a negligible amount, about 50 neutrons/g sec. Trace chemical impurities may also reduce the melting point of final fuel forms, but insufficient data are available yet to permit setting of specifications.

All of the fission products have isotopic diluents that are also formed during fuel exposure. For example, [147]Pm must be allowed to decay about one half-life so that the troublesome [148m]Pm isotopic contaminant decays to negligible level. However, delay prior to chemical processing of fuel is usually sufficient to permit decay of unwanted radiation contaminants for most of the other fission product mixtures. Nonradioactive isotopic dilution of fission products was covered in Section II.

Finally, decay product buildup occurs with all radionuclides. The most troublesome features of this phenomenon are the chemical changes that occur. For example, curium $\alpha$-decay leads to a buildup of plutonium, plutonium decays to uranium, and thus new chemical species are introduced. In addition, $\alpha$-decay builds up helium gas. This presents mechanical problems to heat source designers who must design remedies for potential buildup in gas pressure.

In summary, radionuclides are never pure and always in the process of change. Some changes are quite compatible with the starting material, others create problems requiring remedial action. A high-quality product is one that minimizes the necessity for such remedies.

**8. Coupling with Chemical Separations.** An alternative title for this subsection might be *Yield versus Production*. For many of the radionuclides the final product must be separated chemically before it will be available for source fabrication and application. If a target nuclide is used that is itself in short supply, the rate of production is strongly controlled by the speed with which chemically processed target material is recycled to the reactor for further irradiation. In this case, modest ultimate reactor yield losses could be tolerated if the production rate is increased by a more rapid chemical processing cycle. On the other hand, if the target material is in large or natural supply and could always be made available for irradiation when needed, then reactor yield becomes more important because production rate is a function only of total reactor capacity and, aside from possible inventory charges, chemical processing speed has less value. Further, if target supply is very rare, for example $^{226}$Ra, yield considerations of the $^{227}$Ac product might be the overwhelming consideration regardless of production rate. An exception to these generalizations is a rapidly decaying product, such as $^{210}$Po in irradiated bismuth, where speed of chemical separation can strongly affect the deliverable amount of product. The potential reactor yield of $^{210}$Po ($\tau_{1/2} = 138$ days) is the lowest of any of the neutron produced nuclides (Table 2.3) but the amount of $^{210}$Po produced per neutron absorbed in target compared in thermal watts is significant and the amount of delivered product is obviously affected by the rate of chemical separation of $^{210}$Po from bismuth target.

In all cases involving chemical processing, close coupling or linking of large-scale chemical facilities and reactor irradiation operations are required for maximum production. In many cases the yield, i.e., atoms of product per neutron absorbed in the target, can be sacrificed to increase the production rate. The following examples illustrate the general principles involved.

$^{238}$Pu is produced by irradiating $^{237}$Np. The target can be irradiated over a wide range of neutron flux levels and percent burnup of $^{237}$Np per irradiation. At the higher fluxes the burnup of $^{237}$Np occurs more rapidly, but the amount of $^{237}$Np that can be irradiated at a given time is limited by the need for an adequate multiplication constant in the reactor, and the yield is reduced by increased fission and neutron capture losses in intermediate $^{238}$Np ($\tau_{1/2} = 2.1$ days). At lower neutron fluxes the time spent in the reactor for a given burnup of target is proportionately longer. If carried to lower flux, e.g., $\sim 3 \times 10^{13}$n/cm$^2$-sec typical of nuclear power plants, the production rate would decline substantially, especially since supply of this target is currently limited. Thus for optimum production of $^{238}$Pu, target availability and chemical processing recycle times must be related to available neutron flux to determine maximum production rate. For a product purity of about 80% $^{238}$Pu, yields of about 70% of $^{238}$Pu per atom of $^{237}$Np burned up are usually calculated (20a). With thermal neutron fluxes about 25% of the $^{237}$Np target is burned up in each irradiation cycle to produce the 80% product. Losses occur in $^{238}$Pu product burnup to higher isotopes and $^{238}$Np intermediate burnup. Less target burnup at lower flux increases yield per target atom destroyed, but reduces the production rate, particularly if chemical processing times cannot be reduced.

Recirculating loops of fluids containing $^{237}$Np and irradiation products have been considered as a means of improving the yield while maintaining production rates at high levels (21). $^{238}$Pu product would be removed external to the reactor and neptunium recycled through the reactor loop. Unfortunately the relatively long half-life of $^{238}$Np ($\tau_{1/2} = 2.1$ days) in target $^{237}$Np requires a comparatively long holdup ($\sim 10$ days) of neptunium outside the reactor to permit chemical separation of all $^{238}$Pu. Otherwise continuous loop circulation results in losses to neutron capture in $^{238}$Np similar to that in the conventional batch operation. Potential gains in yield are thus small, of the order 10%. In addition recirculating loops offer operating reactor safety problems for large-scale irradiations where composition of the material in the many loops would control a substantial portion of reactivity of the reactor. Loops offer greater advantage if irradiation samples are in very small supply and, therefore, do not affect reactor operation, and if the primary irradiation product decays rapidly, with a half-life of the order of a few hours, to a desired product. The product can then be separated, without prolonged hold-up, before absorbing an additional neutron. Examples of possible systems can be found in the higher transcurium nuclides, e.g., the $^{249}$Bk–$^{250}$Cf system ($^{250}$Bk $\tau_{1/2} = 3.2$ hr) and for the $^{226}$Ra–$^{227}$Ac system ($^{227}$Ra $\tau_{1/2} = 6.1$ hr) where the intermediate beta-decay precursors have acceptably short half-lives.

Production of $^{210}$Po by irradiating bismuth is enhanced at high flux for two reasons. First, the decay of $^{210}$Po already produced is kept to a minimum by using short irradiation cycles. Second, the concentration of $^{210}$Po can be increased to a level, $\sim 50$ g/ton (22), that makes rapid chemical separation feasible and of reasonable unit cost. The rapid separation means higher output because a delay of only about 4 months after reactor shutdown, of little significance to longer-lived nuclides, would reduce the ratio of $^{210}$Po ($\tau_{1/2} = 138$ days) delivered to that available at reactor discharge by one half, thus doubling unit cost.

It is evident that for optimum production of many radionuclides, close coupling or linking is required between the chemical separation and reactor irradiation facilities. Product loss caused by delay in chemical processing can be significant in reducing the rate of production or reducing the amount of product already produced.

### D. Partial Reactor Loadings or Simultaneous Production of Several Products

Any of the reactor types listed in Section IV can be used to irradiate partial or limited loadings of target material within the reactor core to make radionuclides of interest. For example $^{60}$Co has been made in U.S. AEC production reactors and at the Big Rock Point (23) power reactor, $^{252}$Cf in the HFIR from $^{242}$Pu target made at Savannah River (24), $^{60}$Co commercially at GETR and in Canada. Test production of gram quantities of $^{227}$Ac is planned by $^{226}$Ra irradiation at the test reactor at Mol, Belgium. The production rate for these partial loadings relates directly to the product of the neutron flux, effective cross section, and time of irradiation. Normally partial loadings do not have a large effect on reactivity. They can be considered as sample irradiations. For such situations production estimation has more variables and is subject to larger uncertainties than a full reactor operation run entirely for full-scale production of a single isotope. For example, the flux and effective cross section, which are required to make production estimates, can be determined only if detailed reactor physics cell calculations are made. These would require knowledge of flux ratios between target and fuel, target self-shielding, neutron temperature, sample position in the reactor, neutron spectrum—all factors which have a relatively lesser effect on calculation of the output of full-scale target loadings of reactors where neutron utilization information is sufficient. The required information is derived from experiment or calculations normalized to experiment to assure a higher accuracy of prediction.

Other methods for introducing partial target loadings into reactors for production of radioisotopes are as follows: blankets of productive absorbing material surround the reactor, capturing leakage neutrons; control rods made of productive targets; bismuth inserted in an existing reactor, where the small percentage absorption of neutrons allows bismuth irradiation to ride "piggy back" on other operations, instead of using a

special high-flux full-scale operation designed expressly for $^{210}$Po prcduc-
tion. Irradiation of bismuth is a unique exception and no other target can
be substituted to obtain the same advantage.

Partial loadings of a reactor are useful for less than full-scale production
of a particular isotope. Simultaneous production of many radionuclides in
a single reactor, i.e., multiple partial loadings, also offers advantages when
full reactor quantities are not needed; if carried out on a large scale it is in
effect the same kind of operation as the full, large-scale operation discussed in Section III. In this case targets designed by experiment and calculation are usually matched to absorb close to the same fraction of
neutrons for each assembly to keep the perturbation of reactor flux shapes
to a minimum.

## V.  ECONOMICS OF RADIOISOTOPES

### A.  Competition with Other Energy Sources

The gradual acceptance of radioisotopes for large-scale applications
meets competition from many quarters. For example, radioisotopes for
use as energy sources in outer space compete with solar cells in long-term
applications of the order of years, with chemical batteries and fuel cells
for shorter applications of the order of months. They must compete not
only in initial capital cost but in launch cost; in the tightly designed space
systems each unit of weight to be placed in space has a significant associated unit launch cost, currently between $500 and $1000/lb. Weight is
usually a less important consideration for terrestrial or undersea energy
source applications, but cost comparisons must also include conventional
fossil fuel systems. Costs related to maintenance, reliability, and safety
also must be considered in each case before a given energy source is finally
selected.

Radioisotopes for use as sources for radiation processing must compete with machine accelerators. Generally speaking, sources consisting of
the $\gamma$-emitting isotopes $^{60}$Co and $^{137}$Cs afford deeper penetration of the material being processed. Machines, for example those emitting high-energy
electrons, are more efficient for near-surface or thin-film processing. Substantial argument about the virtues of each type of radiation source has
occurred (25). A complementary as well as a competitive role for each is
predicted for the future. Competition between machines and radioisotopes is most significant where both give rise to comparable radiation.
Under these conditions competition in terms of capital cost, maintenance,

availability, safety, portability, and ease of use must all be weighed in making a selection. This subject is discussed more fully in Chapter 7.

Gamma emitters such as [60]Co and [137]Cs can also be used for radiography, and for this purpose compete directly with industrial X-ray machines. High intensity [60]Co, $>400$ Ci/g, makes a very efficient source which competes in performance and cost in radiography requiring deep penetration of large units of heavy material.

Finally, [252]Cf which emits neutrons by spontaneous fission finds $(\alpha, n)$ sources and neutron-emitting machines already on the market. In the 1970s, direct competition in this field would be limited since [252]Cf has unique application as a physically small neutron source that can be used in otherwise inaccessible regions. A further look into the future shows that [252]Cf production could increase as a result of the growing availability of its target precursors in power fuel residues (Fig. 2.1). [252]Cf might then become the most economical of all neutron sources in the $10^{10}$–$10^{12}$ n/sec source range.

The future development of applications of radioisotopes on a large commercial scale depends primarily on favorable economic comparison with other energy sources. There will probably always be unique applications to justify small-scale efforts.

## B. Cost Projections

The cost of neutron-produced radioisotopes is primarily the cost of producing neutrons, since the cost of target material is usually small. In contrast, the cost of fission products and radioactinide target material is primarily the cost of their chemical separation from power reactor fuel residues.

In a radioisotope production plant the major factors which govern the cost of neutrons are: reactor fuel and associated costs; plant depreciation including interest charges; and salaries, taxes, maintenance, and general operating costs. The unit cost of radioisotope products is also a function of the plant output because the sum of the plant costs listed above would remain fairly constant over a wide range of output, with fuel costs being the major variant. Plant output is determined by the now familiar production parameters: reactor power, operating efficiency, and neutron utilization. Total neutron unit cost must also include cost of target material. Compared to neutron costs, costs associated with naturally occurring targets normally would be low. This is true for cobalt in the production of [60]Co where the current cost of cobalt at $\sim$\$20/lb adds a trivial 0.04 ¢/Ci to product containing 100 Ci/g. However, to assure that this will hold true for $^{210}$Po production from natural $^{209}$Bi, the bismuth target material should be recycled. Even at a concentration of 50 g $^{210}$Po/ton of bismuth that could be generated by high flux reactor operation, discarding bismuth at its current price of $9000/ton after only a single irradiation would add a minimum of $180/g to the cost of final $^{210}$Po product. Final cost would depend on how rapidly $^{210}$Po produced in a reactor is separated for use following discharge. At lower $^{210}$Po concentrations the loss of bismuth would add a proportionately higher cost factor. For $^{170}$Tm, the current price of $\sim$$5/g for natural $^{169}$Tm target could add significantly to product unit cost, depending of course on the $^{170}$Tm/$^{169}$Tm ratio in the delivered product; e.g., with product containing about 2 W/g from high-flux irradiation, the thulium would add $\sim$$5/W, a significant amount.

For large-scale radioactinide production in the 1970s and beyond, the price of target material will be determined primarily by costs associated with chemical separation from power reactor fuel residues. This also will be true for fission products. Estimates of unit recovery costs extrapolated to the mid-seventies for actinide targets and fission products are listed below (*12*):

COMPARISON OF CHEMICAL RECOVERY COSTS

| Actinide Targets | | Fission Products | |
|---|---|---|---|
| $^{237}$Np | $\sim$$15/g | $^{137}$Cs | $\sim$$10/g ($0.10/Ci) |
| $^{241,243}$Am | $\sim$$31/g | $^{90}$Sr | $\sim$$16/g ($0.11/Ci) |
| $^{242,244}$Cm | $\sim$$81/g | $^{147}$Pm | $\sim$$10/g ($0.011/Ci) |

As stated in the reference document, "these costs *are not to be construed as selling prices* but do indicate the magnitude of possible incremental separation plant production costs." As available quantities increase in the late seventies with the growth of nuclear power generation, and if a need for *all* recoverable materials is established, unit recovery costs could be reduced further. For example, $^{144}$Ce ($\tau_{1/2} = 285$ days), because of its relatively short half-life, would not be recovered unless a market develops. However, its removal is a prerequisite for recovery of $^{147}$Pm, $^{241}$Am–$^{243}$Am and $^{242}$Cm–$^{244}$Cm. Sale of $^{144}$Ce would therefore tend to reduce unit costs of these other nuclides. Encapsulation cost is included for $^{137}$Cs and $^{90}$Sr in the above tabulation and is estimated to add $5/g for $^{237}$Np in the same time period. This unit cost should be fairly typical for encapsulating the other actinide products.

The unit cost of producing neutrons can be estimated from information now available in the open literature and the bases for such estimates are developed in the following discussion.

**1.   Fuel Cost.**   The U.S. AEC has announced a price schedule (*26*) for uranium fuel. This schedule shows that in the range of current interest for power reactor fuel, the cost of enrichment including the cost of yellow-cake raw material is: \$240/kg at 3% $^{235}$U enrichment and \$190/kg at 2.5% $^{235}$U enrichment.

For a potential production reactor fuel, where $^{238}$U concentration is kept to a minimum, 90% $^{235}$U would sell for \$10,000/kg. Calculated to an equivalent basis for the $^{235}$U alone, the cost for both types of fuel is:

|  | $^{235}$U content (%) | $^{235}$U (\$/kg) |
|---|---|---|
| Power reactor | 2.5 | 7,600 |
| enrichments | 3.0 | 8,000 |
| Production | | |
| reactor enrichment | 90.0 | 11,100 |

This indicates that the cost of $^{235}$U burnup increases by only ∼50% as $^{235}$U enrichment increases 36-fold. The highest charge for $^{235}$U burnup is used in the following cost calculation.

Experience plus extrapolations to the future have led to estimates that, in addition to enrichment costs, fabrication of power reactor fuel accounts for about 40% of the total fuel cost (*27*) and chemical reprocessing for about 15%. However, these factors applied directly to so-called highly enriched "production" fuel add only about \$250/kg to the fuel cost, which is small (∼2%) compared with fuel enrichment costs. Therefore, because enrichment cost is the major cost factor for highly enriched fuel a simplification of the cost picture can be made which still provides a conservative cost estimate; the unit cost of neutrons is calculated using $^{235}$U burnup as the *sole* criterion of fuel and associated costs, and the $^{235}$U value is increased from \$11,100/kg enrichment price to a conservative \$15,000/kg to account for the variables associated with fabrication, chemical processing, and losses, regardless of percent burnup and utilization of a particular fuel charge. Simplifying the cost estimation in this manner introduces uncertainties of no more than 10% in estimating the cost of neutrons. Specific details of a particular reactor operation should always be used in calculations to arrive at actual costs.

**2.   Depreciation of Capital.**   How much should a reactor cost and how much depreciation should be charged each year? A fortunate coincidence can be used to simplify this picture: Heavy water–natural uranium and light water–enriched uranium reactors cost about the same (*28*). For the example that will be used here, a 500 MW$_e$ or ~1700 MW$_t$ reactor, the range in total investment covers \$80 to 100 × 10$^6$ for both types. An average of \$90 × 10$^6$ was selected for this cost analysis. The reason nuclear power plant costs do not reflect strongly the differences in the reactors is that the direct reactor associated costs are only about 15% of the total investment. It is also assumed that total investment is not significantly affected by whether the fission energy is used for generating electrical power, desalting sea water, or is removed by cooling water. A depreciation charge of 14% per annum is used, which is consistent with privately financed utility operation.

3. **Salaries, Maintenance, Taxes, Etc.**    This is taken to be 15% of the total cost, a factor consistent with practical experience and the conclusions drawn from many studies of nuclear power plant operation (29).

4. **Calculation of Unit Costs of Neutrons.**    Factors needed for calculation are as follows:

| | |
|---|---|
| Reactor power | 1700 MW$_t$ |
| | 500 MW$_e$ |
| Plant investment | \$90 × 10$^6$ |
| Depreciation rate | 14% *per annum* |
| Operating cost | 15% of total cost |
| Fuel burnup charge | \$15/g $^{235}$U destroyed |
| Maximum number of neutrons | 1.04 neutrons/fission |
| available for production | ($^{235}$U) |
| 1 Megawatt thermal | 3.1 × 10$^{16}$ fissions/sec |
| Plant operating efficiency | 83.5% |

The maximum number of productive neutron absorptions in one day can be calculated as

(1700 MW) (3.16 × 10$^{16}$ fiss/sec MW) (1.04 neutron absorptions/fiss) (8.64 × 10$^4$ sec/day) = 48.2 × 10$^{23}$ abs/day.

Since there are 6.02 × 10$^{23}$ neutrons per gram, 8 g of neutrons are available each day for productive absorptions. To make 8 grams of neutrons, 2140 grams of $^{235}$U are destroyed by fission and capture each day (~1.24 g/MWD). At the \$15/g $^{235}$U burnup charge, this amounts to \$32,100 per day. The \$90 × 10$^6$ investment depreciated at 14% per annum amounts to a charge of

(\$90 × 10$^6$) (0.14)/365 = \$34,600 per day.

Continuing with the 15% factor of the total for operating costs alone, the total daily cost is calculated to be \$66,700/0.85 = \$80,000/day or

$10,000/g of neutrons. If profit is included the unit cost would increase. If salable power is generated in the reactor, the assigned cost could be lower. The reader can assign his own qualifications to this type of calculation for the specific reactor considered. The final dollar assignment per neutron is $12,000/g assuming combined net efficiency for neutron utilization and reactor operation of 83.5%. Efficiency of operation is also subject to variation, depending on the specific reactor, and a more refined calculation of cost should include actual operating efficiencies.

Back-calculating from the projected electrical generating cost of about 6 mills/kWh for a 500 MW$_e$ nuclear plant gives an average daily operating cost of about $60,000 compared with the $80,000 derived previously. The unit cost of neutrons, derived in this subsection based on the higher, more conservative daily operating cost, is used to calculate the unit costs of neutron-produced radioisotopes in Section VI.

One additional consideration is reactor power. Over the power range from 300 to 1000 MW$_e$ which includes the reactor size chosen for this discussion, the unit cost of electrical power and/or steam is calculated to drop as reactor power is increased. A general rule developed in one study (28) is that the unit cost of the desired reactor output is inversely proportional to the power, i.e., $P^{-0.4}$, at least to within $\pm 20\%$.

This type of relationship is useful to project relative unit cost of neutrons to reactor conditions that differ from the example chosen in this subsection. Extrapolation to the very large 10,000 MW$_t$ dual-purpose reactors that might be used for electrical generation and desalting water follows approximately $P^{-0.33}$ (29).

## C.  Cost versus Price

Cost and price are not synonymous. The unit cost of neutron-produced radioisotopes is primarily the unit cost of neutrons. As shown previously in Section IV, unit costs are reduced as reactor power, neutron utilization, and reactor operating efficiency are increased. The cost of the several actinide target materials and fission products is primarily the incremental or added cost of chemical separation at a fuel reprocessing plant.

However, in commercial situations the selling price reflects other factors such as profit; competition from other energy sources; the byproduct nature of a radioisotope; the supply and demand picture, especially for short-lived products; the uniqueness of the application of a particular isotope; or the ratio of isotope cost to total cost of an application device.

The field of radiography illustrates some of these factors. In this application, $^{60}$Co competes with X-ray and betatron machines. A comparison of radiographs shows that $^{60}$Co sources, properly collimated, provide radiograph quality as good as the machines (30). The principal advantage of a cobalt device is lower cost; the principal disadvantage is the general requirement for longer radiographic exposure time. Since current MeV X-ray machines are priced above $100,000, a competive source of $^{60}$Co ($\sim$1000–1500 Ci) could range in price from 50¢ to $10/Ci without seriously affecting the cost advantage of a radiography unit containing a cobalt source. Thus the use of 600 Ci/g $^{60}$Co, even though a factor of ten higher in cost than 30 Ci/g material, currently available at about 50¢/Ci, would still have advantage because the higher activity permits reduction of the exposure time required to make a $^{60}$Co radiograph by at least a factor of 3 (30). This is discussed more fully in Chapter 4. In addition, radioisotope radiography can be used in remote or normally inaccessible places, e.g., a $^{170}$Tm source of less than 1-mm focal spot size was used for radiographing welds of a thin-walled, one inch diameter, stainless steel pipe *in situ*. The radiographic examination would have been impossible with existing machines, thus making the radioisotope unique to this application. Again the selling price of the $^{170}$Tm would be judged against the utility and need for the radiographic examination of the welds and its value to the user would have to be well above the cost. For similar small-source radiography with $^{60}$Co it is estimated that only 5 Ci of $^{60}$Co at 600 Ci/g would be needed to develop a usable 1-mm focal spot. Compared with operating and installation costs, the cost of the $^{60}$Co would be trivial at any of the projected prices and the price acceptable to a customer would be established mainly by the need for the application and the cost of the device that would contain the $^{60}$Co.

Fission product costs have been estimated by assuming that they can be obtained by special chemical processing in facilities added to nuclear power fuel reprocessing plants. Costs would depend on whether single or multiple isotope products deliveries were required. Prices would depend on such factors as demand, products wanted, throughput, encapsulation costs, and profit. Fission products cannot be made on demand and consequently for efficient economic utilization of product, application needs would have to match a relatively well-known but inflexible supply. If more product is required, the user would have to wait. If too much product builds up in inventory, the chemical processor's profit would decrease. If fission product $^{144}$Ce ($\tau_{1/2} = 285$ days) is considered as a final product, a special case can be considered since its removal is a prerequisite for recovery of potentially marketable $^{147}$Pm, Am, and Cm. Even though $^{144}$Ce has a relatively short half-life, any possible utilization of this isotope would provide a means for reducing costs for the other nuclides, and consequently would have a potentially beneficial effect on their selling price or the seller's profit.

There are many other factors such as quantity, quality, and availability that affect the desirability of a given radioisotope and as a consequence affect the difference between the cost of manufacture and the potential selling price. The cost estimates developed in Section VI serve as guides to indicate an approach to valid economic estimates of product costs and selling prices.

### D. Interaction of Market Development on Long-Range Economics

The supply of many of the radionuclides depends, in large measure, on the growth of nuclear power generation. The exceptions are $^{60}$Co, $^{210}$Po, $^{204}$Tl, $^{171}$Tm, $^{170}$Tm, and $^{227}$Ac, all of which have naturally occurring target materials. These latter isotopes can be produced today about as cheaply as in the future. Their unit costs depend primarily on the cost of neutrons or reactor operation, which for large-scale operations would not be expected to decrease much with time. Since $^{226}$Ra is in limited supply and expensive, the cost of $^{227}$Ac per gram is quite closely tied to the selling price of radium (currently about \$15,000/g in milligram quantities). The irradiation and chemical separation costs are less significant per gram than for the other products, and also more difficult to evaluate because of the comparatively smaller scale of this operation. The other radionuclides all depend on the chemical processing of nuclear power fuel for a truly large-scale supply and consequently relatively low-cost starting materials.

The actinide target materials $^{241}$Am, $^{243}$Am, $^{244}$Cm, and $^{237}$Np along with fission products $^{90}$Sr, $^{137}$Cs, $^{144}$Ce, and $^{147}$Pm are chemically separable from power reactor fuel residues. The unit cost of separating these nuclides is projected to drop by a factor of about 7 over a seven-year period starting in 1969 (12), because the concentration and amount of the nuclides in the processed fuel will increase by substantial amounts in this time period. This cost reduction will occur if adequate chemical separation facilities are available as needed.

All of these factors will have a strong beneficial effect on both cost and availability, and new applications requiring lower cost radioisotopes would be encouraged.

$^{252}$Cf could eventually be produced with a rapid growth rate, starting with targets such as the transplutonium actinides, because of the time delay required for the large number of required neutron additions, and because of the projected rapid increase in availability of actinide target materials such as the americium and curium isotope mixtures in nuclear power fuel residues (Fig. 2.1). With these combined rapid growth rates, the unit cost could be expected to fall significantly with time, thus making this unique source of neutrons an attractive competitive product. The costs might be expected to drop from millions of dollars per gram to the range of \$100,000/g in the 1980s. As applications are developed, lower costs would encourage expanded commercial use (25a).

In terms of total energy available from the longer-lived radioisotopes, $^{60}$Co will be the leader for at least two decades since hundreds of megacuries can be manufactured in the United States today (1). This amounts (at 65 Ci/W) to a potential of several millions of watts of isotopic power annually. It will be late in the 1970s before the combined total of $^{90}$Sr and $^{137}$Cs generated wattage is that great (Fig. 2.4). Costs for $^{60}$Co as low as 10¢/Ci have been predicted for large quantities (31). Commercial selling prices for megacurie quantities range between 35 and 65¢/Ci. A test of these theories will be afforded if the availability and price of $^{60}$Co encourages the growth of large-scale applications. These qualitative observations serve as a reminder that future markets will depend strongly on future costs and selling prices.

## VI.  ESTIMATING REACTOR PRODUCTION AND UNIT COSTS OF RADIONUCLIDES

Approximate unit costs of reactor-produced radionuclides can be derived from ultimate yields in Table 2.3, using the unit cost of neutrons of \$12,000/g given in Section V. The yields and costs are listed in Table 2.9. The absorption of one gram of neutrons in a target material would produce one gram atomic weight of product, if no burnup or decay occurred. The ultimate yields include an approximate allowance for burnup and decay losses for general or typical irradiations. The discussion that follows presents additional factors, which cause variations in yield and hence inverse variations in unit cost. These variations result from the necessarily different reactor operating conditions that are required to achieve optimum production for particular radionuclides.

The typical ultimate yield estimates and approximate unit costs in Table 2.9 indicate some important general facts:

(1)   The unit cost per gram for each of the actinides are about the same,

TABLE 2.9

APPROXIMATE UNIT COSTS OF LARGE-SCALE REACTOR PRODUCTION OF RADIONUCLIDES

| Radionuclide | Ultimate yield (g) | Unit cost | | |
|---|---|---|---|---|
| | | ($/g) | ($/W) | ($/W-yr) |
| $^{238}$Pu | 167 | 72 | 126 | 1.0 |
| $^{227}$Ac | 170 | 70.50 | 4.93 | 0.16 |
| $^{244}$Cm | 220 | 54.50 | 19.20 | 0.75 |
| $^{242}$Cm | 157 | 76.50 | 0.64 | 1.0 |
| $^{210}$Po | 7 | 1700 | 12.20 | 22.3 |
| $^{204}$Tl | 190 | 63 | 86.30 | 15.7 |
| $^{171}$Tm | 144 | 83 | 374 | 135.0 |
| $^{170}$Tm | 85 | 141 | 10.80 | 23.7 |
| $^{60}$Co | 55 | 218 | 12.60 | 1.85 |
| $^{252}$Cf | 0.25 | a | a | a |

[a] Unit cost not derivable in this manner because of multiple neutron capture required in target. See previous page for unit cost estimates.

but the unit costs per watt differ by a factor of ∼200 and unit costs per watt-year by a factor of ∼140 because of wide differences in specific activity and energy per disintegration.

(2) The extremely high unit cost of $^{210}$Po per gram, because of low reactor yield, is compensated in the power unit cost only because of its high specific activity.

(3) $^{60}$Co, $^{170}$Tm, and $^{210}$Po have coincidentally about the same neutron-associated unit cost per unit of initial power.

(4) $^{171}$Tm is inherently a costly radionuclide to produce because of its low beta energy per disintegration while $^{242}$Cm is comparatively inexpensive because of its high yield, short half-life, and high energy per disintegration.

A more detailed discussion of factors affecting production and unit costs is given in the following section.

## A. Product Losses

Radionuclide products made by neutron absorption in targets can be lost by radioactive decay and destroyed by further neutron absorption in the product. These factors are determined by the neutron flux, spectrum, cross sections, and time of irradiation. Production of $^{60}$Co supplies a good example to illustrate radioactive decay loss.

Figure 2.9 shows calculated $^{60}$Co specific activities as functions of the

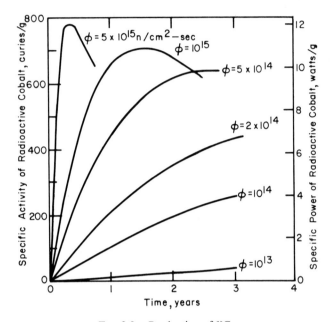

FIG. 2.9.   Production of $^{60}$Co.

neutron flux and irradiation time. The "saturation," observable at the higher fluxes and calculable for all fluxes for longer irradiation, means that eventually the production rate due to neutron absorption in $^{59}$Co equals the loss rate due primarily to decay of $^{60}$Co. Similar variations in production rate owing to decay loss can be calculated for $^{170}$Tm and $^{210}$Po using half-lives in Table 2.1 and cross sections in Table 2.11. The nominal loss of $^{60}$Co selected for Table 2.9 was 10%, which is reasonable for a typical 2-year irradiation to make 100–200 Ci/g $^{60}$Co. Decay losses should be calculated for each particular cobalt target irradiation. The loss implies a higher unit cost because a neutron absorbed to produce a product is considered wasted if the product is not deliverable.

If, however, neutron absorption losses are large compared to decay, as in the case of $^{238}$Pu and $^{244}$Cm burnup during production, then a more careful evaluation of the neutron absorption process must be made before assigning unit cost solely on the basis of the unit cost of absorbed neutrons. In the case of $^{238}$Pu, production can be evaluated in terms of product isotopic purity. This fact can be developed from the following observations: To a close approximation, one neutron is needed to convert an atom of $^{237}$Np to $^{238}$Pu; however, for the standard isotopic purity of

~80% (Table 2.8), neutrons are absorbed to make higher plutonium isotopes; thus in addition to losing desired product, extra neutrons are used nonproductively; alpha decay is negligible for typical irradiation; however, neutrons are also "produced" when $^{239}$Pu and $^{238}$Np undergo fission; thus the net number of neutrons produced and lost is nearly constant, and the yield ratio of $^{238}$Pu can be fairly calculated by determining the ratio of $^{238}$Pu to (Total Pu + Fission), which is about 0.7 for typical 80% product. This ratio was used to calculate ultimate yield in Table 2.9. A consistent set of cross sections derived from Table 2.11 can be used to calculate $^{238}$Pu yields at other isotopic purities or irradiation conditions as shown in Fig. 2.10. Losses are less for higher isotopic purity and for irradiations at lower flux. Similar evaluations apply to $^{244}$Cm production where burnup losses also predominate over decay.

If the resultant products of additional neutron absorption in the desired product do not yield neutrons, these extra absorptions would have to be included in the estimate of the neutron-associated unit cost of product. This can be illustrated by the situation where $^{171}$Tm is produced by burn-through from $^{169}$Tm via $^{170}$Tm ($\tau_{1/2} = 130$ days). Ideally only two neutrons are required, but $^{170}$Tm decays substantially during a real irradiation, thus the net $^{171}$Tm production per total neutrons absorbed in target is reduced

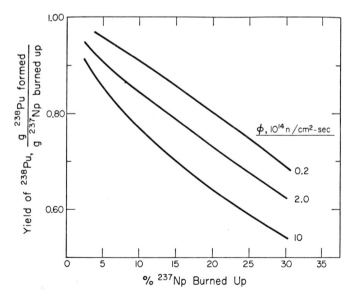

FIG. 2.10.   Yield of $^{238}$Pu.

by the amount of [170]Tm which decays prior to the second neutron absorption and by the amount of [171]Tm which decays or burns up prior to delivery. The absorption of more than two neutrons per delivered product atom is thus required for all available neutron fluxes. Calculations for a product containing predominantly [171]Tm, i.e., after about 90% [169]Tm burnup, and using cross sections developed from Table 2.11 give the relationship in Fig. 2.11 between flux and neutron utilization efficiency. At neutron fluxes below $\sim$2 $\times$ $10^{14}$n/cm$^2$-sec, the production process becomes impractical because the concentration of [171]Tm becomes too low for efficient heat source application.

Another type of product loss factor, which was considered in estimating [242]Cm yields, is the branching ratio of [241]Am where a neutron absorption can produce either of two products, only one of which is wanted. In this case, [242]Am and [242m]Am are formed and the desired [242]Am isotope ($\tau_{1/2} =$ 16 hr) decays by two routes, only $\sim$82% going to [242]Cm by alpha decay; the remainder to [242]Pu by electron capture. The combination of the two branching losses accounts for the lowered yield estimate of [242]Cm from [241]Am, or for [238]Pu that is eventually formed from [242]Cm $\alpha$-decay if [242]Cm is not used when available. Principles involved in optimizing these processes have been studied in detail (7a, 32).

Product decay loss after reactor shutdown is simple to calculate and must also be incorporated into a "practical" yield determination, particularly for materials with short half-lives because the deliverable isotopic power is what the user will pay for.

[252]Cf provides still another kind of product loss situation. First, [252]Cf is made by multiple and sequential neutron absorptions starting with any of its potential target materials. Perhaps the simplest way to consider ulti-

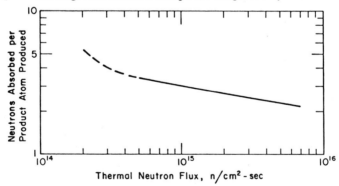

FIG. 2.11. [171]Tm production from [169]Tm target.

mate yield is to calculate the accumulation of fission losses for fissionable $^{244}$Cm, $^{245}$Cm, $^{247}$Cm, and $^{251}$Cf in the production chain from $^{242}$Pu to $^{252}$Cf (Fig. 2.5). At thermal neutron energies the product of the four capture-to-total absorption ratios is about $1.4 \times 10^{-2}$ (Table 2.11); the product yield estimated for the resonance integral capture-to-total absorption ratios is $1.6 \times 10^{-2}$. The ultimate yield for irradiation in a real reactor spectrum would be expected to fall between these two yields assuming that the cross sections are correct. Next, to produce $^{252}$Cf in concentrations that would be efficient to recover by chemical processing requires a thermal neutron flux $\geqslant 10^{15}$n/cm$^2$ sec. The ultimate yield shown in Tables 2.3 and 2.9 is calculated assuming a high thermal flux irradiation in which product alpha decay is negligible.

Figure 2.12 shows how the actual yield of $^{252}$Cf changed with exposure in a Savannah River High Flux operation (33a). This calculation does include alpha decay. Figure 2.12 also shows that much of the burnup products of $^{242}$Pu is held up as intermediates and that the actual $^{252}$Cf yield is below the ultimate yield range as defined in Section III. This emphasizes that for a practical program where $^{252}$Cf is separated at regular intervals for delivery, the ultimate yield has practical meaning only when a steady supply of target is available and the ultimate $^{252}$Cf yield is the anticipated steady-state output. When all the target is burned up, some intermediates in the pipeline are still not converted and to this extent the ultimate yield is never reached. Loss of $^{252}$Cf by alpha decay prevents actual yields from reaching the ultimate and the loss is an inverse function of the neutron flux. The lower flux limit for considering practical $^{252}$Cf production is set by limits imposed by the feasibility of recovering trace quantities of $^{252}$Cf from target residues, and a competition between the neutron absorption production rate and the alpha-decay rate ($\lambda \approx 10^{-8}$ sec$^{-1}$).

## B. High Flux and Unit Costs

As thermal neutron flux is increased, the productivity of a reactor decreases (Fig. 2.8) approaching zero at some maximum flux. The unit cost of available neutrons consequently would increase according to the inverse function to infinity.

Again $^{60}$Co provides a good example to illustrate these effects. The calculated relative unit cost of producing $^{60}$Co, taking into consideration the increase in costs from higher flux inefficiencies, product decay losses, and reduced operating time at high flux, is shown in Fig. 2.13 for a variety of specific activities, neutron fluxes, and irradiation times. Similar infor-

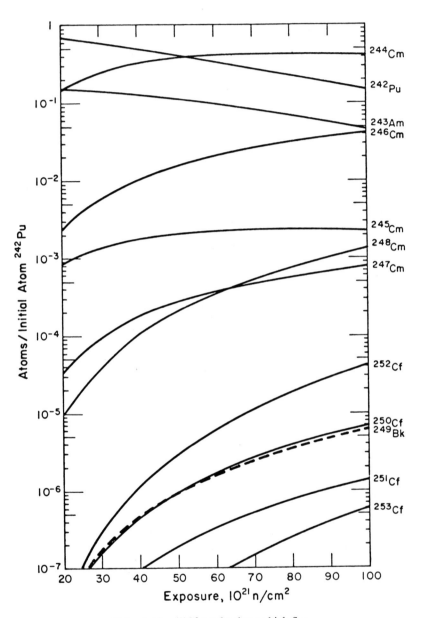

FIG. 2.12.   $^{252}$Cf production at high flux.

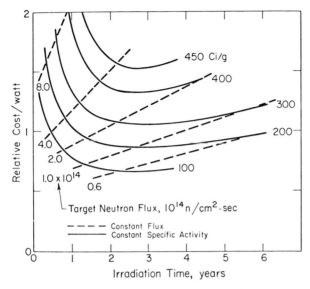

FIG. 2.13. $^{60}$Co production cost estimates.

mation for other radioisotopes can be developed from cross section information in Table 2.11 and the change in neutron unit cost shown in Fig. 2.14. This latter information was derived from the reactor operating relationships developed in Table 2.11 and the neutron utilization efficiencies obtainable in Fig. 2.8. These relationships are approximate but are useful representations of the combined variation of factors affecting the cost of neutrons and hence the cost of product.

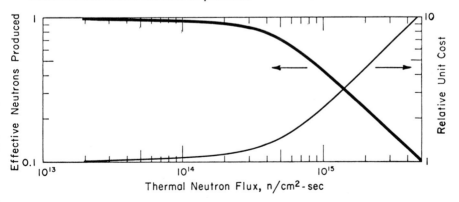

FIG. 2.14. Relative production and unit cost of neutrons.

$^{210}$Po provides an exception because bismuth has such a low neutron absorption potential that a reactor fueled to the proper reactivity with only bismuth present as an absorbing target is already limited to a lightly loaded high flux fuel charge. Bismuth adds so little absorber that, if space is available, it can be added to any operating reactor to produce $^{210}$Po with a minimum effect on reactivity. A high unit cost of grams of $^{210}$Po is inherent, however, because for minimum cost it must be made at a high flux to be chemically separable efficiently from bismuth and the unit cost of the high flux neutrons is inherently high. Losses are also increased in $^{238}$Pu production as a function of flux as already shown in Fig. 2.10 because of $^{238}$Np burnup.

The requirement of high flux for $^{252}$Cf production plus its low ultimate yield indicates a high anticipated unit cost. Only detailed specific $^{252}$Cf studies have meaning and production programs of any consequence extend over a decade or more (*10a*). $^{252}$Cf studies also require information on availability of target material and production facilities (*33b*).

### C.  Special Power Reactor Considerations

The current generation of light-water cooled power reactors are not designed for radioisotope production. They operate at a low neutron flux, $\sim 3 \times 10^{13}$ n/cm$^2$ sec, and have long periods between shutdowns for fuel replacement, typically about 9 months. However, these power reactors can be used to produce $^{60}$Co and other products requiring a single neutron absorption for which low flux is not a deterrent. In deciding how much radioisotopes should cost if made in a reactor primarily paid for by selling electrical power, several considerations should be investigated to determine if the target absorptions introduce economic benefits or deterrents to the overall operation:

(1)  Determine if the expensive fuel cycle is shortened significantly or the reactor power lowered by the presence of target material. If so, sale of radioisotopes must compensate for the extra expense or lost output, in addition to the value of the absorbed neutrons, which otherwise would have produced plutonium-239.

(2)  Determine if a special reactor shutdown is required to remove radioisotope target. The value of the shutdown, in terms of electrical power not generated, would have to be charged against the selling price of the radioisotope product.

(3)  Determine if control rods can be used to absorb productively. This could add useful product output and might provide extra profit.

(4) Determine if specific activity in target is high enough to be useful or if product can be economically recovered by chemical processing. Establish that product purity is acceptable.

(5) Determine if the high operating temperature of power reactors has any harmful effect on production or sets unreasonable limits on target composition and cladding.

Each of these factors must be considered in evaluating whether radionuclide production in nuclear power reactors has value.

### D. Burnup of Fuel and Targets

Much of the discussion on production in this chapter applies to initial conditions of a reactor charge containing targets and fuel, and reference to burnup of fuel and target during the operation of the reactor at power has not been treated in detail. Like the detailed calculations of production discussed in the next section, careful analysis of burnup is required for computing the eventual output of a reactor. A recent survey by Spinrad (*33c*) provides a good summary of methods and a list of references for analysis of reactor burnup. Reference to this work should provide sufficient information to help evaluate the need for precise burnup calculations for a given production goal. As pointed out in the reference article, simple calculational methods seem to do as well as the more elaborate, particularly if the simpler methods can be normalized to an operating condition.

A very simple concept which can be helpful in evaluating the effect on production and production rate of sequential absorption of neutrons in a target distributed in a reactor has been developed. It is derived from the fact that the net production of a radioisotope that results from multiple-sequential neutron absorptions is proportional to $\overline{\phi^n}/\overline{\phi}^n$ where $\overline{\phi^n}$ is the *average of the flux raised to the $n^{th}$ power* and $\overline{\phi}^n$ is the *average flux, raised to the $n^{th}$ power,* where $n$ equals the number of sequential neutron absorptions. This ratio is always greater than unity, unless $\phi$ is a constant, and the amount of a product obtained by multiple-sequential capture will always exceed the amount calculated assuming that the average flux is effective everywhere in the reactor. Modern, sophisticated reactor codes would normally take this effect into account. Point-flux calculations, so often used to estimate radioisotope production, have to be modified according to the above relationship in order to characterize correctly the whole reactor output. Time variation of flux shapes must also be included in a proper analysis.

These observations mean that for products formed by a single neutron absorption, the production and production rate are not affected by the reactor flux shape but only by the magnitude of the flux. If sequential absorptions are required, at the same average flux, gains in production rate can be achieved if the flux is nonuniform, provided the flux shaping does not reduce the average value. The acceleration of multiple neutron capture at a higher flux can be seen by examining Fig. 2.12, where operating results indicate that the production of $^{252}$Cf from $^{242}$Pu was increased by a factor of 10 for only a factor of two in the exposure $\overline{\phi}t$; thus, if similar targets are exposed for the same time, a doubled flux would produce about 10 times the product.

### E. Effect of Chemical Separations and Target Materials on Unit Costs of Radioisotopes

Significant contributions to unit costs of some radionuclides are made by expensive target materials and by the necessary chemical processing and reprocessing. It was shown in Section VB that the contribution of cobalt target cost to $^{60}$Co costs was negligible, but that the contribution of $TmO_2$ target to $^{170}$Tm costs could be substantial. It was emphasized that reactor recycle of bismuth was a requirement for a reasonable cost of $^{210}$Po. $^{226}$Ra costs were also shown to dominate the unit cost of $^{227}$Ac production. At other points in this chapter it has been emphasized that rapid delivery of the short-lived radionuclides can have a benefical effect on the unit cost of the delivered product. In addition, the unit costs of fission products and actinide target material, recovered from nuclear power fuel residues, were shown to depend primarily on costs associated with chemical processing.

However, one important factor related to chemical reprocessing of irradiated targets has not been discussed. This factor is well represented in the production of $^{238}$Pu from $^{237}$Np and $^{244}$Cm from $^{243}$Am.

We know that to produce $^{238}$Pu of acceptable quality from neutron absorption in $^{237}$Np, only about 25% of the $^{237}$Np present in the target is usually burned up. (Some reactor spectra may permit a somewhat higher burnup to obtain the same product quality, but the general observations that follow still apply.) Therefore, the cost of separating and encapsulating all the neptunium in the target must be charged against the $^{238}$Pu output. Assuming again that the yield is about 0.7 g $^{238}$Pu/g $^{237}$Np burned up, a reasonable factor from the curves in Fig. 2.10, about 5.7 times as much $^{237}$Np must be separated and encapsulated as $^{238}$Pu produced. If the cost of separating and encapsulating $^{237}$Np continued to be about \$20/g, as suggested in Section VB, then the target chemical-processing costs associated with the delivered $^{238}$Pu would be about \$114/g, about 58% more than the neutron-associated cost in Table 2.9. Thus, longer burnup of the $^{237}$Np target per irradiation cycle and lower processing costs would be very beneficial for reducing $^{238}$Pu unit costs. Similar factors apply to $^{244}$Cm production, where the americium target material must also be processed and recycled, even though burnup of 50% per cycle is possible. The final separation cost of the radionuclide product from the target remains a small factor, of the order of a few dollars per gram. In contrast, it is possible to burn up nearly 90% $^{241}$Am in a single irradiation, if $^{238}$Pu is the desired final product, thus establishing an efficient overall production operation (7a).

The case for $^{252}$Cf is different. The need for prolonged neutron irradiation of targets in costly high flux or resonance reactors and the relatively infrequent chemical processing attaches most of the cost to reactor operations. The ultimate unit costs are thus inversely proportional to yield and therefore fall in the range of $\geqslant 10^3$ compared with that of the other actinides; "ultimate" being 15 years away.


## VII. DETAILED CALCULATION OF REACTOR PRODUCTION

Detailed calculations of radioisotope production that would pass critical evaluation by reactor physicists are beyond the scope of this chapter. This section contains recommendations of less refined methods that are still adequate for making calculations of radioisotope production. Many powerful reactor physics codes have been developed for the nuclear power industry and good comparison with experiment is well established (34, 35). Heavy water reactor physics has also been developed to a high degree (36), so too has the physics of the other reactor types (37). In fact there is really a plethora of information. For those who want unambiguous, simple but accurate estimates of radioisotope production in a given reactor, the course of action needs some identifying guidelines.

Several nationwide programs are underway to unify basic information used to compute reactor performance, particularly to help with the selection of basic data and calculation methods. The first part is aimed at developing a source of well-defined and universally accepted cross sections to be called the Evaluated Nuclear Data File, ENDF. Calculators of radioisotope production will obtain basic cross section data that have been evaluated and tested by experts throughout the world.

TABLE 2.10

CHARACTERISTICS OF THE EVALUATED NUCLEAR DATA FILES

|  | ENDF/A | ENDF/B |
|---|---|---|
| Basic storage unit | Evaluated point cross section data covering a particular energy range for one reaction type and one material. Highly flexible format. | All evaluated point data for one material needed for a reactor calculation presented in simple format. |
| Type of data included | All reaction types for all incident and final particle types. | Data for neutron-induced reactions required for all reactor calculations. |
| Ordering of data | Data stored in the order received by the ENDF Center. | Ordered by material number, data type, and reaction type. |
| Selection and revision of data | No selection is made. All data are accepted and added to the master files. Hence many alternative evaluations occur. | One complete set of data for a material will be selected and stored. These data will be updated at regular intervals. |
| Main usage | Storage of partial evaluations and alternative or older evaluations used as building blocks to generate complete evaluations. | To provide complete sets of evaluated point data used as direct input to reactor codes or codes to compute multigroup sets of cross sections. |

The characteristics of the data file outlined in Table 2.10 were obtained from an ENDF newsletter. The files are designed primarily for use in reactor codes, but the cross section data are also recoverable directly. Additional reports on work in other countries are also available (38). To complement the availability of evaluated cross sections, efforts are also being made to incorporate the best features of reactor physics codes into modular computational systems (39,39a,40). These combinations would ultimately provide the preferred methods for calculating radioisotope production.

The purpose of the following discussion is to outline principles involved in preparing good production estimates, show some current pitfalls in selecting cross sections, give examples of calculations using current methods, and indicate future developments.

## A. *Effective Cross Sections*

In calculating radioisotope production, it is often convenient to be able to multiply neutron flux and cross section to obtain a specific reaction rate. To do this, it is necessary to characterize the neutron spectrum of the reactor and the cross section dependence on spectrum for the particular target material. Conventions have evolved among users to define "effective" cross section, which can be multiplied by "thermal" neutron flux to obtain a specific reaction rate.

**1. Cutoff Energy.** In order to use cross section conventions, one of the most important factors is knowledge of the ratio of epithermal-to-thermal neutron fluxes, $\phi_{epi}/\phi_{th}$. This factor, which can be obtained from reactor theory calculations or thin-foil irradiation experiments in reactor lattices, is needed to compute the contribution to total neutron absorptions that occurs above thermal because even in "thermal" reactors substantial neutron absorption occurs at the higher neutron energies. The "cutoff" is the energy above which epithermal neutron absorption events take place and below which "thermal" events occur. This energy varies over a small range depending on the source of the neutron cross section information. If the results are based on experimental cadmium ratio measurements (41), the cutoff is usually about 0.5 eV. HAMMER and THERMOS–MUFT calculations, now applied in many reactor computations, use 0.625 eV (34,42). Other calculators have used a variable cutoff energy (43). Particular care in assessing the significance of the cutoff energy is required when an absorption resonance occurs at a nearby energy, e.g., for $^{237}$Np, $^{241}$Am and the plutonium isotopes that exhibit large absorption resonance peaks in the range from 0.3 to 1.0 eV. However, for other nuclides of interest the cross sections vary in the well-defined $1/v$ manner over the narrow energy region and corrections to the resonance absorption cross section can be made easily by determining the contribution of

$$\Delta\sigma = \sigma_1 \int_{E_1}^{E_2} E^{-3/2} \, dE$$

to the cross section for each nuclide; where $E_1$ and $E_2$ are the two cutoff energies.

**2. Neutron Spectrum Distributions in Reactors.** Reactor neutron spectra, as applied to the definition of effective cross section conventions, can be thought of as having two components, thermal and epithermal. The thermal component has a neutron energy distribution that closely approximates the classical Maxwell–Boltzmann distribution law, which was derived for the kinetic theory of gases. The neutrons behave like a dilute gas in thermal equilibrium with its environment. The fraction of neutrons per unit energy interval is represented as

$$\frac{n(E)}{n} = \frac{2E^{1/2}}{(\pi k T_n)^{3/2}} \exp\left(\frac{-E}{k T_n}\right)$$

where $k$ = Boltzmann constant and $T_n$ = effective neutron temperature, °K. Converting energy to neutron velocity the distribution can be represented by

$$\frac{n(v)}{n} = 4\pi \left(\frac{m}{2\pi k T_n}\right)^{3/2} v^2 \exp\left(\frac{-mv^2}{2k T_n}\right)$$

where this equation relates the fraction of thermal neutrons that have a given velocity to the kinetic energy, $1/2\, mv^2$, and the neutron temperature, $T_n$. The most probable speed for neutrons, $\alpha$, is $1.284 \times 10^2\, T_n^{1/2}$ m/sec, and the average speed $\bar{v}$ is $1.128\, \alpha$. The energy at which the flux $nv$ is a maximum is $kT_n$. The average neutron energy is $3/2\, kT_n$. These relationships are used later to define cross section.

The epithermal component of the neutron flux, which is effective in neutron absorption processes, is made up primarily of neutrons that are being slowed down from fission energies. The slowing down process, in which virgin fission neutrons are scattered by nonabsorbing moderating material, imparts a $1/E$ energy distribution to the neutron flux.

The empirical description of the energy spectrum of virgin fission neutrons $n(E) \simeq 0.48\, e^{-E} \sinh (2E)^{1/2}$, where $E$ is energy in MeV, provides information about neutrons which enter into (n, 2n) and high energy fission reactions. The most probable energy of fission neutrons is ~0.7 MeV and the average is ~2 MeV. Except for introducing unwanted impurities, for example $^{237}$Np (n, 2n) reactions to form $^{236}$Pu in $^{238}$Pu, the effect on radioisotope production is relatively small. However, when $^{238}$U is present in large quantity, as in near-natural uranium fuel loadings of power reactors, the fast fission factor $\varepsilon$ contributes about 2–5% to the reactivity $k_{eff}$ (Section III).

The energy range over which epithermal and thermal energy groups merge has been calculated to be between 0.1 and 1.0 eV. The identification of this range helps to understand the "cutoff" energy discussed previously. The virgin fission and epithermal neutron fluxes merge above 100 keV, a region of small significance to thermal reactors and to radioisotope production. Further information on reactor spectrum effects on cross section can be found elsewhere (17, 44).

   3. **Westcott Convention of Neutron Flux and Cross Section.** A widely used method for obtaining "effective" cross sections, involving a semi-empirical separation of thermal and epithermal absorptions, was developed by Westcott (41). The method was originally introduced at the

Geneva Conference in 1958, at a time when high-speed computer capacity was more limited than now. The method was conceived primarily for use with well-thermalized heavy-water moderated reactors, in which Westcott and his Canadian colleagues were most interested. The method has continued to have worldwide application with heavy water and graphite moderated reactors and has been modified for use in evaluating the performance of U.S. light-water power reactors. (15)

Westcott's definition of effective cross section has two components and applies to both fission and absorption as follows:

$$\sigma_{\text{eff}}^{\text{w}} = \sigma_0 \, (g + rs)$$

where $\sigma_0$ = cross section at $v$ = 2200 m/sec; $g$ accounts for deviations from a $1/v$ absorber law in the Maxwellian distribution of thermal neutrons in a typical reactor spectrum ($g = 1$ for a $1/v$ absorber); $s$ accounts for epithermal neutrons and is a measure of absorption, in excess of a $1/v$ absorber, for an epithermal flux that follows the function $1/E$ ($s = 0$ for a $1/v$ absorber); and $r$ is an index of the relative strength of the epithermal-to-thermal components of the reactor neutron spectrum. $g$ and $s$ have been tabulated for many nuclides as a function of the temperature of the neutrons in the thermal Maxwellian distribution (41). $r$ is usually obtained experimentally by cadmium ratio measurements, with thin gold foil being a preferred material for this purpose.

Cadmium ratio, $R_{\text{Cd}}$, which equals the total activity of the bare foil divided by the cadmium-covered activity, can be represented in Westcott notation as

$$R_{\text{Cd}} = [(g + rs)/r]/s + 1/2 \, (T_n/293)^{1/2}.$$

For irradiated thin gold foils,

$$R_{\text{Cd}} = \frac{1.01 + 18r}{18.6r}.$$

Reactor-averaged $r$ usually falls between 0.03 and 0.07 for $D_2O$-moderated reactors. However, $r$ values of about 0.25 have been evaluated for PRWs, 0.18 for BWRs, and 0.18 for HTGRs (43).

Use of Westcott formalisms supplies useful cross-section information for calculating reaction rates in well-moderated reactors. However, this formalism has its limitations. For example, in thermal reactors the neutron spectrum becomes non-Maxwellian, within a strongly absorbing fuel assembly or even in the moderator if sufficient plutonium fuel with its strong absorption resonance at 0.3 eV is present, because thermal neutron absorptions deviate substantially from the simple $1/v$ relationship.

Under these conditions, neutrons are absorbed selectively above and/or below the average neutron temperature, thus distorting the Maxwellian distribution used to define the Westcott parameter $g$. In addition, deviation from the simple $1/E$ distribution of the epithermal flux can also be expected in reactors where moderator-to-fuel ratios are low, as is the case for intermediate or resonance reactors (17). In these and other "nonideal" conditions in reactors where neutron absorption distorts the spectrum, tabulated Westcott parameters would be applied beyond the intended range for calculating reaction rates, and consequently require further adjustments.

The Westcott neutron flux is computed from the following:

$$\text{Reaction rate} = N \, \phi_0 \, \sigma_{\text{eff}}^{\text{W}}$$

where $\phi_0$ is a monoenergetic flux, at a velocity of 2200 m/sec for the reacting neutrons. This is an arbitrary velocity selection made because so many cross section data are reported in the literature for neutrons at the equivalent energy ($\sim$0.0253 eV). Since $\sigma_{\text{eff}}^{\text{W}}$ is composed of $\sigma_0$, the 2200 m/sec cross section, times a function usually greater than unity $(g + rs)$ the Westcott neutron flux for a particular reaction rate is lower than the flux calculated using $\sigma_0$ tabulations. Therefore, great care is needed in combining published neutron flux and cross section data to obtain reaction rates for radioisotope production. Both neutron flux and cross section must have consistent definitions to avoid calculation of ambiguous and possibly misleading results. A convention for defining effective cross section and flux by averaging over the neutron spectrum is presented in the following subsection.

**4. Spectrum-Averaged Effective Cross Sections.** An average or effective cross section can be expressed in the general form

$$\bar{\sigma} = \frac{\int n(v) \, v\sigma(v) \, dv}{\int n(v) \, v \, dv}$$

where $n(v)$ is the actual distribution of neutron density in the energy range of interest and $n(v) \, v$ is the neutron flux.

This cross section convention is an outgrowth of the application of sophisticated reactor calculational methods to the definition of "effective" cross section. The effective cross section is defined here as

$$\sigma_{\text{eff}} = (\bar{\sigma}_{\text{th}}/\sigma_0) \, \sigma_0 + (\bar{\sigma}_{\text{epi}}/I_{\text{eff}}) \, I_{\text{eff}}$$

Both "cross section" ratios are functions of the $\phi_{\text{epi}}/\phi_{\text{th}}$ ratio and this ratio increases with increasing the fuel and target loading of the reactor.

The definition of reaction rate, which also defines flux, appears similar to Westcott's but differs because the "thermal" flux is averaged over the entire thermal spectrum and includes the effect of any deviations from a Maxwellian distribution.

$$\text{Reaction rate} = N \, \phi_{th} \, \sigma_{eff}$$

$\bar{\sigma}_{th}$, the average or effective *thermal* cross section, is calculated using THERMOS *(45)*, a thirty-group reactor code that calculates the thermal flux distribution at neutron energies below 0.625 eV using integral transport theory. Calculated ratios of $\bar{\sigma}_{th}$ to $\sigma_0$, the 2200 m/sec cross section, are shown in Fig. 2.15 as a function of spectrum $\phi_{epi}/\phi_{th}$ for several typical nuclides of interest in a $^{235}$U-fueled $D_2O$-moderated reactor at a temperature of 353°K. The variation of cross section with spectrum change, or its equivalent, the fuel and target loading, is substantial. The average cross section for a $1/v$ absorber is lower than the 2200 m/sec value because it is

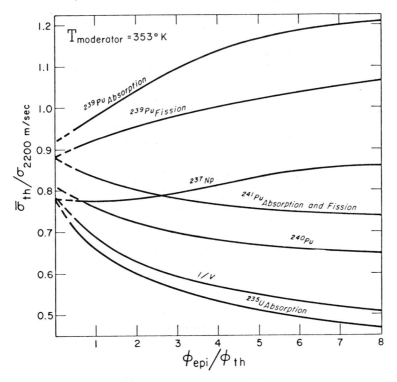

FIG. 2.15.   Change of average thermal cross sections with neutron spectrum.

calculated for the average neutron velocity, which as shown previously for a Maxwellian distribution, is a factor of 1.128 greater than 2200 m/sec. The 80°C (353 °K) moderator temperature results in another approximately 12% reduction in the cross section, according to the function $(T_0/T_{mod})^{1/2}$. Deviations from a Maxwellian distribution are calculated very well by THERMOS; irradiation experiments performed in a large-diameter uranium metal rod compared well with calculations even though the spectrum in the interior of the rod became non-Maxwellian (46). The results are reproduced in Fig. 2.16.

Thermal "resonance" absorption in the actinides increases the average or effective thermal cross section relative to that of a $1/v$ absorber. The parameter $\phi_{epi}/\phi_{th}$ provides a measure of the effect of the $1/E$ spectrum component on "resonance" absorptions below the cutoff energy, further increasing the effective "thermal" absorptions. These "resonance" factors contribute to the different shapes of the "thermal" cross section variations

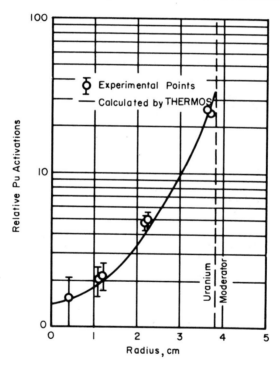

FIG. 2.16. Comparison between measured and calculated Pu foil activations in a uranium metal rod.

with spectrum. Thermal cross sections not shown in Fig. 2.15 are assumed for the most part to obey the $1/v$ law. As detailed data become available for the less-known actinides, possible departure from $1/v$ variation can be estimated by comparison of the new cross section data with that of the better-known nuclides plotted in Fig. 2.15.

The flux ratio $\phi_{epi}/\phi_{th}$ is calculated using HAMMER (42), a composite system of linked reactor physics codes, which includes THERMOS for the thermal flux calculation and HAMLET, a code similar to MUFT (47), but which has improved treatment of resonance absorption. HAMLET is a 54-group program for neutron energies $0.625 \text{ eV} < E < 10 \text{ MeV}$ and a set of three-group cross sections ($10 \text{ MeV}–1.05 \text{ MeV}–9.12 \text{ keV}–0.625 \text{ eV}$) is produced from the 54-group calculation that can be used to compute $\phi_{epi}$ and hence $I_{eff}$, the effective resonance integral for a particular material. $\phi_{epi}/\phi_{th}$ ratios are derivable from the calculation.

In the absence of detailed multigroup calculations, estimates of $\phi_{epi}/\phi_{th}$ in the fuel for $^{235}$U-fueled $D_2O$-moderated reactors of the type discussed in this chapter can be approximated by the following relationship,

$$\phi_{epi}/\phi_{th} \approx 0.008 \sum_i N_i \, \sigma_{0i}$$

$N_i$ equals the concentration, in atoms per foot, of each absorber in a given fuel assembly and $\sigma_{0i}$ equals the corresponding absorption cross section at $v = 2200$ m/sec. Similar empirical relationships could be developed for other reactor types. Calculation of flux ratios in the moderator always requires the more detailed HAMMER-type calculations. The approximate flux ratios are useful for hand calculations or for making rough estimates. Adequate estimates of epithermal events in a target can be made without direct use of HAMMER or any other code once $\phi_{epi}/\phi_{th}$ is determined. The average or effective *epithermal* cross section $\bar{\sigma}_{epi}$ can be expressed as

$$\bar{\sigma}_{epi} = \int_{0.625 \text{ eV}}^{10 \text{ MeV}} I_{eff} \, dE/E$$

and

$$I_{\infty}/I_{eff} \approx [1 + dI_{\infty}\rho/400 \, (\Sigma_s + S/4V)]^{1/2}$$

where $d = 2E/\pi\Gamma$, the self-shielding constant of the single large resonance, $\rho = $ target density, g/cc, $V = $ volume, $S = $ surface, $(\Sigma_s + S/4V)$ equals the geometric cross section of the target assembly. $\Sigma_s$ for typical target and support material is listed below along with $S/4V$ evaluation for possible target shapes.

| Material | $\Sigma_s$ (cm$^{-1}$) | Shape | $S/4V$ (cm$^{-1}$) |
|----------|----------|----------|----------|
| Mg | 0.16 | sphere | $3/4r$ |
| Al | 0.08 | cylinder | $1/2r$ |
| Co | 0.64 | slab | $1/2t$ |
| Bi | 0.26 | | |
| U | 0.40 | | |
| UO$_2$ | 0.37 | | |

Average geometric cross sections for typical materials and for shapes with approximately 1-cm dimensions, equal 1–2 cm$^{-1}$. A nominal value of 1 cm$^{-1}$ was selected for $\Sigma_s + S/4V$ to construct the variation of $I_{\text{eff}}$ with target density shown in Fig. 2.17. These data show how epithermal absorptions are reduced by resonance self-shielding within target material as the target density increases. The variation of the ratio $\bar{\sigma}_{\text{epi}}/I_{\text{eff}}$ with spectrum can also change if the spectrum deviates from $1/E$ dependence. This is shown in Fig. 2.18 where the ratio falls off in the fuel at the higher ratios of $\phi_{\text{epi}}/\phi_{\text{th}}$, showing further the need for detailed HAMMER-type calculations.

Cross section data for use in calculating average or effective cross sections are listed in Table 2.11. This tabulation has been derived from current sources and each value has been selected by the author as the "best available." ENDF/B data are included where available. Effective cross

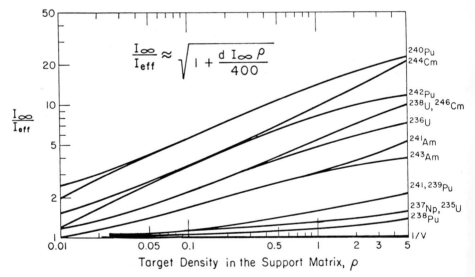

FIG. 2.17. Self-shielding of resonance absorbers.

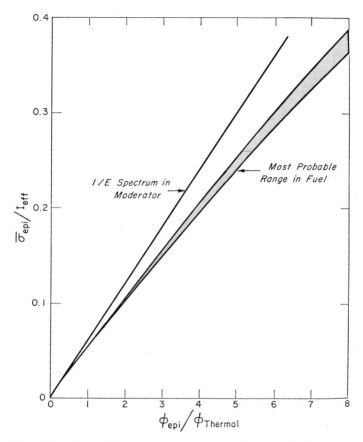

FIG. 2.18.   Effect of non-$1/E$ spectrum on resonance absorption in thermal reactors.

sections calculated with these data give good comparison with results of reactor irradiations.

Examples of how this information can be used to calculate effective cross section are tabulated in Table 2.12. The larger Westcott effective cross sections, derived from very similar input data, illustrate vividly the magnitude of error that improper application of cross section information might cause in production calculations.

It is possible to seek a relation between these two cross section conventions by comparing Westcott's epithermal index $r$ and $\phi_{epi}/\phi_{th}$ as follows:

$$r = \frac{4\,(\overline{E}_n/E_c)\,\phi_{epi}}{\phi_{th}\,\ln\,(E_{max}/E_c) + 2\,(\overline{E}_n/E_c)^{1/2}\,\phi_{epi}},$$

### TABLE 2.11

#### RECOMMENDED CROSS SECTIONS

| Radionuclide | $\sigma_{2200}$ (b) | | Resonance integrals | |
|---|---|---|---|---|
| | Abs | Fiss | Abs | Fiss/Abs |
| $^{59}$Co | 37.1 | | 70 | |
| $^{60m}$Co | 58 | | 230 | |
| $^{60}$Co | 2.2 | | 4.3 | |
| $^{169}$Tm | 120 | | 1625 | |
| $^{170}$Tm | 100 | | 1500 | |
| $^{171}$Tm | <10 | | 120 | |
| $^{168}$Er | 2.3 | | 4.7 | |
| $^{170}$Er | 5.4 | | 43 | |
| $^{171}$Er | 250 | | 250 | |
| $^{203}$Tl | 20 | | 130 | |
| $^{204}$Tl | 30 | | 12 | |
| $^{205}$Tl | 0.11 | | 0.5 | |
| $^{209}$Bi (act) | 0.015 | | 0.1 | |
| (abs) | 0.034 | | − | |
| $^{233}$U | 578 | 524 | 916 | 0.85 |
| $^{234}$U | 95 | 0 | 625 | 0.001 |
| $^{235}$U | 683 | 577 | 410 | 0.67 |
| $^{236}$U | 5 | 0 | 360 | 0.005 |
| $^{237}$U | 478 | 0.4 | 285 | 0.01 |
| $^{238}$U | 2.73 | 0 | 272 | 0.005 |
| $^{237}$Np | 169 | 0.02 | 550 | 0.003 |
| $^{238}$Np | 2200 | 2000 | 900 | 0.9 |
| $^{239}$Np | 60 | 0 | 415 | 0 |
| $^{236}$Pu | 170 | 170 | 68 | 1.0 |
| $^{238}$Pu | 563 | 16.3 | 169 | 0.14 |
| $^{239}$Pu | 1010 | 742 | 460 | 0.61 |
| $^{240}$Pu | 280 | 0.05 | 8500 | 0.001 |
| $^{241}$Pu | 1370 | 1010 | 730 | 0.81 |
| $^{242}$Pu | 20 | 0.05 | 1180 | 0.005 |
| $^{241}$Am | 740 | 3 | 1400 | 0.005 |
| $^{242g}$Am | 2900 | 2900 | 1160 | 0.9 |
| $^{242m}$Am | 8000 | 6600 | 2000 | 0.8 |
| $^{243}$Am | 85 | 0 | 2000 | 0 |
| $^{244}$Am | 2300 | 2300 | 920 | 1 |
| $^{242}$Cm | 20 | 3 | 150 | 0 |
| $^{243}$Cm | 950 | 700 | 2100 | 0.74 |
| $^{244}$Cm | 13.7 | 1.1 | 663 | 0.02 |
| $^{245}$Cm | 2640 | 2200 | 910 | 0.81 |
| $^{246}$Cm | 1.2 | 0 | 121 | 0 |
| $^{247}$Cm | 155 | 100 | 1300 | 0.62 |
| $^{248}$Cm | 1.4 | 0 | 240 | 0 |
| $^{249}$Bk | 1400 | 0 | 1000 | 0 |
| $^{249}$Cf | 1800 | 1550 | 2700 | 0.62 |
| $^{250}$Cf | 1500 | 0 | 5000 | 0 |
| $^{251}$Cf | 6900 | 4900 | 2600 | 0.65 |
| $^{252}$Cf | 28 | 6 | 100 | 0.21 |
| $^{253}$Cf | 2250 | 2235 | 2250 | 0.07 |
| $^{254}$Cf | 100 | 0 | 100 | 0 |

TABLE 2.12

EXAMPLES OF SPECTRUM-AVERAGED EFFECTIVE CROSS SECTIONS[a]

| Radionuclide | $^{237}Np_{abs}$ | $^{239}Pu_{fiss}$ | $^{59}Co_{abs}$ | $^{235}U_{fiss}$ |
|---|---|---|---|---|
| $\rho$ (g/cc) | 1 | 1 | 7 | 1 |
| $\phi_{epi}/\phi_{th}$ | 1 | 1 | 1 | 1 |
| $\sigma_0$ (2200 m/sec) (barns) | 169 | 742 | 37.1 | 577 |
| $RI_\infty$ (barns) | 550 | 280 | 70 | 254 |
| $T_{mod}$ (°C) | 80 | 80 | 80 | 80 |
| $\bar{\sigma}_{th}/\sigma_0$ (Fig. 2.15) | 0.75 | 0.94 | 0.69 | 0.66 |
| $I_\infty/I_{eff}$ (Fig. 2.17) | 1.33 | 1.60 | 1 | 1.33 |
| $\bar{\sigma}_{epi}/I_{eff}$ (1/E) (Fig. 2.18) | 0.06 | 0.06 | 0.06 | 0.057 |
| $\sigma_{eff}$ (barns) | 152 | 712 | 30 | 391 |

[a]Equivalent Westcott (41) cross sections $\sigma_{eff}^{W}$(b) 235, 941, 39, 554, respectively.

where $E_n$ = average energy of thermal neutrons; $E_c$ = cutoff energy of the Westcott convention; $E_{max}$ = 5 MeV, i.e., above this energy, no important neutron absorptions are assumed to occur.

A value of $r$ = 0.29 was reported for the Yankee reference design and $T_n$ was reported to be 402 °C (43). Substituting the equivalent average neutron energy of 0.068 eV, and using $E_c \simeq 4kT_n$ or $\sim$ 0.27 eV as defined by Westcott for the cutoff of the $1/E$ spectrum, $\phi_{epi}/\phi_{th} \approx 6$, using the experimental cadmium cutoff; $E_c$ = 0.5 eV, $\phi_{epi}/\phi_{th} \approx 14$.

Calculated values of $\phi_{epi}/\phi_{th}$, using spectrum-averaging methods (34), are about 11, where $E_c$ = 0.625 eV. Choice of an arbitrary intermediate value of $E_c$ of $\sim$0.4 eV would give an exact equivalence in $\phi_{epi}/\phi_{th}$. Thus there appears to be no simple unambiguous relation between the two conventions. Detailed knowledge of the neutron spectrum is required before an exact equivalence can be established for a particular reactor. If this kind of spectrum information is available, the empirical adjustment of $r$ or $E_c$ to obtain effective cross sections seems unnecessary, especially since the spectrum-averaging method is available and is compatible with current and future systems of computer codes for reactor calculations. Spectrum-averaging involves no such empirical adjustments.

## B. Methods of Calculation

Once effective cross sections and fluxes are established for target nuclei, the rate of neutron absorption processes can, by definition, be calculated directly, where reaction rate = $N\phi_{th}\sigma_{eff}$. Determination of these factors for targets in a particular reactor requires use of sophisticated reactor codes and/or good experiments. The following information about the operating reactor conditions must be included in making accurate production estimates: reactor power; fuel composition and burnup; moderator—type and density; temperatures—fuel, moderator, and target; cladding and support material; control rod positioning and flux shape; and target exposure and self-shielding. The significance of each of these factors on production depends on whether a full reactor charge is being devoted to producing a single radioisotope or whether partial production of many isotopes or of a single isotope is being studied.

An extremely fine analysis of the Yankee PWR is presented in a series of Westinghouse reports (34), showing how spectrum-averaging techniques have been applied to interpret experimental and operational data with particular relevance to radioactinide availability in the fuel.

This treatment is widely used in reactor physics analysis. Portions of the method are similar to the HAMMER computational code mentioned earlier. The general method should be used to obtain precise information about radioisotope production in any reactor. Use of spectrum-averaged cross sections obtained by simpler methods outlined in the previous subsection plus knowledge of the neutron flux determined by calculation or experiment give a good approximation to the more exact theory. However, the simple technique does not generally supply target-to-fuel flux ratios unless the target is adjacent to or part of the fuel. If the reactor lattice has targets interspersed among fuel positions, techniques for calculating the effect of these heterogeneities involve use of still another set of reactor codes. PDQ (48), developed extensively for light-water power reactors, uses multigroup-diffusion theory, and HERESY (49), a source-sink calculation, was developed more for heavy-water reactors. Both can be used to obtain good estimates of target to fuel flux ratios of separated targets. Flux in targets intermixed with fuel can be calculated using the HAMMER method. HAMMER could also be applied above thermal spectrum neutron energies to estimates of intermediate or resonance production of radioisotopes.

In general, when detailed calculations of radioisotope production are required, the complete engineering and physics description of the reactor is required. Anything less than this should be estimated by the approximate method outlined in Section VI or for small samples by use of effective cross sections developed from methods mentioned in this section.

## VIII. POSTIRRADIATION HANDLING OF RADIONUCLIDES

Radionuclides, produced in reactors by neutron capture or as products of fission, progress toward final application in a complex sequence of chemical processing, product fabrication, source handling, and shipping. The ultimate success of radioisotope usage depends to a large extent on how efficiently and economically these processes can be accomplished. This section indicates key factors for consideration in planning postirradiation handling. Many of these factors will be considered in the next chapter (Chapter 3).

### A.  Radiation Shielding and Contamination Control

Shielding and contamination control of large radioisotopic heat, radiation, or neutron sources is a new area for development. Regulations and experience exist that apply to small-scale shipments of radioisotopes but, lacking sufficient real experience, most specifications for postirradiation operations with large sources have to be handled on an individual basis, with the possible exception that large-scale shipments of $^{60}$Co for radiation sources are becoming quite common and may soon be covered by established procedures. Therefore, it is sufficient at this time to indicate some problem areas and to suggest possible solutions.

Shipment of radioactive material within a controlled area where a reactor and associated chemical separations plants are located would create minimum hazard to the general public. However, when radioisotopes are shipped via public transportation to places where they are to be used or processed, extra precautions for shielding and control of radioactivity must be applied.

For $\beta$, $\gamma$-emitting radioisotopes such as $^{60}$Co and $^{170}$Tm, the irradiated product may have been partially prepared for shipment by selection of suitable cladding prior to irradiation in a reactor. Source material might then be shipped in shielded containers without the expense of further processing. However, for $\alpha$-emitting radioisotopes, contamination is the major concern because amounts of penetrating radiation are comparatively small. In this case, it may be necessary to process chemically and then to fabricate the refined product material into a nearly final form, with a primary cladding, before shipment is permitted. A similar situation applies to fission products, which would be separated chemically and then possibly reformed into final shape before shipment in shielded containers. Shipment of irradiated fuel that contains these materials is already done routinely.

A neutron source, such as $^{252}$Cf, must have shielding to slow down and capture neutrons from spontaneous fission, and must be particularly well encapsulated to prevent spread of contamination. Safe performance in handling and shipping operations requires close coordination among personnel involved in reactor operation, chemical processing, and postir-radiation handling.

Heat removal from kilowatt sources is also a design problem in ship-ping and handling. In addition, shipping containers must withstand con-ditions created by external fires, the desert sun, or snow and freezing cold. Accidental drops, immersion in water, and criticality are other factors that must be considered when large radioisotope sources are assembled and shipped. For terrestrial use, the same basic criteria for design of the final application also apply to shipment and handling, with the additional factor that the application is often unattended and hence requires fool-proof safety features.

Aerospace safety requirements are even more stringent. At the present time the Sandia Corporation in Albuquerque, New Mexico, has been given the responsibility by the U.S. AEC for conducting a variety of safety tests in order to develop information for specifying proper source shield-ing and encapsulation criteria in space. These criteria would be more than adequate for terrestrial shipment.

This brief discussion is a reminder that safety problems associated with shipping and using large quantities of radioisotopes are similar and that problem solutions involve long-range planning and testing. Simplifi-cations can result if the selection of proper materials for target fabrica-tion is made prior to irradiation in a reactor or if final fabrication is com-pleted before shipment from the production site. Well-planned and co-ordinated operations throughout the entire phase of radioisotope pro-duction can reduce unnecessary handling and shipping expense and this cost control would contribute to making radioisotopes more attractive in economic comparisons with competitive forms of energy.

### B.  Critical Mass Considerations

Many actinide nuclides have substantial thermal fission cross sections, as shown in Table 2.11, and hence can achieve criticality if assembled in sufficient amounts. However, the only product radionuclides for which criticality in a "thermal" system could occur, are $^{238}$Pu that contains fis-sionable $^{239}$Pu as an impurity, $^{244}$Cm that contains fissionable $^{245}$Cm, and $^{252}$Cf that contains sufficient target precursor, $^{251}$Cf. The entire world's supply of californium over the next decade will probably not exceed 100 g̊, which would contain less than the 10–20 g $^{251}$Cf required for criticality. $^{238}$Pu and $^{244}$Cm criticality cannot be dismissed as easily. Conservative calculations for mixtures of $^{238}$Pu and $^{239}$Pu in a thermal neutron system show that above about 70% $^{238}$Pu criticality cannot be achieved. However, for isotopic purities less than 70% $^{238}$Pu, achieved either in production or by decay during extended use, the possibility of criticality should be evaluated for each particular power source design or for any handling or shipping operation. Because of the very low potential critical mass of $^{245}$Cm ($\sim$40 g), the possibility of "thermal" criticality should always be anticipated and avoided when $^{244}$Cm product contains in excess of about 40 g $^{245}$Cm. For example, the "safe mass" for the standard product listed, in Table 2.8, which contains only 1% $^{245}$Cm, is estimated to be about 10 kg curium, showing that only a minor safety margin is contributed by the other curium isotopes.

Freedom from criticality problems does not apply for large heat source applications of compact metallic or oxide fuel forms of $^{238}$Pu and $^{244}$Cm where "fast" critical conditions are approximated. Considerable theoretical and experimental work on criticality shows that for spherical compacts $^{238}$Pu is slightly more reactive than $^{239}$Pu and $^{244}$Cm is only slightly less reactive. The results are plotted over a range of densities in Fig. 2.19. The theoretical investigations are primarily the work of Keshishian and his co-workers at Atomics International (50). Experiments were performed in fast criticals, such as JEZEBEL, at Los Alamos (51). For an actual power source, structural and cladding material within and sur-

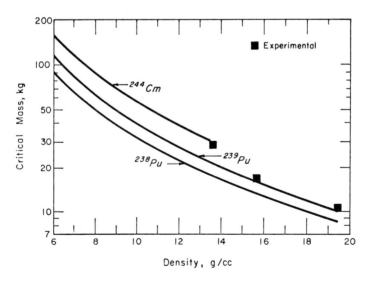

FIG. 2.19.   Critical mass of unreflected $^{244}$Cm and $^{238}$Pu spheres.

rounding the heat source would tend to increase the minimum critical mass above the values in Fig. 2.19, but evaluation of criticality for quantities in excess of the minimum critical mass must include careful analysis of the specific design features of the source to assure that the system is below criticality for all conceivable situations.

## C. Heat Removal

Radioactive nuclides generate heat; during postirradiation handling, the heat must be removed so that temperatures do not exceed prescribed limits. For radioactive material with high specific heat generation, heat removal during chemical processing is usually avoided by diluting process solutions or by use of cooling coils. For solid product material, heat removal problems vary, depending on the step in the source fabrication process that is being considered.

For radioisotopes that are preformed prior to irradiation, temperatures must not exceed limits where oxidation, physical phase changes, thermal cracking, or melting of the product might occur. As several finished source components are assembled to make a larger unit, heat removal requirements approach those of the final application. For fission products and the other chemically processed radionuclides, similar restrictions apply once the source components are fabricated into final form.

Means for cooling can be quite conventional, within the limitation that materials are highly radioactive and require shielding and containment. Water is an ideal cooling and shielding material. Metal heat sinks, i.e., large metal shapes that absorb and dissipate heat from the source, are useful for storing finished sources. Sources may be suspended if air cooling is calculated to be sufficient. Boiling liquids with associated condensers could also be used and have been considered specifically for heat removal prior to and during the launch of aerospace power sources.

With proper design of equipment and adequate preplanning of operations, heat removal during postirradiation handling is not a major problem. As large-scale production and use increase, it will, however, always remain as an important and persistent consideration in planning overall production operations.

## D. Accountability and Assay

Methods for accounting or assaying radionuclides can be categorized as measurements of one or more of the following properties: radioactivity, heat generation, isotopic purity, and weight. These measurements are needed to control chemical processing, to assure product quality, to verify reactor irradiation conditions and product yields, to control conditions and provide assurance that fabricated sources meet specifications set by users and to establish means of accounting for shipment and receipt of product.

The most widespread assay method is the measurement of radioactivity. Standards for $\alpha$, $\beta$, $\gamma$, and neutron sources are readily available or can be created, and are easily interchanged among laboratories to assure calibration of monitoring equipment.

However, for large assembled sources, calorimetric measurement may have substantial advantage over all other methods because, in many cases, heat generation is the intended application and calorimetry provides the ultimate verification of source output. The technology of calorimetry is well established and modifications to protect against radiation should be easy to make.

Mass spectrometry measurement of isotopic purity is an excellent monitor of product quality for many radioisotopes. Combined with measurements of radioactivity the results give confirming evidence of production yield and quality. Since they are independent but related measurements, they tend to resolve ambiguities which often result when a series of analytical measurements of a single type are made. This technique is well established in the analysis of the performance of irradiated nuclear fuels (34) and is having equal success for assaying the radionuclides of interest.

The weight of purified radionuclides is also a potentially accurate assay method, if measurements of isotopic purity provide corrections for impurities. For large-scale operations, large-scale assay methods are needed. Once processes are established, all assay methods will probably be used but calorimetry may ultimately become the most reliable and desirable method.

## IX.  OTHER RADIOISOTOPES WITH PROMISE

With the whole chart of the nuclides in view, it is suspected that there must be other radioisotopes that might also become "large-scale," if the need arises. The following is a brief review of eight neutron-produced radionuclides and additional fission products that show some promise and have a demonstrated or understandable potential.

### A. Scandium-46

$^{46}$Sc ($\tau_{1/2} = 84$ days) is made by irradiating naturally occurring, isotopically pure $^{45}$Sc. It can be produced in high specific activity $\sim$1000 Ci/g and consequently would make a good source for radiography, limited in strength by a low metal density of only $\sim$3 g/cc. $^{46}$Sc also has application as a materials radiation source with its 1.12 and 0.89 MeV gamma radiation.

### B. Europium-152

$^{152}$Eu ($\tau_{1/2} = 12.4$ yr) can be made by irradiating natural europium (47.82% $^{151}$Eu). It can be produced with a specific activity of only $\sim$25 Ci/g, which is intensified slightly by a metal density of $\sim$5.2 g/cc. Even so, $^{152}$Eu may have utility as a source for gamma irradiation with its multitude of gamma rays ranging in energy from 0.4 to about 1.4 MeV.

### C. Ytterbium-169

$^{169}$Yb ($\tau_{1/2} = 32$ days) is made by irradiating natural ytterbium (0.0135% $^{168}$Yb). It has been used for industrial radiography at activities as high as 1000 Ci/g. For this specific activity, isotopic enrichment of the $^{168}$Yb prior to irradiation was required.

### D. Tantalum-182

$^{182}$Ta ($\tau_{1/2} = 115$ days) is made by irradiating natural tantalum ($\sim$99. 988 % $^{181}$Ta). It can be produced in specific activity of several hundred curies per gram, which is also intensified by its high density of $\sim$16.5 g/cc. $^{182}$Ta could be used for radiography.

### E. Iridium-192

$^{192}$Ir ($\tau_{1/2} = 74$ days) is produced by irradiating natural iridium (37% $^{191}$Ir). It can also be produced in high specific activity $\sim$1000 Ci/g which is intensified by its very high metal density of $\sim$22 g/cc. $^{192}$Ir is valuable for radiography of objects up to a thickness equivalent of 3 in. of steel and is used widely for this purpose.

### F. Uranium-232

$^{232}$U ($\tau_{1/2} = 72$ yr) can be produced by neutron absorption in relatively stable $^{231}$Pa ($\tau_{1/2} = 32{,}480$ yr) followed by rapid beta decay of $^{232}$Pa. $^{231}$Pa is a trace byproduct of the irradiation of $^{232}$Th to produce $^{233}$U. $^{232}$U decays by a five-step alpha-cascade to $^{208}$Tl, which at equilibrium provides a long-lived source of high-energy gammas useful in research. $^{208}$Tl is the unwanted decay impurity in $^{227}$Ac and $^{238}$Pu.

## G. Einsteinium

$^{253}$Es ($\tau_{1/2} = 20$ days) and $^{254}$Es ($\tau_{1/2} = 480$ days) are products of neutron absorption in $^{252}$Cf. These isotopes are paving blocks on the road to higher-mass nuclides; at present they are only of research interest. However, einsteinium would be a byproduct of any large-scale effort to produce $^{252}$Cf and deserves mention since it has been used as target for accelerator production of new elements.

## H. Fission Products

There are fission products, other than the major four listed previously, that have been considered for possible chemical recovery and application. One such is low-activity technetium-99, an element not found in nature, which has possible application in metallurgy for imparting corrosion resistance and improving alloys. Another is stable xenon, with a combined fission yield of xenon isotopes of about 21 %. If recovered, xenon could be sold commercially as a rare gas in direct competition both in quantity and cost with the liquid air byproduct. Another is radioactive krypton-85 ($\tau_{1/2} = 10.8$ yr) which has a fission yield of only 0.3 %. It could be recovered from fission residues along with xenon and then separated. It has unique application in phosphors and has found many uses in radiotracer technology. Noble metals (palladium and rhodium) may also be recovered in useful and significant amounts.

Although probably unlikely to become major products, these fission products deserve mention because chemical recovery may become economically attractive if the other nuclides mentioned previously are also recovered from power fuel residues and the additional cost of recovery can be kept comparatively modest by sharing facilities and manpower.

Of the many excellent sources of information concerning radiation properties, shielding requirements, decay schemes, and general properties of radionuclides, References *52, 53, 54,* and *55* have been found very useful.

## REFERENCES

*1.*   P. C. Aebersold, *Proc. 3rd, U.N. Intern. Conf. Peaceful Uses At. Energy, Geneva, 1964*, **15**, 201 (1965).

*1a.*  "Radioisotopes: Production and Development of Large-Scale Uses," 1, U.S. AEC Rept. WASH 1095 (1968).

*2.*   *The AECL Study for an Intense Neutron Generator, ING Status Report*, AECL-2750, July 1967, Atomic Energy of Canada Limited, Chalk River, Ontario.

*3.*   G. I. Bell, *Phys. Rev.* **139B**, 1207 (1965).

*3a.*  "Forecast of Growth of Nuclear Power, 13," U.S. AEC Rept. WASH 1084 (1967).

*4.*   A. De Troyer and P. Dejonghe, "Production and Application of Actinium-227 for Direct Conversion Sources," *Large Scale Production and Applications of Radioisotopes*, U.S. AEC Rept. DP-1066, **I**, p. III-63 (1966).

*5.*   H. J. Groh et al., *Nucl. Appl.* **1**, 327 (1965).

*6.*   E. J. Hennelly and R. R. Hood, *Radioisotope Production Capabilities of U. S. Power Reactors*, U.S. AEC Rept. DP-1015 (1965).

*7.*   L. W. Lang, "Management of Americium in Power Reactor Fuels to Optimize Production of Alpha-Emitting Isotopes," *Large Scale Production and Applications of Radioisotopes*, U.S. AEC Rept. DP-1066, **II**, p. I-79 (1966).

*7a.*  E. J. Hennelly, *Trans. Am. Nucl. Soc.* **11**, No. 2, 456 (1968).

*8.*   W. C. Perkins, "Chemical Separation of Reactor-Produced $^{171}$Tm," *Large Scale Production and Applications of Radioisotopes*, U.S. AEC Rept. DP-1066, **II**, p. II-65 (1966).

*9.*   G. F. Tape, "Plutonium and Other Radioisotope Sources—Discovery to Demand," *Large Scale Production and Applications of Radioisotopes*, U.S. AEC Rept. DP-1066, **I**, p. 29 (1966).

*10.*  C. P. Ross, *Isotopes Radiation Technol.* **5**, No. 3, 185 (1968).

*10a.* J.L. Crandall, "Tons of Curium and Pounds of Californium," *Proc. Plenary Sessions, International Conference on the Constructive Uses of Atomic Energy, Washgton, D.C., Nov., 1968,* American Nuclear Society, Hinsdale, Illinois, 1969.

*11.*  F. P. Roberts and H. H. Van Tuyl, *Promethium-146, Fission Product and Transuranium Isotope Content of Power Reactor Fuels*, U.S. AEC Rept. BNWL-45 (1965).

*12.*  W. A. Rodger, *Multipurpose Plant for the Recovery of Neptunium and Other Isotopes*, report prepared for New York State Atomic and Space Development Authority, 1967.

*12a.* William G. Davey, *Nucl. Sci. Eng.* **26**, 149 (1966).

*13.*  E. J. Hennelly, *Nucl. News* **8**, No. 6, 19 (1965); and *The Savannah River High Flux Demonstration*, J. L. Crandall, compiler, U.S. AEC Rept. DP-999 (1965).

*14.*  D. J. Hughes, *Pile Neutron Research*, Addison-Wesley, Cambridge, Massachusetts 1953, p. 190.

*15.*  D. E. Deonigi, *Formation of Transuranium Isotopes in Power Reactors*, U.S. AEC Rept. BNWL-140 (Rev. 1) (1966).

*16.*  *The High-Flux Isotope Reactor - A Functional Description*, U.S. AEC Rept. ORNL-3572 (1964).

*17.*  *Reactor Physics Constants*, U.S. AEC Rept. ANL-5800, 2nd ed, July 1963, p. 519; and A. M. Weinberg and E. P. Wigner, *The Physical Theory of Neutron Chain Reactors*, University of Chicago Press, Chicago, 1958, p. 442.

*18.*  A. Prince, *Neutron Cross Sections and Technology, NBS Spec. Pub. 299*, **II**, 951 (1968)

*19.* D. H. Stoddard, *Radiation Properties of* $^{244}Cm$ *Produced for Isotopic Power Generators,* U.S. AEC Rept. DP-939 (1964).

*20.* W. M. Rutherford, G. N. Huffman, and D. L. Coffey, *Trans. Am. Nucl. Soc.* **9**, No. 2, 599 (1966).

*20a.* E.J. Hennelly, W.R. Cornman and N.P. Baumann, *Neutron Cross Sections and Technology, NBS Spec. Publ.* **299**, **II**, 1271 (1968).

*21.* F. T. Binford and W. A. Hartman, $^{238}Pu$ *Production by a Continuous Process,* U.S. AEC Rept. ORNL-4023 (1967).

*22.* A. S. Jennings, J. F. Proctor, and L. P. Fernandez, "The Large Scale Separation of Polonium-210 from Bismuth," *Large Scale Production and Applications of Radioisotopes,* U.S. AEC Rept. DP-1066, **II**. p. II-79 (1966).

*23.* *Nuclear Industry* **14**, No. 11, 30 (November 1967).

*24.* "Transuranium Processing Plant," *Annual Report 1966, Oak Ridge National Laboratory,* p. 10.

*25.* C. Artandi and W. Van Winkle, Jr., *Isotopes Radiation Technol.* **2**, No. 4, 321 (1965).

*25a.* Proceedings of Symposium on $^{252}Cf$, New York Section ANS Oct. 22, 1968, CONF-681032 (1969), Clearinghouse, U.S. Dept, of Commerce.

*26.* Enrichment Charge Schedules, *Nucl. Industry* **14**, No. 12, 6 (1967).

*27.* G. W. Beeman, *Nucl. News* **10**, No. 2, 23 (1967).

*28.* *An Evaluation of Heavy-Water-Moderated Power Reactors — A Status Report as of March 1963*, U.S. AEC Rept. DP-830 (1963).

*29.* *Nuclear Desalination Program - Annual Progress Report on Activities Sponsored by the Atomic Energy Commission for Period Ending October 31, 1966,* U.S. AEC Rept. ORNL-4087 (1967).

*30.* E. W. Coleman, "Radiography," *Large Scale Production and Applications of Radioisotopes,* U.S. AEC Rept. DP-1066, **I**, p. IV-43 (1966).

*31.* *Nucleonics Week* **8**, No. 35, 5/6 (August 31, 1967).

*32.* D. C. Stewart, R. W. Anderson, and J. Milsted, *The Production of Curium by Neutron Irradiation of Am$^{241}$,* U.S. AEC Rept. ANL-6933 (1964).

*33a.* J. A. Smith, *Neutron Cross Sections and Technology,* NBS Spec. Pub. 299, **II**, 1285 (1968). National Bureau of Standards, Washington, D. C., 1968.

*33b.* G. T. Seaborg, *Isotopes Radiation Technol.* **6**, No. 1, 1 (1968).

*33c.* B. I. Spinrad, *Reactor Fuel Reprocessing Technol.* **10**, No. 3, 190 (1967).

*34.* *Yankee Core Evaluation Program - Quarterly Progress Report for the Period Ending September 30, 1966,* U.S. AEC Rept. WCAP-6082 (1967).

*35.* R. L. Hellens and H. C. Honeck, "A Summary and Preliminary Analysis of the BNL Slightly Enriched Uranium, Water Moderated Lattice Measurements," Panel on Light Water Lattices, Vienna, May 28 – June 1, 1962, *IAEA Technical Report Series No. 12,* 1962, pp. 27–71.

*36.* H. C. Honeck and J. L. Crandall, "The Physics of Heavy Water Lattices," *Reactor Technology, Selected Reviews,* U.S. AEC Rept. TID-8541, 1965, p. 1.

*37.* *Reactor Physics Constants,* U.S. AEC Rept. ANL-5800 (1963).

*38.* *Proceedings of A Conference on Neutron Cross Sections and Technology, NBS Spec. Pub. 299,* **I** and **II**, (1968).

*39.* B. J. Toppel, *The Argonne Reactor Computation System, ARC,* U.S. AEC Rept. ANL-7332 (1967).

*39a.* HC Honeck, et al., "JOSHUA - A Reactor Physics Computational System." U.S. AEC Rept., CONF-690401, p. 324. Clearinghouse, U.S. Dept. of Commerce, Springfield, Va., 1969.

*40.* E. D. Reilly and W. H. Turner, *The Automation of Reactor Design Calculations at the Knolls Atomic Power Laboratory,* U.S. AEC Rept. ANL-7050 (1965).

*41.* C. H. Westcott, *Effective Cross Section Values for Well-Moderated Thermal Reactor Spectra,* AECL Report CRRP-960, November 1960, Atomic Energy of Canada Limited, Chalk River, Ontario.

*42.* J. E. Suich and H. C. Honeck, *The HAMMER System,* U.S. AEC Rept. DP-1064 (1967).

*43.* F. G. Dawson, D. E. Deonigi, and E. A. Eschbach, "Plutonium Buildup and Depletion," *Nucleonics* **23**, No. 8, 101 (1965).

*44.* *Proceedings of the Brookhaven Conference on Neutron Thermalization,* April 30 to May 2, 1962, U.S. AEC Rept. BNL-719, Vol. 1-4, November 1962.

*45.* H. C. Honeck, *Nucl. Sci. Eng.* **8**, 193 (1960).

*46.* H. D. Brown and E. J. Hennelly, "Neutron Thermalization Studies at Savannah River," *Proceedings of the Brookhaven Conference on Neutron Thermalization,* April 30 – May 2, 1962, U.S. AEC Rept. BNL-719, III, 1962, p. 879.

*47.* H. Bohl, Jr. et al., *MUFT-4 - Fast Neutron Spectrum Code for the IBM-704,* U.S. AEC Rept. WAPD-TM-72, 1957.

*48.* *Reactor Physics Constants,* U.S. AEC Rept. ANL-5800, 2nd ed. July 1963, p. 781.

*49.* D. R. Finch, *User's Manual for SRL - HERESY I,* U.S. AEC Rept. DP-1027 (1966); and W. E. Graves, F. D. Benton, and R. M. Satterfield, *Nucl. Sci. Eng.* **31**, 57 (1968).

*50.* V. Keshishian, E. H. Ottewitte, and C. L. Dunford, *Trans. Am. Nucl. Soc.* **8**, No. 2, 549 (1965).

*51.* D. M. Barton, *Nucl. Sci. Eng.* **33**, 51 (1968)

*52.* C. M. Lederer, et al., *Table of Isotopes,* 6th ed., Wiley, New York, 1967.

*53.* E. K. Hyde et al., "Detailed Radioactivity of Elements," *The Nuclear Properties of the Heavy Elements, II,* Prentice-Hall, Englewood Cliffs, New Jersey, 1964.

*54.* E. D. Arnold, *Handbook of Shielding Requirements and Radiation Characteristics of Isotopic Power Sources for Terrestrial, Marine, and Space Applications,* U.S. AEC Rept. ORNL-3576, April 1964.

*55.* *Reactor Physics in the Resonance and Thermal Regions,* Proceedings of the National Topical Meeting of American Nuclear Society, San Diego, February 7-9, 1966, **I** and **II**, M.I.T. Press, Cambridge, Massachusetts 1966.

# 3 RADIOACTIVE SOURCE ENCAPSULATION

*KIRK DRUMHELLER*

PACIFIC NORTHWEST LABORATORIES
BATTELLE MEMORIAL INSTITUTE
RICHLAND, WASHINGTON

# I.  INTRODUCTION

The intent of this chapter is to describe some of the general requirements for encapsulation of isotopic heat and radiation sources, and to illustrate the specific requirements for encapsulation of a particular source. While the specific requirements could probably not be applied directly to the encapsulation of any other source, description of these requirements may provide a partial basis for the development of processes for a particular source.

Radioisotopes exist as solids, liquids, and gases. The most common form of a radioisotope is a solid. Regardless of the radioisotope form, it requires encapsulation (cladding) or permanent packaging for any or all of the following purposes:

(1)  To completely contain the radioisotope so as to prevent inadvertent release to the environment.

(2)  To protect the radioisotope from the environment (for example, oxidation, hydration, and nitriding).

(3)  To modify the isotope's radiation or heat producing characteristics, such as to shield out undesirable radiation and to provide improved heat transfer surfaces, more surface area for heat transfer, or to resist heat transfer in order to generate higher internal temperatures, or to serve as a susceptor to convert radiation to heat.

(4)  To aid in the safe and efficient handling of high-temperature, radioactively toxic materials.

(5)  To meet minimum regulatory standards required by the various state and national licensing bodies governing the fabrication, storage, and use of the radioisotope (1).

Generally, encapsulation or cladding techniques have been developed for most isotopes with heat or radiation source potential. To date, most uses for isotopes as either radiation or heat sources have required relatively small quantities. Sources are usually encapsulated in quantities varying from one capsule to a maximum of a few thousand capsules instead of mass production quantities in the millions. As large-scale uses are developed, costs should be greatly reduced.

# II.  DESIGN CONSIDERATIONS

## A.  *Environment*

Isotopic sources may be used in space, terrestrial surface, or oceanographic applications. Such uses require that source encapsulation be designed to withstand severe thermal, chemical, and mechanical environments.

Thermal environments may range from a few degrees above body temperature for a potential heart pump heat source (2) to temperatures as high as 2000 °C (3) for a thermionic heat source. If a heat source is to be used in space, the capsule asssembly may have to withstand reentry temperatures higher than the melting point of the cladding material.

A source may be exposed to pressure environments ranging from the near perfect vacuum of outer space to a pressure of several thousand pounds per square inch encountered at great ocean depths.

By either design or accident, a source may have to withstand underground burial, immersion in the sea, or exposure to Arctic cold. Therefore, all possible extremes of such environments must be anticipated in selection and design of radioisotopic encapsulation.

### B.  Isotope Characteristics

In selecting a radioisotope for a given application, one must consider availability, cost, radiochemical purity, half-life, and any factors in the application which may restrict types of fuel forms which can be used.

There are two principal supply sources for radioisotopes (4, 5). One source is the irradiation of target materials in commercial or government-owned nuclear reactors. The other source is fission products resulting from reprocessing of spent uranium fuel elements.

Considering the plutonium production reactors which are presently in standby condition, radioisotopes made from irradiated targets would seem to be almost unlimited in supply. Production cost for these radioisotopes is likely to be more important than availability. Certain radioisotopes produced by the irradiation of target materials are shown in Table 3.1.

Availability of fission products resulting from spent fuel elements may be limited. The expected availability of a variety of fission products from power reactor fuels in the U.S. is shown in Table 3.2, expressed in terms of available heat output.

Economic considerations in producing encapsulated radioisotopes include the cost of fuel or target fabrication, the cost of irradiation, the cost of separation, the cost of encapsulation, the cost of alternative sources of power or radiation, and in the case of power generators, the cost of placing the generator in its use environment. The estimated costs per kilowatt hour for various isotopes are shown in Table 3.3.

TABLE 3.1

TYPICAL RADIOISOTOPES PRODUCED
BY THE IRRADIATION OF TARGET MATERIALS

| Radioisotope | Half-life (yr) | Target material | Typical potential use of isotope |
|---|---|---|---|
| $^{238}$Pu | 86.4 | $^{237}$Np | Low shielding heat source, space and terrestrial - artificial heart pacemaker. |
| $^{60}$Co | 5.24 | $^{59}$Co | Radiation sources, terrestrial power sources. |
| $^{170}$Tm | 0.35 | $^{169}$Tm | Space power, low shielding terrestrial uses. |
| $^{210}$Po | 0.38 | $^{209}$Bi | Short life space missions. |
| $^{85}$Sr | 0.178 | $^{84}$Sr | Short life radiation, e.g., biosatellite. |

TABLE 3.2

EXPECTED AVAILABILITY of RADIOISOTOPES IN THE U.S. *(6, 7)*
AS A BYPRODUCT OF POWER REACTOR OPERATION
1980 (95,000 MW$_e$ installed reactor power)

| Isotope | Expected annual availability — 1980 (kW$_t$) |
|---|---|
| $^{90}$Sr | 850 |
| $^{137}$Cs | 850 |
| $^{144}$Ce | 10,000 |
| $^{147}$Pm | 40 |

TABLE 3.3

COST PER KILOWATT HOUR FOR ISOTOPIC POWER *(6)*

| Isotope | Cost/kWh$_e$ | Mission life (yr)[a] |
|---|---|---|
| $^{60}$Co | $ 15 | 5 |
| $^{90}$Sr | 6 | 10 |
| $^{137}$Cs | 7 | 10 |
| $^{147}$Pm | 350 | 3 |
| $^{171}$Tm | 1150 | 2 |
| $^{210}$Po | 235 | 0.4 |
| $^{238}$Pu | 138 | 10 |

[a]  Assumes terminal or lowest specific power at 5 % thermal to electrical conversion efficiency for assumed mission life as shown.

TABLE 3.4

TYPICAL STAND-IN MATERIALS FOR ISOTOPE PROCESS DEVELOPMENT

| Isotope | Stand-in (natural) |
|---------|--------------------|
| $^{210}$Po | Te |
| $^{147}$Pm | Sm |
| $^{238}$Pu | Ce |
| $^{137}$Cs | Cs |
| $^{90}$Sr | Sr |
| $^{85}$Sr | Sr |
| $^{60}$Co | Co |
| $^{170}$Tm | Tm |
| $^{171}$Tm | Tm |

Cost is probably the most important single factor in the extensive use of isotopes. Because quantity is low at the present time, unit costs may be quite high. In fact, unit costs are so high in some cases that an increase in quantity is unlikely. However, a thorough analysis prior to beginning production and the application of available nonradioactive chemically and physically similar "stand-in" or "substitute" material technology can in many cases reduce the cost of isotopic sources to much below their present levels. Table 3.4 shows typical stand-in materials.

Radiochemical purity is likely to be a primary concern in heat source materials where low energy radiation is desirable. This applies to such isotopes as $^{238}$Pu and $^{147}$Pm. When these materials are selected for a use in which low shielding is desirable, radioactive impurities must be minimized as they might result in a much higher radiation field. For example, the radiation through uranium shielding from a 1000 W $^{147}$Pm source containing varying amounts of $^{146}$Pm is illustrated in Fig. 3.1 (8). Characterization of $^{147}$Pm containing 0.25 ppm $^{146}$Pm indicated that the following radiation was being emitted by the $^{146}$Pm impurity (9):

| Type | Energy (MeV) | Radiation emission |
|------|--------------|--------------------|
| $\beta$ | 0.78 | $9 \times 10^6$ particles/W sec |
| $\gamma$ | 0.45 | $1.7 \times 10^7$ photons/W sec |
|  | 0.75 |  |
| Brems-X-ray | 0.22 | $2.6 \times 10^4$ photons/W sec |

One of the most important considerations in selecting source materials for various uses is the half-life of the radioisotope. Polonium-210, for example, has a half-life of only 0.38 yr and, therefore, must be used in

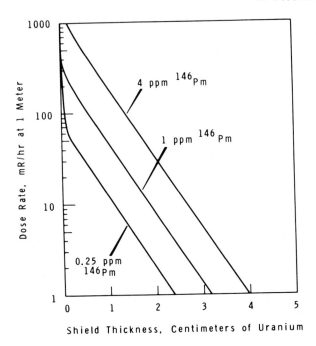

FIG. 3.1.   Dose rates from 1000-W promethium sources with different
¹⁴⁶Pm contents.

applications of relatively short durations. An isotope which is to be used
to power a deep space probe sending signals back for 10 years or more
must have a relatively long half-life. Plutonium-238 with a half-life of
86.4 yr is a likely candidate for such applications *(10)*. An isotope which
is to be used to power an underwater beacon may require a half-life of
ten years or more in order to be economical. For most current applications the overall economics, including factors such as the cost of alternate
power sources, the cost of refueling, and the cost of placing the source
and shielding in its use environment will affect the choice of half life.

In some instances radiation requirements of a radioisotope's intended
application alone may be important enough to dictate the selection of a
radioisotope. For example, isotopes considered for heart pumps must be
of light weight when combined with fairly complete shielding *(11–13)*.
They must have a fairly high power density in order to minimize the volume of material which is to be implanted.

Isotope source materials may be in the form of metals, alloys, ceramics,
cermets, gases, and mixtures or solid solutions. Metals normally provide

TABLE 3.5

PHYSICAL FORMS IN WHICH RADIOISOTOPES ARE COMMONLY USED

| Radioisotope | $^{60}$Co | $^{90}$Sr | $^{137}$Cs | $^{147}$Pm | $^{171}$Tm | $^{238}$Pu | $^{244}$Cm |
|---|---|---|---|---|---|---|---|
| Form | Metal | SrTiO$_3$ | CsCl | Pm$_2$O$_3$ | Tm$_2$O$_3$ | PuO$_2$ | Cm$_2$O$_3$ |

the highest density of isotope. In general, metals are not as resistant to corrosion as ceramics and are more likely to be used in such applications as food irradiators or low power thermoelectric generators which are not likely to be subject to very hostile environments. However, $^{60}$Co is fairly stable *(14)* and is one of the least expensive and most successful isotopes for many applications.

Ceramics provide a very stable source material in general. A ceramic such as strontium titanate has a high degree of resistance to corrosion *(15, 16)*. Typical forms for some isotope sources are shown in Table 3.5.

Cermets are becoming more popular because they combine some of the benefits of ceramic and metallic fuel forms *(3)*. When used in isotopic heat sources, cermets are usually made of spheroidized particles of the source material coated with metal and consolidated into a dense body *(17)*.

## C. Radiation Effects

For some radioisotopic applications, the radiation emitted is the desired product. Such applications include: nondestructive testing of castings and welds; the use of radiation sources for gauging; curing of plastics, plastic-impregnated wood, and paints; the sterilization of surgical materials; food preservation.

Applications for which radiation is not the desired end result, such as heat sources, must consider that most organic materials have only a limited resistance to radiation. For instance, this must be considered in the design of electronic components where organic insulation could deteriorate under radiation and in the design of mechanical components where oils or other lubricants could deteriorate from radiation.

Unwanted radiation exposure to people and environment must be prevented by the use of adequate shielding. Shielding requirements for typical isotope applications are shown in Table 3.6. In general, 6 in. of lead will suitably shield a one kilowatt $^{90}$Sr source; 0.1 in. of lead will shield a 1-kW $^{238}$Pu source when used with an additional several inches of hydrogenous material to shield out the neutrons associated with $^{238}$Pu.

TABLE 3.6

Shielding Requirements for Typical 1 kW$_t$ Isotope Applications

| Isotope | Approximate shielding required (6) to limit beta and gamma radiation to 10 mR/hr at 1 m (inches of lead) |
|---------|-----------|
| $^{60}$Co | 9.5 |
| $^{90}$Sr | 6 |
| $^{137}$Cs | 4.6 |
| $^{147}$Pm | 1.0 |
| $^{170}$Tm | 2.5 |
| $^{210}$Po | 1 |
| $^{238}$Pu | 0.1 |
| $^{244}$Cm | 2 |

Heavy neutron shielding is not necessarily required for Pu sources if the Pu is free of light elements which can given an $\alpha$-n reaction—for example, if the oxygen in $^{238}$PuO$_2$ is depleted in $^{18}$O, neutron emission is greatly reduced.

### D.  Configuration

Configurations in which radioisotope sources may be fabricated include the simple cylinder, tubes, flat plates, thin films, and spheres. The most common and simplest to fabricate is the cylindrical or pin-type configuration which may be used for a large number of applications. A limiting factor in any capsule configuration is the thermal conductivity of the source form and the average capsule surface heat flux. The surface heat flux will determine the surface temperature (as a function of energy dissipation or insulation) and the thermal conductivity of the source form will determine the increase in internal temperature (usually at the center-line of the source core) to sustain the residual surface temperature.

A modification of the pin configuration is the tube configuration in which thermal conductivity problems are reduced by providing coolant flow through the center of the tube. An extension of the tubular concept to minimize the heat flow path results in a honeycomb-type configuration. This configuration can be used to provide a very large mass of source material with short heat flow paths.

The spherical configuration may be used to achieve minimum surface area for a given volume. This offers some advantages in that the maximum amount of heat-producing material may be used with a minimum length of heat path, and the minimum surface area configuration results in minimum shielding requirements. The spherical configuration is also resistant to impact damage *(18)*.

Flat plate configurations are generally used for radiation sources in which it is desired to minimize self-shielding and to spread out the radiation field. Cobalt-60 and cesium-137 are generally considered prime candidates for plate type configurations. Plate configurations are also considered for conversion devices in which a very thin layer of a beta-emitting radioisotope is placed on an emitter plate and a collector plate picks up the emitted electrons to produce an electrical current *(19)*.

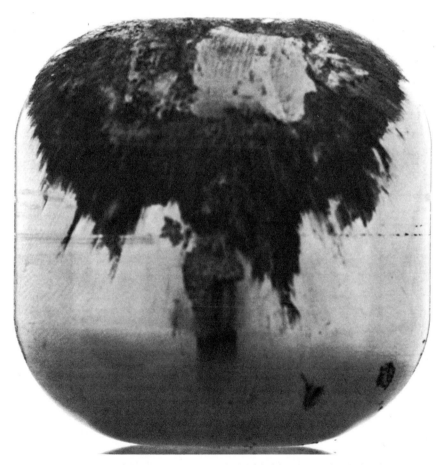

FIG. 3.2. Radioisotope heat source following impact test simulating free fall from 60,000 feet.

### E.  Safety

Safety design considerations *(20)* require that no person could credibly be injured by a radioisotope source. Therefore, the encapsulated radio-isotope must be designed so that no radioactive material could be liberated by any credible accident associated with its use. Encapsulating materials must be selected to withstand high shock resulting from impact or explosion as well as high temperatures resulting from fires or explosions during transportation or actual use. These requirements have dictated the extensive use of graphite, superalloys, refractory metals, stainless steel and high strength steels. Even in applications where a rupture of the encapsulation would not be particularly dangerous, the isotope may require a stringent encapsulation design from transportation considerations alone.

An example of impact resistance which may be expected in a source is shown in Fig. 3.2. This source was built to provide heat for a proposed aircraft inertial guidance unit *(21)*. It was designed to survive a free fall from 60,000 ft with an impact on solid granite. Figure 3.2 illustrates the source following its impact on concrete at a velocity 50% greater than that expected from a 60,000 ft free fall. This particular source was a promethium oxide source encapsulated in tantalum for shielding and Haynes-25 alloy for environmental control and impact resistance.

Power sources to be used in space usually require design for reentry capability *(22)*. These sources must be capable of surviving entry into the earth's atmosphere at velocities that would result in temperatures well above the melting point of the source material if protection by additional ablative or insulating material in addition to the shielding was not provided.

### III.  PROCESSING METHODS

### A.  General

In order to produce a usable radiation source, some processing is usually required to extract it from the irradiation target, to purify and refine it, and to convert it to the form in which it will finally be used. Since the radiation levels of these materials will be high, special precautions must be taken.

Three basic types of processing are used for isotopes and other nuclear materials (see Figs. 3.3, 3.4, and 3.5). These are: (1) contact processing in

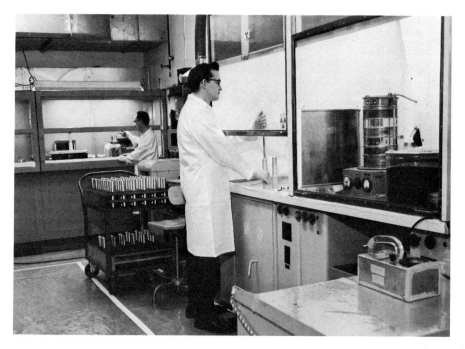

FIG. 3.3. Open faced hood processing.

which source materials may be processed in open-faced hoods with personnel working with them directly or with gloves, (2) glove box processing in which the materials are completely enclosed in an air-tight box (materials are handled only through sealed gloves), and (3) remote processing in which materials are handled only by means of tongs or manipulators inside a shielded cell (23). Processes for encapsulation of a particular source may utilize one or all of these basic process types during different steps.

In addition to the requirements for containment during processing, consideration must be given to the effects of heat from the isotopes on equipment with which the source may come in contact. For example, plastic bags may melt and measuring equipment may be affected by heat. In immersing sources in water tanks for nondestructive testing, consideration must be given to thermal shock on a hot source.

The chemical and physical stability of the source form often dictates the maximum temperature and the environmental conditions (air, inert gas, $H_2$, etc.) which may be used during the encapsulation process. If the

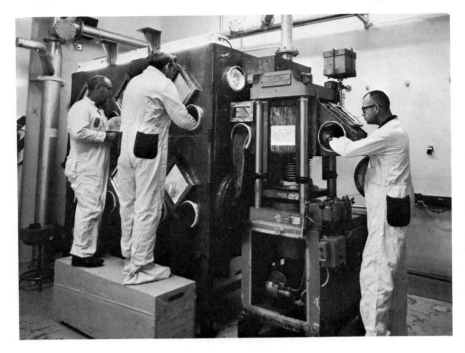

FIG. 3.4.   Glove box processing.

source form is stable, high temperature plasmas *(17)* or casting treatments *(24)* might be employed. If the source form has unstable characteristics which cannot be corrected after processing, lower temperature processing might be employed like sintering *(25)*, cold pressing, high energy impaction *(18)*, or simple vibrational compaction of loose powders or particles.

The environment in which the source is to operate may also dictate processing methods. If the environment is relatively nonhazardous and not likely to result in release of the isotope, a simple powder form may be used. Generally a densification process which produces an insoluble, high integrity core is desirable.

The required density of core material may necessitate specific processing methods. A high density may be necessary to achieve a sufficient energy in a given volume. In general, high density reduces the volume of the source and hence the volume of shielding. The overall system weight and space requirements are thus reduced.

The process yield, the percentage of the starting source material which is finally encapsulated, is particularly important in processes where unit costs are very high. With production quantities of one or two capsules,

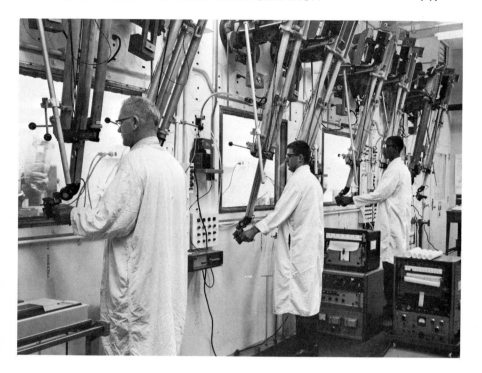

FIG. 3.5. Hot cell processing.

it is not uncommon to consider anything less than 100% yield a complete failure. Since a 100% yield is not very realistic, such complete failures sometimes occur. This can be guarded against to some extent by providing complete nondestructive tests on all components which go into the process up to the final capsule closure steps. For example, all components of the container should be very thoroughly checked before final processing.

The methods of processing vary so much with the source encapsulation material to be used and the end use of the source, that we will only discuss typical processes here. These typical processes which can be used with strontium, cobalt, promethium, plutonium, polonium, and cesium sources can in general also be applied to other materials.

## B. Core Material Preparation

The final source assembly consists of the "core," which is the actual radioisotopic material and the capsule or cladding which shields, protects the core from the environment, and prevents loss of source material. The process by which the material is separated from other fission products is directly related to the form in which it will be used. Typical physical properties of isotopic fuel forms are shown in Table 3.7.

Promethium, which is a byproduct of the nuclear fission production process, must be chemically separated from the total spectrum of nuclear fission products (26). From the acid feed, the rare-earth constituents of the fission products are isolated and stored to allow decay of the $^{145}$Pm isotope. This is followed by a general rare-earth purification, a specific promethium purification, and a final conversion step to the sesquioxide fuel form.

Plutonium-238 is made by the irradiation of a neptunium alloy with subsequent chemical processing which results in an oxide fuel form.

It is usually possible to achieve other forms if desired. Promethium, for example, has been produced in the metal form (27).

### C.  Pretreatment Before Encapsulation

After final processing of materials to the desired form, the sample may require further treatment before encapsulation. For instance, a cesium chloride sample may require the dissolving of the salt and recrystallization under carefully controlled conditions just prior to encapsulation. Such treatment may minimize any moisture pickup. For a number of applications, material which is to operate at a high temperature may be treated above the operating temperature under vacuum conditions just prior to the final encapsulation. Such treatment will remove gases or impurities which might evolve under operating conditions.

Mechanical preparation of powders may include ball milling to increase surface area and provide uniform particle size, pneumatic impaction to obtain high-density, large-size particles for vibrational compaction, or pressing and sintering of preslugged and sized particles to obtain high density particles for plasma fusion.

A "preslugging" operation, consisting of pressing loose powders into compacts followed by breaking the compacts into particles much larger than the original particle size, may be very helpful in achieving desired densities. This operation is usually carried out with sources which are to be consolidated by powder metallurgy techniques such as pressing, sintering, and compacting (21). This effectively reduces the final energy input required by forming together some of the fine particles which do not have to be recombined during the regular consolidation process step.

TABLE 3.7

TYPICAL PHYSICAL PROPERTIES OF ISOTOPIC FUEL FORMS

| Fuel form | Melting point (°C) | Thermal expansion coefficient (per °C) | Thermal conductivity (cal sec⁻¹ cm⁻¹ °C⁻¹) | Specific heat (cal g⁻¹ °C⁻¹) | Electrical resistivity (ohm cm) | Density (g cm⁻³) |
|---|---|---|---|---|---|---|
| Co | 1495 | $1.2$ to $1.8 \times 10^{-5}$ | $0.13 - 0.17$ at 30°C | $\sim 0.103$ | $6 \times 10^{-5}$ at 800°C | 8.7 |
| SrTiO₃ | ~1900 | $1.12 \times 10^{-5}$ | $0.013-0.017$ at 30°C | $0.16$ at 600°C | $10^{10}$ at 100°C $10^{6}$ at 500°C | 5.0 |
| CsCl | 646 | | | | | 3.99 |
| Pm₂O₃ | 2130 | $10.8 \times 10^{-6}$ (30-740°C) | $\sim 0.006$ at 150°C | $0.0944$ (0-1000°C) | $3 \times 10^{8}$ at 25°C 100 at 700°C | 7.43 |
| Tm₂O₃ | | $7.7 \times 10^{-6}$ (400-800°C) | | | | 8.6 |
| PuO₂ | 2280 | $9 \times 10^{-6}$ (25-1000°C) | $0.0056$ at 1200°C $(96.5\%\ TD)^{a}$ | $0.0818$ at 700°C | $10^{14}$ at 25°C $10^{2}$ at 1250°C | 11.46 |

ᵃ TD = Theoretical density.

### D.  Core Material Consolidation

Source material may be consolidated as a single-phase material or as a cermet in which one phase is enclosed in another phase in such a way that the second phase is continuous.

Conventional pressing and sintering may be applied to a variety of ceramic fuel forms. This type of operation generally consists of cold pressing pellets or other shapes and sintering them at a temperature somewhat below the melting point of the material. Materials are usually cold pressed to a density of about 75% and sintered to 90–95% of theoretical density (TD). Typical cold pressing, sintering temperatures and density for $Pm_2O_3$ are shown in Table 3.8.

TABLE 3.8

TYPICAL COLD PRESSING PRESSURES, SINTERING TEMPERATURES, AND
DENSITY FOR PROMETHIUM OXIDE *(17)*

| Cold pressing pressure | Cold pressed density | Sintering temperature | Final density |
|---|---|---|---|
| 65 tons/sq. in. | 73% TD | 1355 °C | 90% TD |

Promethium oxide can be sintered in air up to temperatures very near the melting point without adverse effects. With some materials, even a brief exposure to air at room temperature may produce undesirable effects. For instance, a hygroscopic material such as cesium chloride can pick up enough moisture in a few hours to undesirably affect subsequent processing.

The temperature ranges for pressing and sintering of several isotopic materials are shown in Table 3.9. Because of relatively limited data

TABLE 3.9

APPROXIMATE SINTERING TEMPERATURES FOR ISOTOPIC MATERIALS

| Isotope compounds | Sintering temperature range (°C) | Refs. |
|---|---|---|
| $SrTiO_3$ | 1300 | *28* |
| $Pm_2O_3$ | 1300 | *17* |
| $Tm_2O_3$ | 1700 | *29* |
| $PuO_2$ | 1400 | |

available so far, we do not feel that these temperatures are optimum at the present time.

Dies and lubricants suitable for powder metallurgy type fabrication of conventional materials under comparable conditions may not be suitable for the fabrication of isotopes. For example, in pressing an isotopic heat source, a lubricant that might be suitable for conventional ceramic pellets

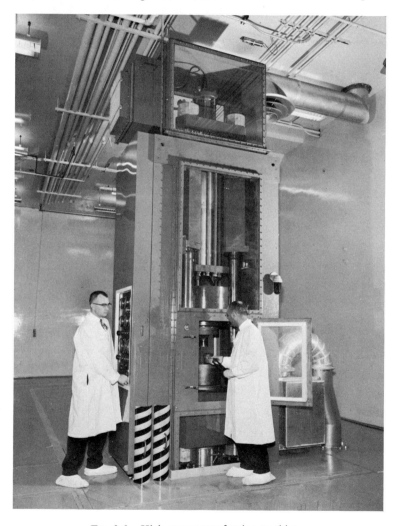

FIG. 3.6.   High energy rate forging machine.

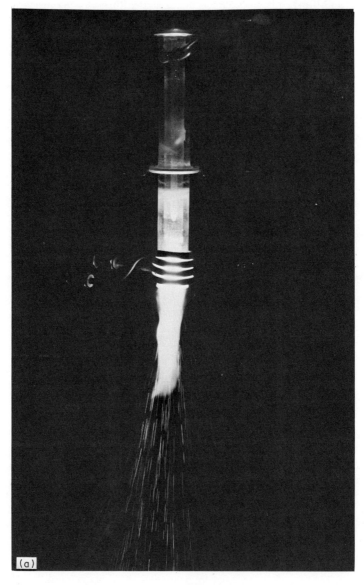

(a)

FIG. 3.7a.   Plasma torch.

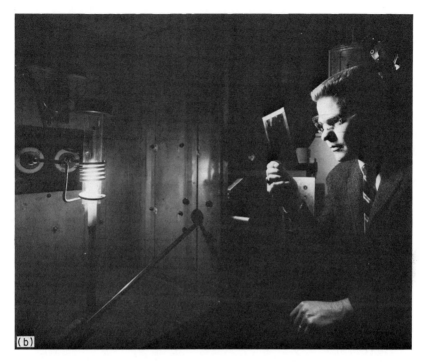

(b)

FIG. 3.7b.    Plasma torch—detail.

could boil off due to the heat of the isotope before full pressure is applied.

Consideration must also be given to thermal stresses which may arise from self-heat of the core material.

Pneumatic impaction is a process which uses a high energy-rate forging machine *(18)* (Fig. 3.6.). Materials are generally encapsulated in a cylindrical can. The can is dropped into a die, and the machine is fired. The punch presses the material in the die with pressures up to 400,000 psi. The density of most pneumatically impacted materials is greater than 95% of theoretical and usually will be almost 100% of theoretical density. This process may be used to obtain high-density particles for other types of processing, or it may be used for direct encapsulation and densification.

Plasma spheroidizing is a process in which particles are densified and spheroidized *(3,30)*. It has been a primary method for the fabrication of plutonium oxide heat sources because the particles produced are relatively stable. It is also used to achieve a high density particle for later coating and consolidation into a cermet. In this process, small particles, usually

50–300 microns in diameter, are dropped through an inductively heated plasma torch (Fig. 3.7.). The temperature in the plasma may reach 17,000 °C. The particles melt and, after they drop through the plasma, they cool to form high density spheroids. The operation is much the same as that used to make round lead shot.

Hot pressing has been used successfully on promethium oxide and other isotope compounds (31). This process may achieve higher density than conventional pressing and sintering and may also result in closer dimensional tolerances. During this process the material is heated to a high temperature at the same time that pressure is being applied. In this process, the promethium oxide is heated to a temperature of about 1590 °C and pressed at a pressure in the 5000-psi neighborhood.

Melting or casting may be used with cesium chloride. The material can be melted and simply poured into a mold or final container. However, because cooling contraction of cesium chloride can be 15 to 20%, it is usually preferable to pour only a small amount at a time and allow that amount to solidify before pouring more.

Some representative temperatures for processes other than pressing and sintering are shown in Table 3.10.

A simplified process was used in the fabrication of a biosatellite radiation source (32). The source used $^{85}Sr$ in the form of strontium nitrate. The material was simply poured into the container, the lid decontaminated, and the cap inserted and welded.

Vacuum vapor deposition, chemical vapor deposition, and sputtering may be used to coat small particles or to coat the inside or outside of containers to ensure electrochemical compatibility or to make thin layers of isotopes for direct conversion devices (19).

Vacuum vapor deposition is a process in which materials are placed in a vacuum and heated to the point where they vaporize (33), and subsequently deposit on the objects to be coated. Vacuum vapor deposition equipment is shown in Fig. 3.8a.

Chemical vapor deposition usually refers to a thermal decomposition process in which a mixture of gases such as tungsten hexafluoride and hydrogen is passed through a heated fluidized bed of particles (Fig. 3.8 b.). The heat results in reaction of the tungsten hexafluoride with hydrogen, forming tungsten and hydrogen fluoride gas. The tungsten is deposited on the particles.

Sputtering is a process for coating objects with material ejected from a target bombarded by a beam of high velocity inert gas ions.

TABLE 3.10

REPRESENTATIVE PROCESSING TEMPERATURES FOR ISOTOPE PROCESSING

| Source fuel form | Typical process | Processing temperature (°C) |
|---|---|---|
| Co | Rolling | 950 – 1100 |
| $SrTiO_3$ | Pneumatic impaction | 1200 |
| CsCl | Fusion casting | 650 |
| $Pm_2O_3$ | Pressing and sintering | 1500 |
| $Pm_2O_3$ | Hot pressing | 1700 |
| $PuO_2$ | Plasma fusion | to 20,000 |

### E. Clad Material Processing

Many different methods of forming may be used for isotope cladding. In fact, virtually all conventional techniques may be applied. Selection of a particular process depends on the degree of dimensional control required, the type of cladding or combination of types and configurations, the use to which the source is to be put, and the environment in which the source is to operate.

Materials used in isotope encapsulation may vary from conventional steel alloys to such materials as high strength alloys and refractory metals. With beta emitters, materials such as tantalum or tungsten may be desirable to provide shielding both from any gamma-emitting impurities and from bremsstrahlung radiation. The refractory metals have excellent high temperature compatibility with some isotope materials.

Typical encapsulation requirements call for compatibility with the core material, adequate shielding, compatibility with the environment, and perhaps compatibility between various adjacent materials which are required to meet a combination of other requirements. For example, a material that may be compatible with the core may not be useful as a shielding material. A good shielding material may not be compatible with the core or the environment. Another material may be compatible with the environment but not with the core clad material. One could conceivably thus have a requirement for three different cladding materials in the encapsulation.

In most cases, conventional processes may be used for forming cladding for heat or radiation sources. However, the forming processes for some clad materials may be somewhat less than conventional because some of the materials used are unique. Rhenium as a clad material may

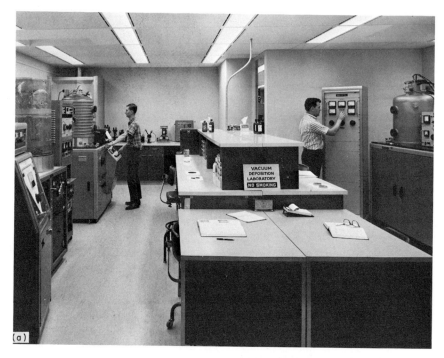

FIG. 3.8a.   Vacuum vapor deposition equipment.

be made by pressing and sintering with subsequent rolling and welding. Tungsten-rhenium alloys may be made by vapor deposition.

Capsule materials currently being considered for high temperature use (up to 1000 °C) with $^{60}$Co are TD nickel, TD nickel chromium, Inconel* 600, Hastelloy† C, Hastelloy† X, Nickel 270, and Haynes† Alloy 25 *(35)*.

## F.   Closure

Two welding processes are most frequently used for enclosing an isotopic source within its capsule. These are: (1) arc welding using a tungsten electrode shielded with an inert gas (gas tungsten arc welding GTAW) *(36)* and (2) electron beam welding *(21)* (Figs. 3.9 and 3.10).

Other processes with potentially desirable characteristics are magnetic

---

\* Trademark of International Nickel Company, Inc.
† Trademark of Union Carbide Corporation.

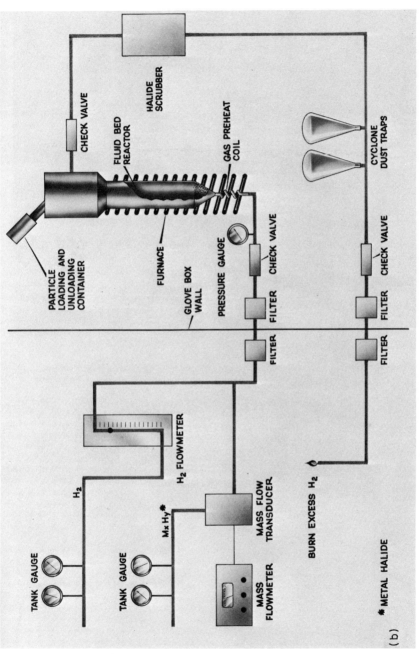

Fig. 3.8b. Chemical vapor deposition.

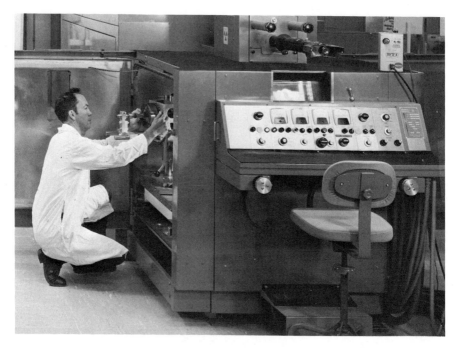

FIG. 3.9.   Electron beam welder.

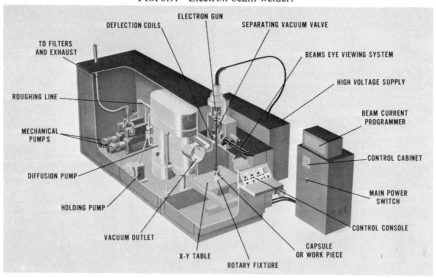

FIG. 3.10.   Schematic illustrating components of an electron beam welder.

force welding *(37)*, ultrasonic welding, pneumatic impaction welding, and pressure bonding.

GTAW welding of source material capsules is popular for two reasons: first, it uses available, low-cost equipment; and second, it can be used in any mode of operation from fully manual to fully automatic. Other welding processes do not generally offer this latter advantage. Gas tungsten arc welding is covered here in some detail because of its widespread application and use.

GTAW welding of source capsules is performed in inert gas chambers (Fig. 3.11). The inert gas chamber not only contains the inert gas used for welding, it also serves as a radiation shield and as a gloved hood for containing contaminating particles. Where very reactive or refractory metal capsule cladding is to be welded, high purity, inert gas chambers are used which can be evacuated to a high vacuum before being backfilled with inert gas.

In typical GTAW welding operations, cylindrically shaped capsules

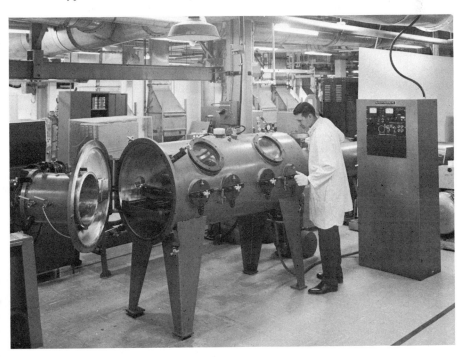

FIG. 3.11. Gas tungsten arc welding equipment.

are almost always rotated while the torch is held stationary. Many light-weight rotary weld fixtures are available for capsule rotation.

At least two manufacturers are producing a unit with a small welding head which incorporates a rotating tungsten electrode that can be used for closure welding of cylindrical capsules. These, however, could only be used in a semiautomatic operation.

Generally, where capsules are not cylindrical in form, the welding torch is manually moved over the joint.

In order to prevent damage to rotary welding fixtures and to keep capsule temperatures reasonably constant, chill blocks are commonly used to cool hot capsules. In some instances water-cooled rotary fixtures have been used.

The weld joint must be very clean for a successful GTAW weld closure. This is most important because a foreign particle could cause a small inclusion or crater in the closure joint which would jeopardize the seal and thus the entire capsule. The weld joint must not only be free of scale, grease, oil, and dirt, it must be free of source material as well. Depending on the type of source material used, decontamination of the weld joint may be required to extremely low levels. Where such decontamination is difficult, double or even triple layers of encapsulation may be required.

The GTAW weld closure method may be used on an unlimited number of joint designs although it is generally used on the simple radial and butt joint designs.

While GTAW welding is suitable for use with most cladding material, electron beam welding may be particularly desirable in applications where a vacuum is desired inside the capsule. It may also be particularly applicable where low heat input and deep weld penetration are desired.

Magnetic force welding (Fig. 3.12) may prove particularly applicable for two reasons. First, it is an inherently higher speed process than GTAW or electron beam welding, and second, it can produce a satisfactory closure with a minimum heat input. This may be advantageous for the closure of sources with a low melting point or a low-temperature vapor point. Equipment for magnetic force welding of closures is well developed.

Ultrasonic welding may be desirable for the same reasons as magnetic force welding, but processes for closures of this type require more development.

A potential application for magnetic force or ultrasonic welding would be the enclosure of a cesium chloride source within its capsule. GTAW or electron beam welding with their high heat input could possibly damage

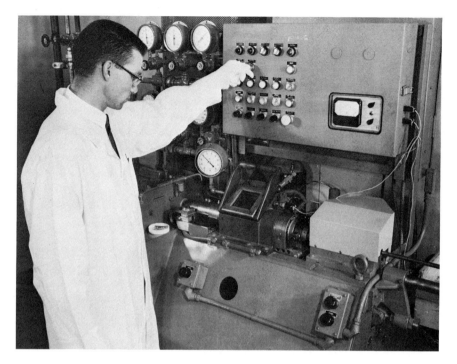

FIG. 3.12. Magnetic force welding equipment.

the source because cesium chloride melts or vaporizes at relatively low temperatures. (However, these latter two methods can be used where an intermittent welding process is employed that does not cause excessive heat buildup.)

## G. Scale-Up Potential

Although initial development work may require only one or two capsules, the potential for scale-up for larger production runs should be carefully considered in any process development. Such scale-up may still involve relatively few capsules.

Most processes have a good potential for production scale-up. For instance, some people consider the plasma fusion spheroidization coating compaction processes to be uneconomical. However through one plasma facility costing $20,000, it is possible to process 300 to 400 grams of $^{147}Pm_2O_3$ per eight-hour shift. Particles can be coated in an apparatus costing only a few hundred dollars at a rate of several hundred grams per eight-hour shift. These processes could readily be scaled-up to produce several kilograms per day.

## IV.  EVALUATION

The cost of high-activity sources and the complexity of manufacture require the use of very rigid inspection tests. Some of these tests are applied immediately after assembly. Others may have to be repeated at intervals throughout the useful life of the sources to check the dimensional stability and continued integrity. Sources may be evaluated by both nondestructive and destructive testing.

Nondestructive tests include ultrasonic *(38)*, eddy current, radiography, neutron radiography, dye penetrant, and acoustic emission tests. Ultrasonic and eddy current tests are normally applied for the detection of weld voids or cracks or voids in the cladding. A typical ultrasonic test station for isotope capsules is shown in Fig. 3.13. Radiography is used to detect such anomalies as weld defects, potential cladding defects, and uniformity of source configuration. Neutron radiography may be particularly applicable in those cases where source radiation would essentially obliterate the results from conventional radiography. Dye penetrant tests are used to detect weld porosity and potential cracks much the same as they are used in conventional weld inspections.

Acoustic emission is presently being developed as a means of detecting flaws as they occur *(39)*. This provides the potential for improved welding techniques, improved quality, and reduced fabrication costs.

### A.   Mechanical Properties

The extent of mechanical testing needed for source and cladding materials depends on the requirements of the source. For example, in a heat source which utilizes an alpha emitter, the pressure resulting from helium buildup can be very significant. An advantageous set of circumstances does exist in that as helium builds up the thermal output decays; it is still necessary to perform creep tests under normal operating conditions.

### B.   Environmental Tests

Stability at operating temperatures is one of the main characteristics to be looked for in evaluating isotopic heat sources. A source can normally be evaluated for this capability by testing it at or above the expected

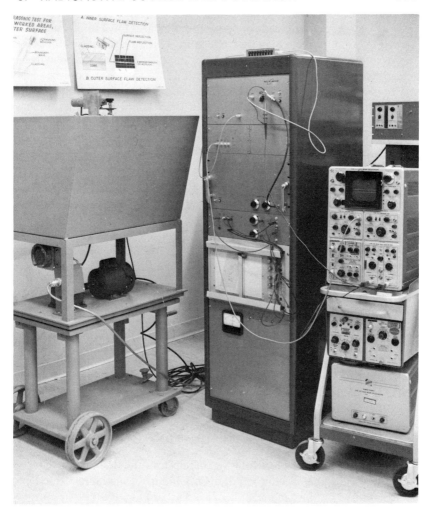

Fig. 3.13.   Ultrasonic test station for isotope capsules.

operating temperature in an environment comparable to that in which it is expected to survive.

If a heat source is to be operated under cyclic thermal conditions, evaluation must include effects of thermal cycling on source and cladding materials. Materials which may be compatible (nonreactive) under steady-state high temperature conditions may not be compatible under temperature cycling conditions.

Tests on sources intended for space use may also have to include simulation of conditions encountered in reentry. Thus, the source may require testing under high temperature service. For space applications, environmental tests also may include test operation in a vacuum chamber.

Compatibility tests between the clad and its environment should include tests under simulated conditions of time, temperature, and atmosphere. In some cases, materials which apparently survive a one-month test may not survive a twelve-month test because of long-range effects of radiation, corrosion, and some other long-term degradative process.

Compatibility tests should include tests under operating conditions, tests under maximum conditions which could conceivably be reached, and tests under conditions approaching the life-time of the source.

In some cases, although corrosion may seem to be nonexistent at the operating temperature for a substantial portion of the source's lifetime, it may then become catastrophically severe, causing earlier termination of the useful life of the source.

Compatibility tests must also cover any unusual conditions that the source could encounter such as a fire in jet fluid, reentry conditions, or effects of sea life.

### C. Destructive Tests

Destructive tests to evaluate the performance of source and clad materials selected include metallography, microprobe analysis, chemical tests, and chemical analysis. One of the most frequently used destructive tests is metallography.

## V. DESIGN AND ENCAPSULATION PROCEDURES

To illustrate the procedure followed in selecting and designing a suitable source capsule, the specific requirements for a promethium oxide heat source will be used as an example (21). This section outlines the capsule design, the fabrication process, and the quality control plan for the encapsulation of a 65-W promethium sesquioxide heat source. Included are the encapsulation process from the receipt of the promethium oxide through the shipment of the final capsule. A promethium source fabrication facility is shown in Fig. 3.14.

### A. Capsule Design

A promethium-147 heat source capsule was fabricated for the Air Force to be used in a thermal preconditioning unit (TPU) within an advanced

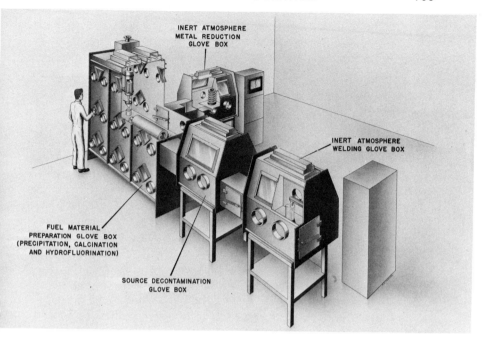

FIG. 3.14. Promethium source fabrication facility.

aircraft. The TPU, a piece of auxiliary support equipment for an inertial measuring unit (IMU) was designed to provide an improved navigation system reaction capability. The TPU reduces the time interval between the application of power to the navigation system and the attainment of specified performance by maintaining the navigation system at an elevated temperature. To accomplish this function, a promethium-147 source of 65 thermal watts initial power was designed, developed, and flight qualified.

The basic capsule dimensions were fixed by the TPU design, while the shape, including the dome ends, was designed to optimize impact resistance (Fig. 3.15). Promethium-147 met the basic requirements of geometry, weight, and safety for the application and was considered a desirable isotope due to:

(1) A very low external dose rate with only minimal shielding (beta emitter).
(2) Appropriate half-life.
(3) Adequate power density of the stable sesquioxide fuel form.

(4)  Minimal design problems due largely to a demonstrated capability
     of producing heat sources of this size.
(5)  Projected availability for potential scale-up requirements.

Tantalum, because of its shielding characteristics and its relative ease
of fabrication was selected as the inner cladding. Tantalum radiation
shielding 0.060 in. in thickness reduced the dose rate to 10 to 30 mR/hr
at 1 m. A uniform 0.200 in. thick wall of L-605 alloy for the secondary
outer cladding was selected to maximize impact strength within limits
dictated by the total capsule size, by the fuel core volume, and by shielding requirements. This high strength cobalt alloy has outstanding corrosion resistance.

Another pertinent consideration in the capsule design was the weld
location. The primary and secondary welds were offset from each other
to minimize any possible shear plane of weakness through the capsule
(Fig. 3.15). The primary weld, intended only as a contamination seal, was
offset from the center of the capsule. The secondary weld, which required
the optimum impact resistance, was located at the center of the longi-
tudinal axis of the capsule. This center location, because of the capsule's
dome end shape, afforded the greatest protection regardless of impact
attitude.

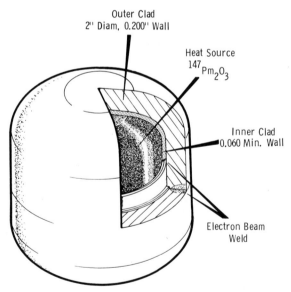

FIG. 3.15.  Promethium oxide heat source.

This particular design resulted in an overall capsule size 2 in. in diameter and 2 in. long, with dome ends on a 0.645 in. outside radius. Dimensions of the inner capsule were chosen to allow adequate radiation protection and sufficient clearance for easy assembly while providing the maximum practical fuel volume. The resulting volume for the isotope, approximately 37 cm³, was adequate to provide the specified 65 W of thermal power using freshly purified promethium-147 oxide at a density of 90 to 95% of theoretical density.

## B. Process Description

The process selected to meet the above specifications is shown in flowsheet form in Fig. 3.16. The three horizontal sequences deal with the three main stages of the process, namely, fabrication of the source material, fabrication and loading of the inner capsules, and preparation, loading, and finishing of the outer container. The more important stages are discussed in detail below.

## C. Promethium Oxide Preparation

The isotopic purity of the $^{147}$Pm fuel material is determined by radiochemical techniques after the chemical purification process but before the oxalate precipitation and oxide conversion procedures. The presence and amount of $^{146}$Pm, $^{148m}$Pm, $^{154}$Eu, and $^{144}$Ce are determined.

After the oxalate precipitation and oxide conversion steps, the final step is a calcination at 1100 °C in $H_2$ to obtain a purified monoclinic $Pm_2O_3$ phase; then the $Pm_2O_3$ is subjected to a prepressing consolidation and crushing step to increase the bulk density of the powder. The additional powder preparation treatment (Fig. 3.16, process steps 3–6) makes the oxide more suitable for pressing to the optimum green (prior to sintering) density. The powder is weighed accurately to assure the exact initial material required for the heat source.

## D. Pressing and Sintering

A punch and die set including a special tempered, tapered and split sleeve is used in dry pressing the oxide powder (Fig. 3.17). This die design with the periphery release sleeve, makes possible the ejection of a rounded dense, integral pellet of optimum green density (75–80% TD). The purpose of the release sleeve is to provide a simultaneous release of radial pressure rather than a continuous release as the pellet is ejected from the

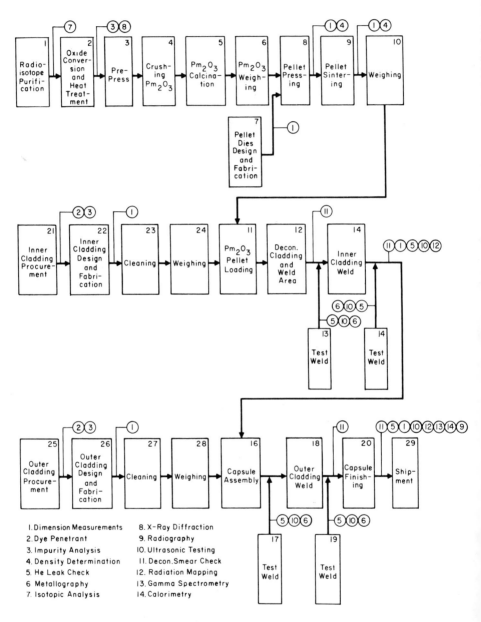

FIG. 3.16.   Typical Pm₂O₃ radioisotope encapsulation process.

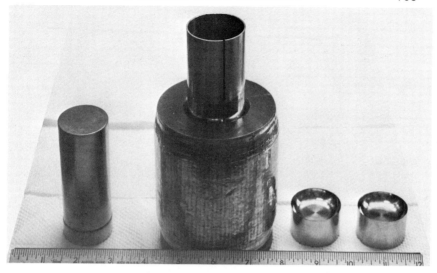

FIG. 3.17.   Punch and die set for pressing promethium oxide pellets.

die. Under the conditions used, there is significant expansion of the green pellet when pressure is released. If the pellet expands continuously as it is ejected, laminations can result. The powder is carefully weighed, placed in the die cavity, and pressed under approximately 150,000 psi. A radius-shaped backup plug and radius-shaped punch are used to obtain the required dome ends. The pellet is handled remotely with special tongs. The pressed pellet is weighed, the as-pressed dimensions are determined and the pressed density is calculated.

The green pellet is heated slowly (12 hr minimum) to a sintering temperature of 1350–1450°C, held for a minimum of 16 hr, and allowed to cool slowly over a period of 12–16 hr. The weight and dimensions are determined to calculate sintered density and to assure assembly into the capsule. These steps are noted on the process flow diagram (Fig. 3.16), steps 7-10.

### E.  Inner Capsule Assembly

A dye penetrant test and a chemical analysis are made on the electron beam melted tantalum bar stock prior to capsule fabrication. The inner capsule is machined directly from the bar stock (Fig. 3.18). The machined capsule is checked for adherence to dimensions and is inspected for flaws using radiographic and ultrasonic techniques. The capsule

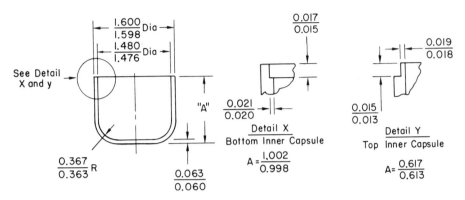

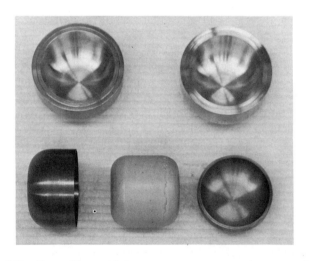

FIG. 3.18.  Promethium oxide inner capsule design.

components are cleaned ultrasonically and weighed prior to the fuel-
cladding assembly (Fig. 3.16, process steps 21–24).

The $Pm_2O_3$ pellet loading (process step 11) is a critical operation. Components prior to assembly are shown in Fig. 3.19. It is necessary to minimize any contamination of the capsule weld surfaces. The lower portion
of the inner capsule is protected from $Pm_2O_3$ powder contamination on
the entire outer surface and on the weld joint surfaces by an aluminum
foil jacket. The foil is removed after the pellet is loaded in the capsule.
The capsule weld joint is smeared to test for contamination and decon-

FIG. 3.19.  Promethium oxide heat source components prior to assembly.

taminated as required. The upper portion of the capsule is then clamped into position.

### F. Inner Capsule Welding

Welding is done with an electron beam welder, Fig. 3.10, followed by nondestructive examination. Welding conditions are verified prior to and immediately after the welding of the fueled capsule. The test welds (Fig. 3.16, process steps 13 and 15) are subjected to the same nondestructive testing as the fueled capsule plus a metallographic examination. The destructive examination of these test welds directly before and after the welding of the fueled capsule will confirm the degree of quality assurance indicated by the ultrasonic flaw testing of the fueled capsule. Other nondestructive examinations prior to assembling the fueled inner capsule into the outer cladding include: a smear test, dimensional checks, a helium leak test, and radiation mapping.

Typical parameters to achieve the weld shown in Fig. 3.20 were:

| Beam potential (kV) | Beam current | Transverse beam deflection | Face speed |
|---|---|---|---|
| 135 (no load) | 7.5 mA | 16 mils | 30 in./min |

This inner capsule weld is maintained at a low penetration because strength is not required and it is not desirable to allow penetration of the

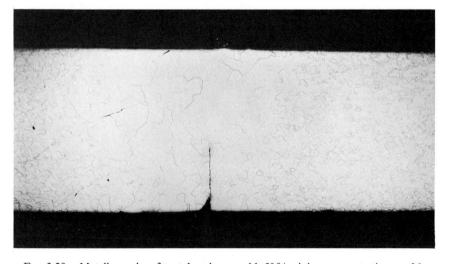

FIG. 3.20.   Metallography of tantalum inner weld, 50% minimum penetration. × 36.

electron beam to the promethium oxide. This might result in vaporization of the promethium oxide with resulting contamination of the system.

### G.  Outer Capsule Assembly

A dye penetrant test and a chemical analysis are made on the hot rolled, solution treated alloy L-605 bar stock. The outer capsule is machined directly from the bar stock (Fig. 3.21) checked for adherence to dimensions, and inspected for flaws using radiographic and ultrasonic techniques. The capsule components are cleaned ultrasonically and weighed prior to the inner capsule-outer capsule assembly (Fig. 3.16, process steps 25–28).

### H.  Outer Capsule Welding

The procedure for welding the outer capsule is a duplication of the inner welding including test welds (Fig. 3.16, process steps 17–19). Decontamination is accomplished after each welding step for the fueled capsule and after final finishing (processs step 20). The repeated smear testing is required to maintain constant surveillance of the capsule's clean condition previous to any test or following process step. The testing of

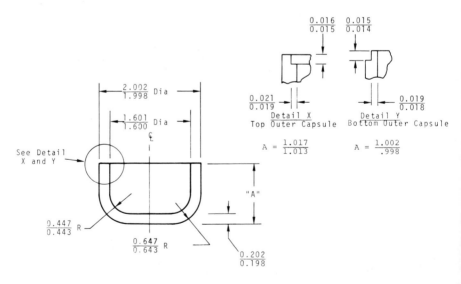

FIG. 3.21.   Promethium oxide outer capsule design.

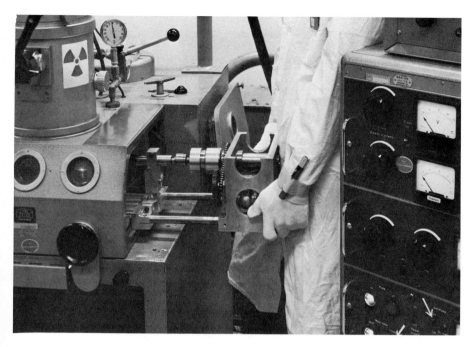

Fɪɢ. 3.22. Tooling for electron beam weld of promethium oxide capsule.

the finished capsule will also include a helium leak test, a dimensional check, ultrasonic testing of the weld, gamma spectrometry, calorimetric testing, and radiation mapping.

Optimized parameters for Phase II electron beam welding of L-605 alloy were:

| Beam potential (kV) | Beam current | Transverse beam deflection | Face speed |
|---|---|---|---|
| 142.5 (no load) | 13.5 mA | 0.016 in. | 24 in./min |

Tooling for this weld is shown in Fig. 3.22. (This is a smaller beam welder than that shown in Fig. 3.9.) Weld metallography is shown in Fig. 3.23. Since strength was a primary requirement for the outer capsule, a minimum penetration of 90% was required. Since the inner capsule was already sealed, there was no danger of contamination resulting from slight over penetration.

Handling of the completed source is illustrated in Fig. 3.24. While the radiation from this source is relatively low, it is still too radioactively and

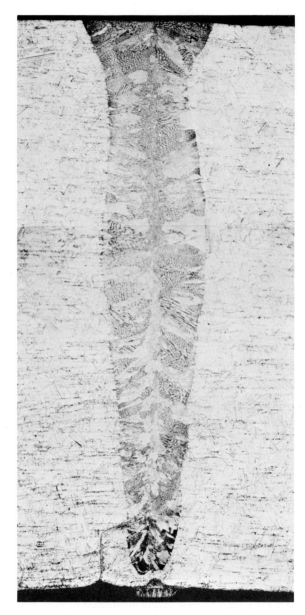

Fig. 3.23.   Metallography of full penetration electron beam weld.

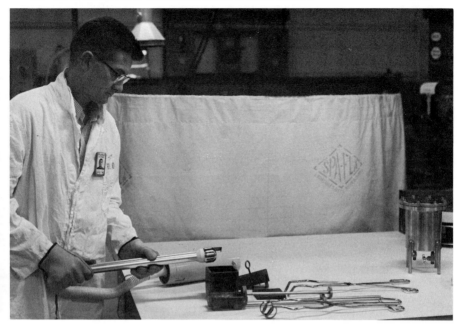

FIG. 3.24.    Handling of fully assembled promethium oxide heat source.

thermally hot for direct contact handling. The vacuum cleaner attachment provided a simple means of handling and also made it possible to withdraw the source from cylindrical containers with ease.

### I.  Quality Control Plan

The details of the quality control plan are outlined in the following sections.

1.  Flow Diagram.    The process flow diagram (Fig. 3.16) shows the stations at which various test are made and the type of test that will be carried out.

Table 3.11 contains a description of tests and illustrates the variety and complexity of test equipment required.

2.  Records of Inspection and Tests.    An inspection or test report is made covering each test or inspection performed. This report contains the following information: (a) type of test; (b) identification of the part tested; (c) time and place of the test; (d) equipment identification; (e) brief description of test method; (f) calibration standards used; (g) results of test or inspection (in case of dimensional inspection, all dimensions

TABLE 3.11

TEST DESCRIPTIONS

| | |
|---|---|
| 1. Radioactive contamination smear test | Wipe capsule with a dry cotton swab and measure the contamination level with a mica window (beta detection) GM counter. Decontamination is effected by wiping with moistened cotton swabs. |
| 2. Helium leak test | Helium leak detector, chamber containing the capsule evacuated to 0.05 torr and held for 30 min, backfilled with helium to 15 psi and held for 5 min; leak detection sensitivity checked before and after capsule leak check. Minimum detectable leak $< 7 \times 10^{-7}$ std cc/sec helium. |
| 3. Dye penetrant test | Zy Glo-Post Emulsifier technique (Magnaflux Corp.); viewed under ultraviolet light. |
| 4. Ultrasonic integrity test | Hanford-developed broad band ultrasonic tester, 15 MH$_z$ Li$_2$SO$_4$ transducer 3/4 in. spherically focused with a mechanical system calibrated to $\pm 0.001$ in. |
| 5. Radiography | GE OX250 X-ray machine; Kodak type M film; viewed under high intensity illumination. |
| 6. Metallography | Four sections per weld; polished and etched. |
| 7. Radiation mapping | CP dose rate meter calibrated with a known source. |
| 8. Gamma spectrometry | 2 in. by 2 in. NaI (Tl) detector with 400 channel analyzer. |
| 9. Calorimetry | Thermal gradient calorimeter with thermopile output having a 223 $\mu$V/W sensitivity at 60 W, electrical heater calibration before and after each measurement. |

measured will be recorded); (h) person or persons performing the test or inspection and signature of the person confirming test.

3. Nonconforming Parts. Parts that do not conform to requirements are held and identified as such. Parts may be repaired and retested or inspected with the program director's approval. Material from rejected parts is salvaged where possible.

4. Process Control. Records of process steps and process variables are kept on each part fabricated. The keeping of the process records is done by the person responsible for the processing step involved.

## J. General Requirements

1. Safety. All established safety rules in handling materials and fabrication equipment are followed. No work of either fabrication, assembly or testing will proceed until all questions regarding any possible unsafe methods or equipment are resolved.

2. Radiation Control. Radiation work procedures are prepared and

approved to cover all steps of the fabrication process and testing where promethium oxide is to be handled. All work involving contamination is done in hoods.

Protective equipment required includes: film badge, self-reading pencils, finger rings, coveralls, shoe covers, and surgeons gloves. Continuous monitoring by a radiation monitor is required. Protective clothing is surveyed periodically and personnel are surveyed when leaving the work zone.

Special instructions and hazards are noted below:

(1) Radiation hazards: Approximately 25 R/hr at surface, 3 R/hr at 2 in., low-energy X-ray and intermediate-energy gamma radiation, gross low-energy beta contamination potential if capsule is ruptured.

(2) Thermal hazard: Pellet as pressed or assembled approximately 370 °C in air.

(3) Special handling tongs must be used during handling to minimize radiation exposure.

(4) Radiation Monitoring will determine dose rate in work positions and tag all areas as well as movement of material.

(5) Hood gloves shall be surveyed frequently during work.

(6) A personnel survey including at least hands and shoe covering shall be completed with a mica-window GM probe when leaving work area.

(7) Any abnormal condition; Radiation Monitoring will specify any changes to these special instructions.

(8) The capsule is to be checked for smearable contamination and is to be <1000 counts/min before transfer between buildings.

(9) While the capsule is in storage or during sintering no special monitoring precautions are necessary under normal conditions.

(10) Responsible personnel are to be in attendance at all times, when pellet or capsule is outside storage container.

(11) Transfer and/or storage container to be designed to effect protection by minimum of 2 in. spacing from surface of bare pellet as well as 0.5 in. lead. Capsule to be placed in this container to minimize thermal retention.

3. Cleanliness, Handling. Cleanliness of parts shall be maintained to the extent that no dust, oil, grease, rust, or other extraneous material on parts are visible to the unaided eye. All work areas will be kept clean and procedures developed to prevent contamination of the promethium sesquioxide with any other material.

All radioactive and nonradioactive parts shall be handled with clean tongs or gloves throughout the process.

4. Storage. In the event that fabrication assembly or testing is delayed, an interim storage place and method will be selected and used in accord with maintaining cleanliness of parts, minimizing hazards from radiological effects, elimination of possible mechanical damage to parts, and oxidation or corrosion from the atmosphere in which storage is made. Identification of all parts will be maintained particularly while in storage.

## ACKNOWLEDGMENTS

While many persons contributed greatly to this effort, special thanks are due to R. K. Robinson, D. W. Brite, N. C. Davis, R. F. Boolen, H. H. Van Tuyl, and H. T. Fullam.

## REFERENCES

1.  Division of Materials Licensing, *How to Get a License to Use Radioisotopes,* Superintendent of Documents, U.S. Government Printing Office, Washington, D.C., 1967.
2.  J.R. Lance and A. Selz, *Isotopes Radiation Technol.,* **7**, 184 (1969).
3.  R. S. Cooper, R. L. Andelin, and R. K. Robinson, *ANS Transactions,* **10**, 453 (Nov. 1967).
4.  U.S. Atomic Energy Commission, *Radioisotopes - Production and Development of Large-Scale Uses,* U.S. AEC Rept. WASH 1095, May 1968, p. 7.
5.  George Y. Jordy, W. J. Lindsey, and J. A. Powers, *Nuclear Metallurgy,* Vol. **14**, Symposium on Materials for Radioisotope Heat Sources, Proceedings of the 1968 Nuclear Metallurgy Symposium held in Gatlinburg, Tenn., Oct. 2-4, 1968, p. 71.
6.  C. A. Rohrmann, *Chart of Characteristics of Radioisotopic Heat Sources,* extension of Table VI, HW-76323, Rev. 1, March 1, 1967, p. 52.
7.  D. E. Deonigi, R. W. McKee, and D. R. Haffner, *Isotope Production and Availability from Power Reactors,* BNWL-716, July 1968.
8.  F. P. Roberts and H. H. Van Tuyl, *Promethium-146, Fission Product, and Transuranium Isotope Content of Power Reactor Fuels—Comprehensive Chemical Analyses,* BNWL-45, March 1965, p.11.
9.  H. T. Fullam and H. H. Van Tuyl, *Promethium Isotopic Power Data Sheets,* BNWL-363, February 1967, p. 2-3.
10. H. J. Schwartz, et al., *Space Power Systems Advanced Technology Conference,* NASA SP-131, Lewis Research Center, Cleveland, Ohio, August 23-24, 1966, p. 74.
11. L. J. Mullins and J. A. Leary, *Isotopes Radiation Technol.* **7**, 197 (1969).
12. J. K. Poggenburg, *Isotopes Radiation Technol.* **7**, 222 (1969).
13. F. T. Cross and J. C. Sheppard, *Isotopes Radiation Technol.* **7**, 231 (1969).
14. W. C. Windley, Jr., *Properties of* $^{60}Co$ *and Cobalt Metal Fuel Forms,* DP-1051 (Rev. 1), Oct. 1966.
15. J. L. Bloom, *Production of Strontium-Titanate Radioisotope Fuel for SNAP-7B Thermoelectric Generator,* MND-P-2977, April 15, 1963, p. 3.

*16.* M. G. Lai, et al., *Radioactivity Release from Radionuclide Power Sources. VIII. Release from Fully Fueled Strontium Titanate and Strontium Oxide to Seawater,* NRDL-TR-68-135, August 23, 1968.

*17.* K. Drumheller, "Properties and Fabrication of Promethium Fuel Forms," same book as Ref., *5*, p. 156.

*18.* C. Berglund, V. L. Hammond, and B. M. Johnson, *The Densification and Encapsulation of Isotopic Fuels by High Energy Pneumatic Impaction - Final Report,* BNWL-381, June 1967, p. 21.

*19.* W. R. Mikelsen, *Basic Design Considerations for Radioisotope Electro-generators,* The Dane Company, Ft. Collins, Colorado. Paper presented at 3rd Intersociety Energy Conversion Engineering Conference, Boulder, Colorado, August 13-16, 1968.

*20.* Report of the Ad Hoc Committee on the Nuclear Space Program, *An Evaluation of Information on the Nuclear Space Systems,* Atomic Industrial Forum, Inc., 850 Third Avenue, New York, New York.

*21.* N. C. Davis and D. W. Brite, *Promethium-147 Radioisotope Application Program AMSA Heat Source Final Report,* BNWL-994, March 1969, p. 32.

*22.* S. McAlees, Jr., "Effects of the Reentry Environment of Radioisotope Heat Sources," same book as Ref. *5,* p. 281.

*23.* M. J. Gaitanis and L. F. Tripp, *Operational Experience at the Quehanna, Penn., Facility: A Two-Megacurie $^{90}Sr$ Conversion and Encapsulation Plant,* Proceedings of 14th Conference on Remote Systems Technology, 1966.

*24.* H. T. Fullam, *Slip Casting of Rare Earth Oxides,* BNWL-437, June 1967.

*25.* H. T. Fullam and L. J. Kirby, *Cold Pressing and Sintering of Rare Earth Oxides,* BNWL-386, April 1967.

*26.* E. J. Wheelwright, et al., *Ion-Exchange Separation of Kilocurie Quantities of High Purity Promethium,* BNWL-318, Dec. 1966.

*27.* E. J. Wheelwright, *J. Phys. Chem.* **73**, 2867 (1969).

*28.* J. Cochran and G. Pierson, *Quehanna Pilot Plant First Generation Process Operations,* MND-3062-22, May 1965.

*29.* J. R. Keski and P. K. Smith, "Properties and Fabrication of Thulium-170 Oxide Targets," same book as Ref. *5,* p. 176.

*30.* S. G. Abrahamson, "Properties and Fabrication of Plutonium Fuel Forms," same book as Ref. *5,* p. 99.

*31.* H. T. Fullam and C. J. Mitchell, *Hot Pressing of Rare Earth Oxides,* BNWL-448, June 1967.

*32.* C. H. Allen, "Radiation Sources for the NASA-Ames Biosatellite Program," same presentation as Ref. *3,* p. 453.

*33.* W. J. Coleman, *Downward Vacuum Vapor Deposition of Rare Earths onto Hollow Microspheres,* BNWL-1288, February 1970.

*34.* W. J. Coleman, *Fail Safe Installation of a Vacuum System for Sputtering Applications in a Glove Box,* BNWL-1287, February 1970.

*35.* C. P. Ross, *Isotopes Radiation Technol.* **5**, 185-194 (1968).

*36.* J. P. Faraci, *Experimental $^{60}Co$ Heat Source Capsules,* DP-1145, May 1968.

*37.* R. F. Boolen, *Magnetic Force Welding Applications at Battelle-Northwest,* BNWL-422, May 1967.

*38.* R. W. Steffens, F. M. Coffman, *Nondestructive Testing of Isotope Containment Capsules: Remote Ultrasonic Test Station UT-40,* BNWL-918, Nov. 1968.

*39.* W. D. Jolly, *An In Situ Weld Defect Detector - Acoustic Emission,* BNWL-817, September 1968.

# 4   DESIGN OF TELETHERAPY UNITS

*ALEXANDER SHEWCHENKO*

ATOMIC ENERGY OF CANADA LIMITED
OTTAWA, ONTARIO, CANADA

## I.   INTRODUCTION

Interest in the use of radiation for the treatment of various human diseases began at the turn of the century, shortly after the discovery of X rays. This interest revolved about radium since it was the first source of energy with a stable output. Although radium was costly and had a low output, advantages were noted in the treatment of cancer by the use of this form of radiation.

Radiotherapy is one of the major forms of cancer treatment. Currently, at least one-half of all cancer patients at some time during the course of their disease have received radiotherapy. The biological response of tissue

*181*

to ionizing radiation is the basis for radiotherapy. Exposed tissue is inflamed; the degree of reaction depends on the dosage of radiation. It has been noted that malignant cells are more sensitive to radiation than normal tissue cells, though this effect may also depend to a large extent on the amount of oxygen present.

To provide good radiotherapy for the treatment of cancer a variety of techniques are used, one of which is teletherapy. The apparatus used for beam therapy is one which directs radiation in the form of a collimated beam to the treatment area, the source of energy being some distance away. There are many sources of energy available for the use of beam therapy; one of the first was radium-226.

After World War I enough radium bromide was accumulated to allow the manufacture of a "radium bomb." This device was a lead-lined brass box, with one end fitted with a conical beam-former. This beam of radiation was applied to the skin for about eight hours, causing some traumatic effects to the skin, but also causing the disappearance of nodules of carcinoma. Unfortunately, the low dose rate and the high cost of radium prevented its popular use.

Before World War II, the requirement for higher outputs led to the design of conventional tube-type therapy machines, in which X rays are produced by the impact of electrons from a hot filament impinging on the anode. Those units operated at 300 kV energy levels, which still did not permit the delivery of effective tumor doses. Units were developed to operate at higher energy levels but proved to have unstable output.

World War II ended and developments resulting from research carried out during the war made possible the production of radiation of considerably higher energy. One of the approaches was the adaptation of electron accelerators for clinical use. An example of such a machine is the linear accelerator. It produces a beam by accelerating electrons in a straight line by a traveling high-frequency radiowave. Generally, these machines have proved costly and required skilled maintenance, allowing only the most affluent hospitals to use such devices.

During the same period development work in nuclear energy made available other radioisotopes besides radium-226 and radon. In the 1950s many people (1–4) realized the potential of radioisotopes emitting gamma rays as sources of supervoltage radiation. Cobalt-60 was quickly selected as the most readily available radioisotope with the required high energy level (12), and possessing attractive production and cost features. The design of cobalt-60 therapy machines began. In Canada during the summer of 1951 two cobalt sources were produced in the NRX reactor in

Chalk River, Ontario. The radiation output of these sources was considerably better than for an equivalent amount of radium. For the first time it was feasible to use a reactor-produced radioisotope that had the advantage of emulating the characteristics of a generating supervoltage machine. The initial cobalt units were similar in design to the old teleradium units.

In view of their importance and the wide-spread use of collimated radiation sources this chapter will discuss the design of cobalt-60 teletherapy systems and machines.

## II. DEFINITION OF TERMS

There are many terms which are peculiar to radiotherapy. Most of them will be used throughout the chapter to describe the characteristics of the cobalt teletherapy machines or will be found in references on the subject. A brief description of the more common terms is given. Additional definitions will be found in Appendix A at the end of the book.

*Source-to-Skin Distance (SSD):* The source-to-skin distance refers to the distance from the leading surface of the isotopic source of radiation to the point of entry of the beam at the patient's skin. For diagnostic roentgen-ray machines and other ray-emitting machines the terms FSD or TSD for *focal* and *target skin distance,* respectively, are used.

*Exposure:* Exposure, the measurement of radiation output from a teletherapy unit at a specified distance, with given collimation; exposure is expressed in *roentgens* (R).

*Teletherapy:* The form of radiation treatment in which an external beam of radiation is directed toward the tumor site in the body.

*Rad:* An energy absorption of 100 ergs per gram of absorber material is defined as 1 *rad,* which is the unit of absorbed dose.

*Integral Dose:* The total energy absorbed from radiation beams by the patient. The unit of integral absorbed dose is the *gram-rad.*

*Gram-Rad:* The amount of energy absorbed in 1 gram of material by the absorption of 1 rad.

*Given Dose:* The *given dose* is the absorbed dose at the maximum point at the beam axis. All therapy prescriptions are usually written in *rads* of absorbed dose.

*Isodose Curves:* Lines of equal absorbed dose within a patient or tissue-equivalent medium (usually water). These are normally presented as a group of curves for a certain field size in the form of an isodose chart.

*Penumbra:* Penumbra is the radiation field outside the design area of the full beam. It arises from scattering of the radiation at the collimator walls and in the target material; the ideal would be a point source requiring no collimation. In common usage the radiation outside the beam from all causes is usually called *penumbra*.

*Field Size:*   The area covered by the beam of radiation. Because of the finite size of the source, the effect of penumbra can make definition of the field size ambiguous. When field sizes are quoted, it is necessary to define them. Usually the field as determined by the 50% geometrical penumbra line is used.

*Half Value Layer (HVL):*   The thickness of any material which reduces the intensity of a narrow beam of radiation at a given energy by a factor of two.

### III.   COMPARISON OF SUPERVOLTAGE AND COBALT TELETHERAPY MACHINES

The use of cobalt-60 as a source of supervoltage radiation has proved to be reliable and inexpensive. As a source of high energy it has replaced in many cases the earlier X-ray machines (5) and competes with electrical high-energy machines. Table 4.1 lists a few of the high-energy devices.

The use of cobalt-60 is normally associated with the treatment of deepseated lesions (6). Treatment plans using X rays ranging from 2 to 35 MV or gamma rays from cobalt-60 are similar, the major objective being the delivery of an adequate cancerocidal dose of sufficient uniformity to the lesion. Some clinicians have felt that energies of 10 to 25 MeV offer some advantages in special situations but this has not been the rule. Although cobalt-60 gamma rays give an equivalent of a monochromatic gamma ray of 1.25 MeV, in actual treatment use the characteristics of the radiation are equivalent to those produced by a 2–3 MV machine. The production of energies greater than 30 MeV is possible with an X-ray generator such as a linear accelerator; however, there appears to be no significant therapeutic advantage. In fact the lower linear energy transfer (LET) rates at very high energy make it difficult to obtain good localization of exposure. Therefore, the only real factors for comparison of an isotope machine and an X-ray generator in the 3-MeV range are: reliability, ease of maintenance, capital cost, and operating cost.

An economic evaluation of such equipment with respect to a complete treatment facility has been made in a joint meeting of the International Atomic Energy Agency and the World Health Organization. The report of this meeting has been published as World Health Organization Technical

TABLE 4.1

HIGH ENERGY MACHINES

| | Source of energy | Remarks |
| --- | --- | --- |
| 200-400 kV X-ray machine | Conventional X-ray tube, high-energy electrons strike tungsten anode producing X-rays | Inferior treatment to that capable by supervoltage equipment. Skin reaction and small depth dose. Maintenance problems in hot and humid climates. |
| Resonance generator | High voltage obtained using a circuit tuned to its own capacity and inductance. | Energies of up to 2 MeV possible. Machines generally reliable but are very large, especially machines that operate at the 2 MeV level. |
| Van de Graaff generator | A high voltage is maintained by conveying charged particles from ground potential to high voltage terminal with a moving insulating belt. | Energies of up to 2–4 MeV possible. These machines are generally large. To maintain operation skilled maintenance is required. |
| Betatron | Electrons are accelerated in orbit by a changing magnetic field. The electron is kept in orbit by increasing magnetic field. | Energies of 15 to 30 MeV possible. High outputs are also possible. These machines are very expensive and require skilled maintenance and are therefore used in large centers only. |
| Linear accelerator | Electrons are accelerated in a straight line by a traveling high-frequency radiowave. | Machines with energies of 4 to 30 MeV are produced. These machines are generally expensive, requiring skilled servicing. |
| Cobalt-60 machine | Cobalt-60 used as source of gamma rays. | Units generally simple, do not require complex electronics. Capable of producing same results as higher energy machines. |

Report Series No. 328 *(7)*. This comparison is of supervoltage machines for the treatment of deep-seated lesions. The machines compared were cobalt-60 teletherapy units, resonant transformers, Van de Graaff generators, linear accelerators and betatrons. (See Fig. 4.1 for distribution of different machines in the world.)

It is generally acknowledged that the two most reliable sources of supervoltage radiation are the resonant transformer and the cobalt-60 teletherapy unit. Both have been known to operate for almost a decade without major overhaul. The other machines listed require a program of preventive maintenance and the services of a highly qualified maintenance

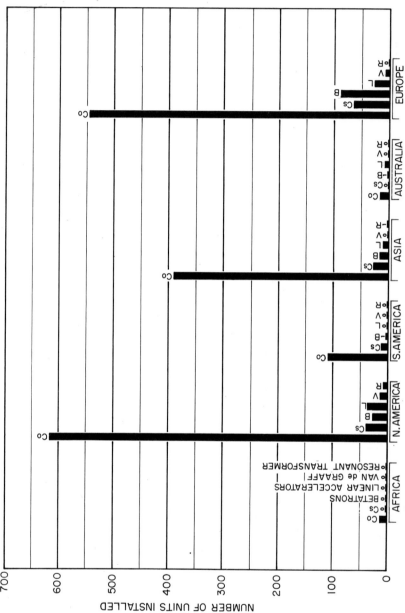

FIG. 4.1.   Distribution of various high-energy teletherapy equipment by continent (1968).

technician. This is an important consideration, since reliability is a chief factor in the installation of radiotherapy facilities, particularly in the developing nations, where trained technicians are expensive and scarce. The report claims that a vertically mounted cobalt-60 unit is easier to maintain than a rotational one. With a large variety of reliable electrical and mechanical components available any differences in the difficulty of maintenance can be virtually eliminated.

The most telling comparison is therefore in the economics of operating such equipment in a clinic. Table 4.2 is an analysis of the economics of operation of various supervoltage equipment types. The following assumptions have been made:

(1)   All units are operated under conditions of full use during a treatment day.
(2)   Same or comparable source-surface distances used.
(3)   Constant set-up time of 10 min.
(4)   200 rad tumor dose at 10 cm.
(5)   Cost of operating personnel excluded, due to the large variations in different parts of the world.

It is evident from Table 4.2 that the capital costs and cost per patient with the cobalt therapy unit are greatly superior to that for comparable high-voltage machines. Until the cost of electronic equipment is substantially reduced and the reliability of operation improved, this will be unchanged.

## IV.   COBALT TELETHERAPY SOURCE

The radioactive isotope commonly used for supervoltage radiation therapy is cobalt-60. It is readily produced by the neutron irradiation of cobalt-59 in an atomic reactor. The maximum theoretical specific activity of cobalt-60 is approximately 1200 Ci/g. The time needed to produce cobalt to a specific activity depends on the thermal flux and irradiation efficiency. The thermal flux is usually set by the reactor design and the cobalt loading positions available. The irradiation efficiency depends on the target thickness, day to day variation in the flux due to material in adjacent reactor positions, impurities in the target, and unscheduled variation in the reactor power levels. For teletherapy cobalt, the irradiation time varies from one to three years. When saturation level is reached the rate of production of cobalt-60 is balanced by its decay and burn-up rate of the target. Acceptable specific activities range from 100 to 300 Ci/g

TABLE 4.2

ECONOMICS OF SUPERVOLTAGE EQUIPMENT FOR RADIATION THERAPY (FROM REF. 7)

| | Cobalt-60 unit[a] | | | | 2-MV Van de Graaff machine | 2-MV resonant transformer machine | 6-MV linear accelerator | 25-MV betatron |
|---|---|---|---|---|---|---|---|---|
| | A | B | C | D | | | | |
| *Physical factors* | | | | | | | | |
| Radiation output[b] (R/min at 100 cm) | 64.6 | 38.7 | 132[c] | 57[d] | 85 | 108 | 200 | 54 |
| 10-cm depth dose (%) | 58 | 58 | 54 | 56 | 57 | 57 | 67 | 84 |
| 10-cm dose rate | 37.4 | 22.3 | 71.4 | 31.9 | 48.4 | 61.6 | 134 | 45.5 |
| Time to reach 200 R (minutes) | 5.4 | 8.9 | 2.8 | 6.3 | 4.1 | 3.2 | 1.5 | 4.4 |
| Time needed for set-up (minutes) | 10 | 10 | 10 | 10 | 10 | 10 | 10 | 10 |
| Duration of treatment session (minutes) | 15.4 | 18.9 | 12.8 | 16.3 | 14.1 | 13.2 | 11.5 | 14.4 |
| Treatments per year[e] | 8,140 | 6,610 | 9,800 | 7,680 | 8,730 | 9,430 | 10,850 | 8,680 |
| *Capital costs ($)* | | | | | | | | |
| Equipment | 20,000 | 20,000 | 32,000 | 20,000 | 56,000 | 120,000 | 150,000 | 131,000 |
| Source | 32,000 | 17,500 | 32,000 | 15,300 | — | — | — | — |
| Therapy room[f] | 19,200 | 19,200 | 19,200 | 19,200 | 24,000 | 42,000 | 19,200 | 29,000[g] |
| Total | 71,200 | 56,700 | 83,200 | 54,500 | 80,000 | 162,000 | 169,200 | 160,000 |
| *Annual costs ($)* | | | | | | | | |
| Amortization[h] | | | | | | | | |
| Equipment 10% | 2,000 | 2,000 | 3,200 | 2,000 | 5,600 | 12,000 | 15,000 | 13,100 |
| Building 5% | 960 | 960 | 960 | 960 | 1,200 | 2,100 | 960 | 1,450 |
| Source 25% | 8,000 | 4,375 | 8,000 | 3,060[i] | — | — | — | — |
| Interest 5% | 3,560 | 2,835 | 4,160 | 2,725 | 4,000 | 8,000 | 8,460 | 8,000 |

*Maintenance*

| | | | | | | | | |
|---|---|---|---|---|---|---|---|---|
| Parts and service | 500 | 500 | 1,000[j] | 500 | 5,900[k] | 4,500[l] | 4,000[m] | 7,000[n] |
| Exchange of source[o] | 350 | 350 | 0 | 280[i] | 0 | 0 | 0 | 0 |
| Hospital personnel[p] | 0 | 0 | 0 | 0 | 1,000 | 0 | 1,000 | 1,000 |
| Total | 15,370 | 11,020 | 17,670 | 9,525 | 17,700 | 26,600 | 29,420 | 30,550 |
| Cost per treatment ($) | 1.89 | 1.82 | 1.80 | 1.24 | 2.02 | 2.82 | 2.71 | 3.52 |

[a] The four units have the following characteristics:
 A = 5000 Ci 2-cm source with vertical support 100 cm SSD
 B = 3000 Ci 2-cm source with vertical support 100 cm SSD
 C = 5000 Ci 2-cm source with rotational support 80 cm SAD
 D = 3000 Ci 2.5-cm source with vertical support 80 cm SSD
(NOTE: In commercial practice, the output of a teletherapy source is frequently stated in "Rhm," i.e., in R/hr of a distance of 1 meter, As a rough approximation, 1 Ci of cobalt-60 is equivalent to 1 "Rhm.")

[b] For the cobalt sources the mean exposure rate over a 4-year life is quoted (77.5% of initial rate).

[c] Mean exposure rate at 70 cm SSD (80 cm SAD).

[d] Mean exposure rate at 80 cm SSD over a 5-year life (73% of initial rate).

[e] 1 year is 52 weeks at 40 hr per week.

[f] Building costs at $5 per cubic foot of space.

[g] Includes room for power supplies.

[h] Amortization over 10 years for equipment, 20 years for building and 4 years for cobalt-60 sources.

[i] 5-year life in this case.

[j] Inquiries show more maintenance problems with rotational teletherapy units.

[k] 60% of tube life at $6500 per tube+$2000 for service from manufacturer.

[l] $4000 for tube pro rata (assuming 2000-hr life) plus $500 for other maintenance.

[m] 300 hours at $10 per hour for component life+$1000 for service from manufacturer.

[n] $6000 for cost of 1 "doughnut" per year (600-hr life) plus $1000 for other components and service.

[o] Net cost after credit for old source deducted.

[p] No maintenance personnel is assumed for cobalt-60 and resonant transformer equipment; 10% of the time of a maintenance engineer with $10,000 per year salary is assumed for other equipment.

using a flux of approximately $10^{14}$ neutrons per cm² per second. With a much higher flux specific activities up to 800 Ci/g have been obtained.

The target material is prepared by fabricating cobalt metal into various shapes. The common shapes are wafers, slugs, and pellets. Nickel-plated, 1-mm long by 1-mm diameter pellets are most commonly used in the preparation of teletherapy sources of various source diameters. Plating before irradiation prevents cobalt oxidation, reducing contamination during hot-cell handling. The pellets are sealed in a stainless steel welded capsule. This capsule is then decontaminated and sealed into a second stainless steel welded capsule. Once again it is decontaminated to levels specified by the government licensing authorities. Some teletherapy machines use an International Source Container to hold the doubly encapsulated cobalt (Fig. 4.2.) The active source diameters range from 0.5 to 3.0 cm. Because of the large physical size of the International Source Container, which requires a very large source shielding mechanism, most teletherapy units are directly loaded with the doubly encapsulated capsule.

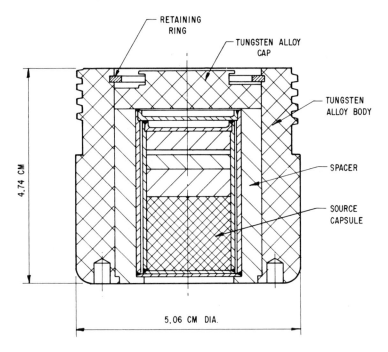

FIG. 4.2.  International source container modified for beam therapy capsule.

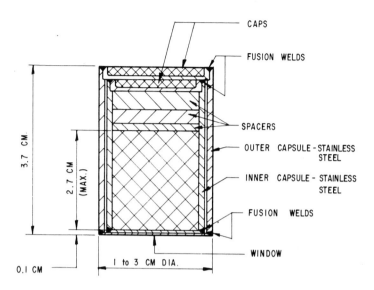

FIG. 4.3.   Typical teletherapy source capsule.

The encapsulation of the cobalt pellets is an art which has been developed over the years by suppliers of sources. The sealing of the source material requires great care to avoid surface contamination due to radioactive particles. The therapy source capsule (Fig. 4.3) must be capable of withstanding mechanical and thermal stresses, pressure, and chemical attack without loss of its integrity. To allow radiation beams to penetrate efficiently through the capsule, the window end is constructed from a very thin stainless steel disc. This window absorbs only 2% of the radiation beam without effect on the spectrum of the beam.

The requirements for maintaining the integrity of the source capsule have been established empirically over the years by source manufacturers. In an attempt to identify these requirements the American National Standards Institute has published standards (see Ref. *16*). The ISO is presently working on a similar document.

Commercially, cobalt sources are specified and sold by output. This is described in terms of *Rmm* (roentgens per minute at one meter). This is essential because the radiotherapist determines the efficacy of treatment by the exposure rate. The source output is dependent on several factors, such as source diameter, specific activity, collimation and other contributors of scatter radiation. The activity of the source may be determined by calculation or measurement.

To determine approximately the output in Rmm, the following equation is a useful approximation:

$$I = KC \frac{(1 - e^{-\mu h})}{\mu h} \qquad (4.1)$$

where $I$ = source output in Rmm, $h$ = source material height; $\mu$ = linear absorption coefficient = 0.245 cm$^{-1}$, $K$ = dose conversion constant, which is 0.022400 Rmm per curie for cobalt-60; $C$ = activity, in curies, of the source, and is determined as follows:

$$C = s\pi D^2 k P$$

where $s$ = specific activity in curies per gram; $k$ = 4.4375; $D$ = source material diameter in centimeters; $P$ = packing density for pellet source = 5.4 g/cm$^3$. This equation is based on actual measurements, and the value of 0.0435 cm$^2$/g is selected as the mass absorption coefficient. No attempt has been made to correlate the output with an actual teletherapy unit. In fact the output of the source in a teletherapy unit will vary for each different combination of source shield and collimator configuration. The actual exposure rate for a specific source must be measured in the therapy machine itself if the source output data are to be used for calculation of treatment dose (8, 10).

There are difficulties in actual measurement or calculation of the source output. In the calculative method the activity of the cobalt source is based on neutron flux in the reactor, the activation cross section of the cobalt, the half-life of cobalt-60 and the duration of the activation. Measurement is at best a comparative process. Because of the difficulty in establishing a value for the self-absorption coefficient, it is difficult to determine the actual amount of activity by measurement. This is probably the other consideration which helped influence the choice of exposure rate as a measure of source output.

Further corrections can be made to Eq. (4.1) to obtain a closer relationship to the actual exposure rate. Allow 2% absorption through the end of the capsule and increase the output 7% to allow for the scatter coefficient of the collimator. Again, the designer should be cautioned that calculating the source output should be used only as a guide to determine the source size for a set of conditions. The final exposure rate must be determined by measurement.

In the design of a cobalt teletherapy unit the configuration of the source has much influence. It not only reflects the economics of the unit but it also influences the basic design of the machine, especially the collimation system.

The cost of a source depends on the combined effect of the following: source diameter, source height, and source material specific activity.

Because of reactor time required for production, the cost per gram of cobalt-60 increases with an increase in specific activity. Figure 4.4 shows a

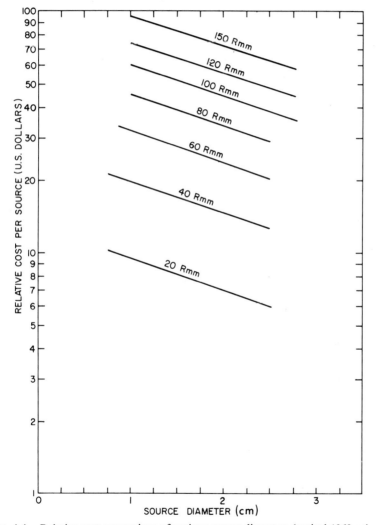

FIG. 4.4.   Relative cost comparison of various source diameters (typical 1968 prices).

typical cost relationship for different outputs and source sizes. As long as the source height is constant, the cost increase is solely a function of the specific activity. Note that all the curves have essentially the same slope.

## V.  COBALT-60 RADIATION TELETHERAPY SYSTEMS

### A.  Introduction

The tool of the radiotherapist is the radiation beam. The major objective of a teletherapy machine is to aim and collimate the beam of radiation so that it can give a lethal dose to the tumor and spare the surrounding healthy tissue. This objective cannot be achieved solely by machine, but is a combination of many skills and machine capabilities. The teletherapy unit is the supporting structure for the source of radiation. During the early 1950s much time was spent on evolving different treatment techniques to achieve better treatment results. The optimum is to produce an even distribution of absorbed energy within the tumor area while producing no energy absorption in the uninvolved tissue surrounding this volume. The radiotherapist, after examination of the patient, estimates the extent of the tumor, making allowance for tumor spread as his experience dictates. He then prescribes a dose of radiation which may have to be delivered over a period of weeks.

As previously indicated there are important advantages in the use of cobalt-60 for a teletherapy machine. The constancy of output and the lack of complex electrical and electronic circuits in the machine provide a reliable therapy system. The selection of a source for a teletherapy machine is dependent on many requirements, such as useful life, energy required, beam penetration, dose rate, source cost. To best determine the cobalt-60 source characteristics, the interaction of the above requirements should be balanced so that the desired treatment system is achieved economically.

### B.  Radiotherapy Treatment System

The design criteria for a teletherapy unit will be discussed within the narrow framework of providing a suitable structure for positioning the beam of radiation emanating from the cobalt source, providing good beam quality, and securing the patient so that he will be accurately positioned to receive the radiation in the correct exposure patterns. The treatment of cancer by radiation depends on many factors. There must be an accurate definition of the treatment area, based upon careful analysis of the patient's tumor, an appreciation of its mode of spread and of its natural history.

The current technique is to treat the tumor area so that the distribution of energy assures that the tumor receives maximum irradiation with the minimum of energy absorbed in the normal surrounding tissue. The treatment plan must be reproduced precisely for each treatment session. To better understand the needs of treatment by cobalt-60 it is important to understand how a typical treatment is processed.

A treatment system can be broken down into four stages: (1) diagnosis, (2) treatment preparation, (3) treatment, and (4) treatment summary.

Referring to Fig. 4.5, a brief description of each stage and its requirements follows:

*Stage 1—Diagnosis:*  Although there is no requirement for therapy equipment at this stage, this is a very important event in the life of a patient. It is at this point that the nature of the illness is determined. Many hospital resources, such as diagnostic X ray and pathology, are brought into play. The accurate determination of the spread of the cancer, its type and the stage of its development will help to establish the type of treatment.

*Stage 2—Treatment Preparation:*  Once the decision has been made that the treatment is to be by radiation, the radiologist requires a treatment plan. This plan is based on past experience and accurate calculation by the hospital physicist of the dose distribution at the treatment site. The techniques and methods of treatment planning are described in more detail in the references on teletherapy *(8-10)*. The primary function is the location and the determination of the tumor volume in relation to the skin surface through which the radiation beam is to be directed. After a suitable plan is devised, the treatment beams must be properly positioned and identified so that their location can be accurately reproduced for each treatment day. There are many methods used to locate the beam accurately during a course of treatments; some of the methods use special beam positioning accessories *(8, 9)*. Other localization methods employ diagnostic X-ray techniques *(10)*. The ideal system would incorporate treatment and tumor localization with computer techniques used to feed the proper information to the teletherapy unit for the set-up of beam direction and exposure rate. Provision for recording the treatment technique, dose, and other pertinent treatment data would be made.

*Stage 3—Treatment:*  In the actual treatment of the patient it is

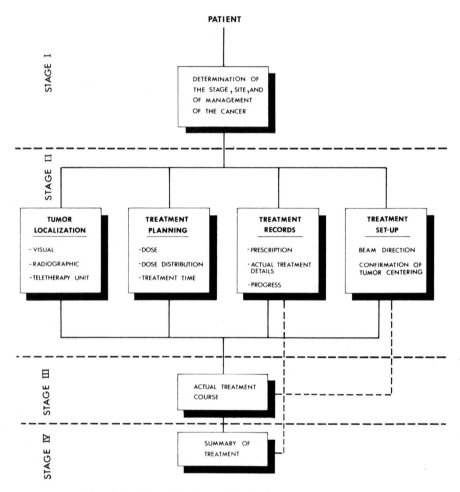

FIG. 4.5.  Schematic diagram of a typical treatment system.

necessary to position him so that the spatial relationships of the patient and the therapy unit are set accurately. Present techniques rely upon mechanical or optical beam positioning devices which are used by the technician to assist in placing the patient into the treatment position. This means that the treating machine is set up manually from the prescription; at best the data are subject to interpretation by the technician. Therefore to assure good therapy the technician must be highly skilled or closely supervised by the radiotherapist.

Any change in location of the patient or of the skin-to-tumor distance will vary the dose absorbed by the target volume. Methods used to maintain beam-to-patient relationship are mechanical immobilization of the patient by the use of straps or the preparation of cast moulds for each patient. Other methods currently being developed use skin marks on the patient as points of reference. Because of the possible change of the patient's physical characteristics, the use of skin marks may require checks during the course of treatment. The relocation of the beam entry positions during a set of treatments is not uncommon *(14)*.

*Stage 4—Treatment Summary:* This is the stage where the data are compiled and made available from use to change treatment or for analysis so that the method of therapy can be used for similar future cases. It is at this point that the storage of this information in a computer can be used to advantage.

## C. Dose Rate

The radiotherapist is interested in the absorbed dose, for it is the measure of his prescription. The increment of the dose obtained over a unit of time is the dose rate. It is usually defined in *rads per minute*. As the biological conditions in the area treated are different in each treatment situation, it has been found better to identify changes in the dose rate by using the exposure rate of the source as a criterion. For this, the unit usually used is *Rmm* (roentgens per minute at one meter).

There are two methods of increasing dose rate; first increasing the source strength, and second, bringing the source closer to the treatment area.

**Illustrative Example 1**

Consider a $^{60}$Co source of 50-Rmm output, treatment dose to be 300 R. What will the treatment time be for the following units:

Unit A — the source located so that the SSD (source-to-skin distance) is 50 cm?

Unit B — the source located so that the SSD is 100 cm? The output is determined by the application of the inverse square law as follows:

$(\text{Exposure rate})_{\text{skin}} = (\text{source exposure rate})_{\text{Rmm}} \times (100/\text{SSD})^2$

Therefore, exposure rates are:

Unit A $= 50 \times (100/50)^2 = 200$ R/min at 50 cm

Unit B $= 50 \times (100/100)^2 = 50$ R/min at 100 cm

The treatment times are:

Unit A $= 300/200 = 1.5$ min

Unit B $= 300/50 = 6$ min

A reduction in the source-to-skin distance will result in shorter treatment time, but there are other factors to be considered such as minimum clearance between the unit and the treatment area. The implication is that a reduction in distance may affect the depth dose, which may be altered unfavorably, thereby diminishing the beneficial effect of gamma radiation. For example, $^{60}$Co teletherapy units designed for source-to-skin distances of 75 to 100 cm give better depth dose distribution, i.e., the point of maximum dose is further below the skin surface. This allows larger dosages to a deep seated tumor without adverse effects to overlying tissue. Use of a teletherapy unit with shorter SSD cannot be discounted; in the treatment of superficially located tumors the point of maximum dose will be closer to the skin surface, thereby allowing a greater dose to be administered to the superficial lesion *(14)*.

A further consideration in the economical operation of a large therapy clinic could favor the use of two separate isotope therapy units in conjunction with one source. The unit with the greater SSD would be fitted with a higher-output source. After the source has decayed for one to two years it could be put to useful service in a unit with a shorter SSD, thereby extending the useful life of the source.

**Illustrative Example 2**

Consider two units, (A) 80-cm SSD (B) 55-cm SSD. Unit A would be initially loaded with a cobalt–60 source having an output of 100 Rmm. After one half-life this source would have an output of 50 Rmm. At this time the source would be placed in Unit B. What is the output of the source in Unit A initially, and its output in Unit B after it has decayed one half-life?

Initial output in Unit A is:

$100 \times (100/80)^2 = 156.3$ R/min at 80 cm

After one half-life, the source now located in Unit B would have an output of:

$50 \times (100/55)^2 = 165.4$ R/min at 55 cm.

## D.   Treatment Set-up Time

An economical study of required sources cannot be made without considering the patient set-up time. As dose rates in excess of 100 rad/min are becoming more common with the use of higher specific activity cobalt in teletherapy sources, the set-up time becomes increasingly important. The number of patients treated per day will be limited by the extra time needed for setting up each patient.

**Illustrative Example 3**

If it is assumed that each patient receives an average dose of 200 rads (it can be assumed that the exposure of 1 R is equivalent to 1 rad absorbed dose) what will be the number of patients treated in a seven-hour work day for the following conditions?

(1)   10 min set-up time and exposure rate of 50 R/min

(2)   10 min set-up time and exposure rate of 150 R/min

 (3) 5 min set-up time and exposure rate of 150 R/min

 (4) 3 min set-up time and exposure rate of 150 R/min.

A plot of the number of patients treated per day versus exposure rate has been prepared (see Fig. 4.6). The data of Fig. 4.6 indicate that for:

 (1) number of patients treated is 30 per day

 (2) number of patients treated is 40 per day

 (3) number of patients treated is 69 per day

 (4) number of patients treated is 102 per day

The above example has illustrated that to increase the number of patients treated each day from 30 to 40 by using a source of a higher output requires three times the increase in source strength. At the current prices of cobalt-60 sources this would be a fourfold increase in source cost to treat 10 more patients each day; however, if the set-up time is decreased the patient throughput per unit can be increased greatly. The example illustrates this point. The same source was used in part (2) and part (4); however, treatment set-up time has been decreased from 10 to 3 min resulting in an increase of the number of patients treated from 40 to 102. This emphasizes the need to consider the design of a teletherapy machine not just as a mechanical design problem but as the design of a treatment

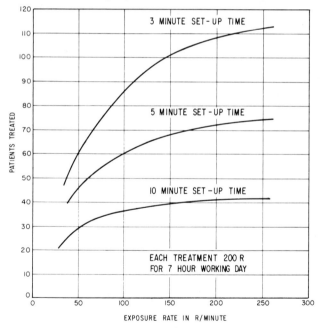

FIG. 4.6. Effect of set-up time on patient throughput for a range of exposure rates.

system for which the major objective is to simplify setting-up procedure. Time saved represents a saving so that the decaying source is utilized
more efficiently. There is, of course, an optimum time limit where the
benefits of systems engineering are lost because accurate alignment will
be unobtainable and the personal contact important in the treatment of
seriously ill patients will be lost.

### E. Penumbra

Although the gamma-ray beam is fairly well collimated by the source
capsule and directional shielding, a certain fraction of the radiation will
still be scattered out of the beam by the collimator sleeve or will penetrate
the shield, though at a highly attenuated level. This stray radiation will
impinge on the areas surrounding the target area delineated by the beam
geometry. This penumbra, the irradiated region outside the treatment
field, is of prime clinical importance. The amount of penumbral radiation
will determine the design of the collimation system and cost of the source.
Total penumbra is due to the combined effect of several components,
namely: the geometrical effect due to source diameter, transmission penumbra through the collimator shield, and scatter from the collimator.

Once a given degree of permitted tolerance can be established with the
radiotherapist, an analysis of source cost can be made. To simplify this
analysis the effect of geometrical penumbra only will be considered. Ellis
*(17)* established a numerical criterion for this. He called it the *area efficiency factor.* It is defined as the ratio of the useful dose over the area of
cross section of the beam to the total integral dose, including the penumbra. Referring to Fig. 4.3.

$$A = U/W \tag{4.2}$$

where $A$ is the area efficiency factor, $U$ is the useful integral area dose,
ignoring dose due to penumbra, $U = xy$ is the nominal dose area, and
$W = 2p(x + y) + xy$ is the total effective dose area.

It should be noted that the corner penumbral areas $(4p^2)$ are assumed
to be negligible compared with $U$.

**Illustrative Example 4**
Determine the value on the area efficiency factor for the following units:
Unit A        80-cm source-to-skin distance (SSD)
              (a)   65-cm source to definer distance (SDD)
              (b)   45-cm SDD
Unit B        60-cm SSD
              (a)   45-cm SDD
              (b)   27.6-cm SDD

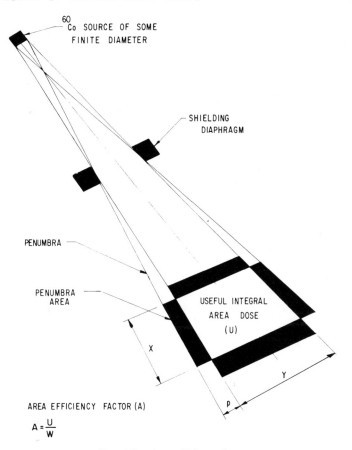

FIG. 4.7.   Area efficiency factor.

Unit C      75-cm SSD
            27-cm SDD

A plot is prepared (see Fig. 4.8), using geometrical penumbra values from Eq. (4.2) shown in the collimator design section for each unit. This plot indicates that for all conditions depicted by the examples a reduction in source diameter will increase the area efficiency factor, However, as will be shown later, a premium must be paid for small source diameters. It is obvious that the closer the defining edge of the diaphragm is to the skin the greater the area efficiency factor becomes. In the case of Unit A it is seen from Fig. 4.8 that the efficiency has increased from about 20 to 48 % by bringing the defining edge 20 cm closer to the skin.

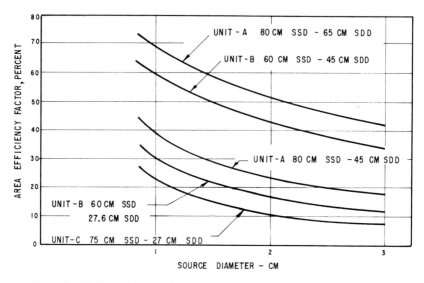

FIG. 4.8.  Variation of area efficiency factor for various source diameters and geometries.

There are limitations to bringing the defining edge close to the skin; the major problem is the dose build-up at the skin surface caused by electron scatter off the definer. For protection of the skin from excessive exposure, the collimator's defining edge must be at least 15 cm away from the skin. Before a small diameter source is selected at great expense, the collimator or diaphragm design of the unit must be carefully considered to assure that it provides the maximum efficiency possible.

## VI.  COBALT-60 TELETHERAPY UNIT DESIGN

### A.  Description of a Teletherapy Unit

A teletherapy unit is a machine which is capable of positioning and aiming a beam of radiation emitted from a source, such as an isotope like cobalt-60 or an X-ray tube. As previously discussed this beam of radiation is used to treat human cancer by directing a cancerocidal dose of radiation to the tumor while sparing healthy tissue.

The therapy unit itself may be broken down into five functional parts:

The *radiation source* which emits the necessary beam of radiation. The nature of the source has already been discussed in Section IV.4. To protect the operators and other people in the area from harmful radiation the source must be stored safely when it is not in use. The *source housing,* which consists of lead or some other heavy metal used as a shield, provides this protection. Some means must be provided to expose and interrupt the beam of radiation to treat a patient or to safely conceal the source; this is achieved by the *source exposure mechanism.*

The beam of radiation emitted by a source must be defined so that the cross section of the useful beam is properly shaped to fit the treatment volume without spurious radiation. The *collimator system* must limit the beam cross section both in area and in shape providing a sharply defined beam to achieve the above requirements. Since the combination of the functional parts may result in a machine of large proportions and great weight, special attention must be given to the *support structure;* it determines the manner in which the beam of radiation can be employed.

The accuracy and flexibility of the treatment set-up is determined by the support structure. If a cobalt-60 teletherapy machine is to be properly considered as part of a treatment system, the location of the patient must be achieved easily with maximum patient comfort; therefore, thought must be given to the design of a *patient positioning device.* This can be in the form of a simple stretcher, or a specially developed unit integral with the therapy machine, depending on the flexibility desired.

## B. Source Housing

**1. Introduction.** The function of the source housing is to provide adequate shielding around the source so that personnel are protected from radiation during the patient set-up period. To ensure that operating personnel do not receive more than the maximum permissible levels of radiation, many nations have prepared standards which must be adhered to before permission to use the therapy machine is obtained. Most of these national regulations have been based on the recommendations of the International Commission on Radiological Protection (ICRP) *(18).*

To provide protection from radiation exposure inadvertently caused by accident, the design of the source housing should provide for the possibility of fire or other hazards.

**2. Structural Design of the Source Housing.** The design currently adopted by most manufacturers of cobalt-60 therapy machines is a welded construction or cast steel container filled with lead. To decrease the overall size of the housing, tungsten or depleted uranium are used as part of the shielding.

The source housing should be constructed so that the integrity of the shield is preserved in a fire. With the variety of the shielding materials available there can be different approaches to the solution of this problem. In the case of a lead shield it would be recommended that a steel housing be used. There should not be any structural weakness in the housing which could allow molten lead to escape. To relieve the high stresses which could result in a fire of the intensity to melt the lead, a void to allow the expansion of the lead should be designed into the housing. A void of about 10% of the shield volume would be adequate. The use of depleted uranium as a shield presents a unique problem in that the uranium metal possesses adequate structural strength; however, its rate of oxidization will rapidly increase in the heat of a major fire, diminishing the radiation protection. A steel jacket around the uranium shield would probably provide adequate protection in the event of a serious fire.

An alternative solution would be the use of a uranium alloy which would be more corrosion resistant. An alloy such as one containing 2 to 8% of molybdenum is currently available from suppliers of depleted uranium. (This is the uranium left over after the extraction of [235]U in the enrichment process, or it can be extracted from spent reactor fuel rods.)

**3. Selection of Shielding Material.** To provide protection from the radiation source, it is generally required that the housing be constructed so that the exposure rates at 1 m from the source in any direction do not exceed a maximum of 10 mR/hr nor the average of 2 mR/hr. To assure that an adequate shield is provided it is best to calculate the shielding thickness using the exposure rate of 2 mR/hr at one meter. It should be noted that certain national authorities further stipulate that the radiation levels at 5 cm from the outer surface of the housing do not exceed 10 times the values previously stated (19). When a heavy metal material such as depleted uranium is contemplated for use as the sole shielding medium, care must be taken to consider the exposure rates.

The calculation of the thickness of shielding material involves the physical processes which occur when a beam of radiation interacts with the shielding material. To adequately cover all the processes, any calculations made to determine the shielding thickness must consider broad-beam geometry. Apart from attenuation due to scatter and absorption, a beam of radiation diminishes in intensity proportional to the inverse square of the distance from the source. Assuming a point source the following equation provides the first approximation to design a source housing:

$$I_i = I_o \, B \, e^{-\mu x} \, (d_o/d_i)^2 \qquad (4.3)$$

where $I_i$ is the intensity at the point of measurement, which is usually

1m from the center of the source, or in the case of surface radiation the shield thickness plus 5 cm; $I_o$ is the initial intensity of radiation in the absence of a shield expressed in Rmm. $B$ is the build-up factor, the ratio of the measured gamma-ray flux to that which would be calculated using a simple exponential attenuation (for values, refer to references); $d_o$ is the distance to the point of measurement of $I_o$ (1m); $d_i$ is the distance from the source to the point of measurement of $I_i$; $\mu$ is the linear absorption coefficient (see Table 1.7 for typical values).

**4.  Composite Shields.**  Optimization of the source shield may favor the combined use of several materials. A very successful combination is the use of a heavy metal, such as tungsten or depleted uranium near the source. Lead is then used to bring the shield up to requirements of protection. To determine approximately the amount of shielding materials required, Eq. (4.3) becomes

$$I_i = (d_o/d_i)^2 \; B_t \; e^{-(\mu_1 \, x_1 \, + \, \mu_2 \, x_2)} \qquad (4.4)$$

for two materials, where:

$$B_t = \frac{B_1 \, \mu_1 \, x_1 \; + \; B_2 \, \mu_2 \, x_2}{\mu_1 \, x_1 \; + \; \mu_2 \, x_2} \qquad (4.5)$$

$B_1$, $B_2$ are the build-up factors of the two materials for the total thickness $(x_1 + x_2)$.

**5.  Source "ON" Position Shielding.**  Since the shielding geometry may be altered when the cobalt-60 source is in the irradiating position, protection will be required to reduce the total integral dose to the patient.

The maximum exposure rate of the leakage radiation is not to exceed 0.1% of the useful beam exposure rate at 1 m from the source shield which includes the collimator. Consideration should be given to the values at 0.05% of the useful beam dose rate, since a reduction of the leakage rate below this value can result in more economical secondary protection of the treatment room, and it will further minimize the total integral dose to the patient.

**6.  Source Exposure Mechanism.**  The shutter mechanism is a device which performs the function of interrupting the beam of radiation, thus allowing safe storage of the source between treatments. This mechanism must not disturb the source shield geometry at any time. It must always return the source to the safe 'OFF' position. The device must be capable of reproducing accurately the length of the exposure time repeatedly. Therefore, a high order of reliability must be incorporated into the design of the shutter mechanism. To establish some guidelines on this subject, a report has been prepared by the International Commission on Radiological Protection (ICRP Publication 3) *(18)*. The codes of practice outlined in this report have been adopted by most national regulatory bodies. Parts of the report applicable to shutter mechanism design are as follows:

"(146) The beam control mechanism shall be constructed so that it is capable of acting in any orientation of the housing. In addition to an automatic closing device the apparatus should be so constructed that it can be turned off manually with a minimum risk of exposure.
(148) The beam control mechanism shall be provided with a timer that automatically terminates the exposure after a pre-set time.
(149) Warning devices that plainly indicate whether the apparatus is 'ON' or 'OFF' shall be provided at the source housing, on the control panel, and at the entrance to the radiation room."

Further to the above, consideration should be given to all requirements which would aid to ensure the safety of the source exposure mechanism. The design must consider the reliability of the mechanism to consistently return to the same exposure position. The system should also be capable of returning to the safe position in the event of any breakdown or interruption of the activating force.

There are a variety of mechanisms that can be made to meet successfully the above requirements. Three of the types most commonly used in teletherapy machines are illustrated in Figure 4.9. Each of these systems has its own advantages and disadvantages (see Table 4.3). The selection of a shutter mechanism is influenced by the collimation system, source geometry, source shield, or even the type of isotope used. If a curved-movement multivane collimator is used, the necessity (see Section VI.C on collimators) of having the source close to the apex of the collimation device will discourage the use of a shutter block. The use of a dense shielding material such as uranium will encourage the design of a compact beam control device so as to take full advantage of the shield material selection.

Figure 4.9a illustrates a typical sliding shutter block mechanism. The source is in a stationary position above the collimator and the block provides the necessary protection in the "OFF" position. The thickness of the block must meet the requirements for radiation protection in the "OFF" position. The sliding block can be moved by a linear mechanism

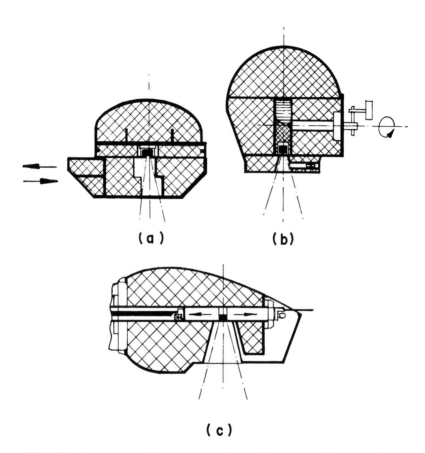

( a ) ( b )

( c )

FIG. 4.9. Three types of shutter systems for radiotherapy machines: (a) sliding shutter block; (b) rotating source wheel; (c) sliding source drawer,

actuated by a pneumatic cylinder or a rack and pinion powered by an electric motor. In shielding for cobalt or for higher-energy radiation, the maximum feasible thickness of the block may be a limiting factor. It will keep the source and collimator substantially apart, thereby discouraging the use of a penumbra-reducing collimator system which requires the source to be at the apex of the collimator. The physical size of the shutter block will require a robust mechanism to move the shutter back and forth. The problem is further increased by the necessity of avoiding the use of a lubricant to reduce friction.

TABLE 4.3

Source Exposure Mechanisms for Cobalt-60 Teletherapy Machines

| Type | Description | Advantages | Disadvantages |
|------|-------------|------------|---------------|
| Sliding shutter block (Fig. 4.9a) | Source stationary; part of source shielding, the shutter block slides to provide aperture between source and diaphragm. | Accurate source diaphragm alignment assuring properly shaped beam of radiation. Speed of closure relatively unimportant because of short travel distance. No special mechanism required to keep block from jarring during closure as the source is separate; this is also advantageous for source exchange. | Heavy shutter block slides in machined ways which are difficult to lubricate because of radiation breakdown of lubricants. Requires frequent checkup. Manual closure can be difficult because of shutter block weight. Close tolerances and step cracks required to reduce radiation leakage. |
| Rotating source wheel (Fig. 4.9b) | Source contained in wheel which is part of the inner shield of the source housing. | Relatively simple, close machining tolerances no. required. Allows source housing to be sized near optimum for best weight size for shielding requirements. | Source wheel presents problem in aligning source to collimating device. Dampers required to decelerate shutter wheel to prevent shock loads which may disturb source locating mechanisms. Source transfer requires elaborate source holding system which can be remotely actuated to transfer source into shipping container. |

| | | | |
|---|---|---|---|
| Sliding source drawer (Fig. 4.9c) | Source drawer moves linearly from "on" to "off" position. | Simple exposure mechanism; close machining tolerances not required to reduce leakage radiation. Source exchange simple as complete source-shutter can be exchanged by sliding into shipping container. | Source housing may be larger because of shielding requirements in the "on" position. Care must be taken to assure proper source alignment. |
| Rotating shutter block | Source located in housing with aperture below it. | See Rotating source wheel for advantages. | Extra shielding required because source is above shutter block |
| Mercury shutter | Shutter is a pool of mercury which is pumped out into a reservoir for radiation. | Mercury offers good protection because of its density. Source is unaffected by shutter movement assuring alignment. | Elaborate syphon pressure system required to move mercury. Sealing problems; possibility of not removing all the mercury from the shutter area. |

Despite this problem, sliding block systems have been made to operate satisfactorily in commercial units that are still operating after a decade of continuous use.

Figure 4.9b shows a rotating source wheel mechanism. The heavy metal source wheel rotates 180° from the "OFF" to "ON" positions. This system probably allows the greatest flexibility in collimator design; however, a complex mechanism is required to locate the source accurately in its "beam-on" position. Because this arrangement can be almost completely enclosed within the primary source housing, leakage of radiation can be kept to a minimum. This system can be satisfactorily actuated with a rotary mechanism, such as a gear reducer electric motor combination. This eliminates the need to transfer rotary to linear motions, thereby allowing a compact arrangement for the drive.

The third method, illustrated in Fig. 4.9c, depicts a sliding source drawer. The source is contained in a plug which moves to the irradiating position from its storage location in the protective housing. A linear drive mechanism such as a hydraulic or pneumatic cylinder can effectively control the source. This system has similar advantages to the rotating wheel system, with the advantage of having a simple source transfer system.

There is also a variation on the rotating source wheel, where the source remains stationary above the rotating wheel. This system has advantages in that source location is undisturbed; however, the disadvantage is the need to provide more shielding material to effect the same protection.

A shutter system, in which compressed air forces mercury out of the cone-shaped shutter cavity thus allowing the beam to emerge, has also been developed. The principle of this system is very simple; however, the difficulty of completely evacuating the mercury must be considered. Care must be taken to assure leak-tight containment of the mercury to avoid leakage of toxic fumes.

### C.  Collimator System

**1.  Introduction.**  The major role of the system is to produce a sharply defined beam with as little penumbra as possible. Originally, fixed cones of different sizes and shapes were used. Because of the thickness of the absorbing material required, the weight of these cones was excessive. Current practice has preferred the use of square or rectangular fields. By providing continuously variable collimator systems, the radiotherapist can choose any field size that suits the problem on hand. Because the fields are rectangular, the cataloguing of isodose distributions is simple with the added advantage that the same information will be applicable to all collimators of the same design. Any changes to the radiation field to provide other than rectangular shape is achieved by the use of secondary shielding blocks which can readily be attached to the collimator.

At present there is only one practical method of shaping the radiation beam to fit the treatment volume, that is by the use of radiation absorbing material. These absorbers are assembled to be controlled by mechanisms to produce the required rectangular radiation fields or, if required, circular fields.

**2. Collimator Mechanism.** There are many arrangements that can be used to provide collimation. The simplest is a set of interchangeable cones previously described. Another method is the use of four pieces of heavy metal moving in one plane with respect to each other in order to describe rectangular or square fields. This system is shown in Fig. 4.10. Unfortunately, the system is large and awkward. To keep the size reasonable it must be located close to the source, thereby creating problems due to geometrical penumbra.

Another system, shown in Fig. 4.11, uses a number of moving heavy metal bars arranged so that their leading edges lie on a line drawn through the edge of the source. Opposite sets of these bars interlock for smaller fields thereby keeping the overall dimensions reasonable. A variation of this system is depicted schematically in Fig. 4.12. In this system the bars are held together on a common spine the apex of which is pivoted at or near the edge of the source face. This system has the advantages of the system previously discussed with the added feature of the possibility of a simpler field changing mechanism.

Because of the need to use brute force by the application of beam absorbers, there are certain problems associated with the design of a collimation system capable of producing a sharply defined field; they are: transmission, penumbra through the absorbers; field penumbra; and electron contamination.

**3. Penumbra**

*a.* TRANSMISSION. The radiation transmission through the diaphragm cones should be kept to a minimum so that the useful total integral dose will be high and unwanted exposure is minimized. There are no calculative methods of arriving at a value of allowable transmission; however, advisory and regulatory bodies have made recommendations and rules. These can be found in Table 4.4.

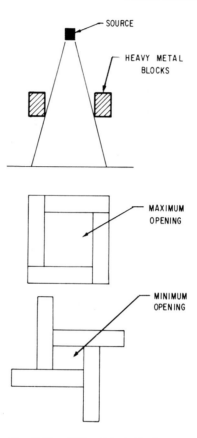

FIG. 4.10.  Sliding block diaphragm

Care should be taken when using the maximum permissible values as excessive stray transmission will result in penumbra that will destroy the definition of the field. With the use of higher specific-activity sources and smaller source diameters, the resultant decrease in geometrical penumbra may accentuate the transmission penumbra.

*b.* FIELD PENUMBRA.  The shaping of a beam of radiation from a finite diameter source results in penumbra, i.e., an irradiated area surrounding the desired target area. The penumbra destroys the sharpness of the field, compared for instance to an ideal field produced by a point source. The disadvantage of using a beam with a large penumbra is the potential damage to healthy tissues surrounding the selected treatment area.

TABLE 4.4

ALLOWABLE COLLIMATOR LEAKAGE

| Organization | Allowable transmission through collimator cone (percent of useful beam) |
|---|---|
| ICRP | 5 |
| NCRP | 5 |
| United Kingdom Authorities | 2 |

Since the source has finite dimensions, the edges of the collimator do not define the beam sharply, as radiation from one side of the source will contribute a different amount of radiation than the opposing side collimator edge (Fig. 4.13). The magnitude of the geometrical penumbra

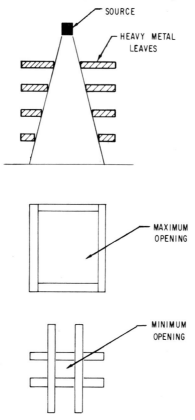

FIG. 4.11. Sliding vane collimator.

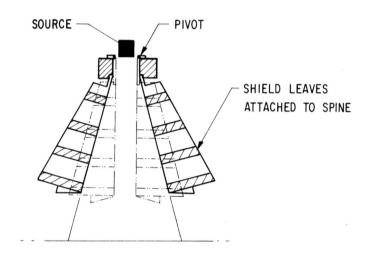

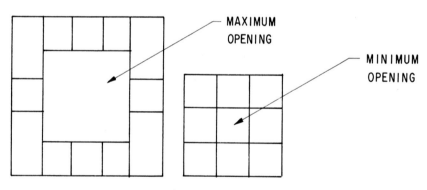

FIG. 4.12. Pivoted sloping-sided wheel.

depends upon the source diameter, the source-to-collimator distance, and the collimator-to-surface distance. From simple geometry of similar triangles,

$$P/D = (b-a)/a;$$

therefore,

$$P = D\ (b-a)/a. \tag{4.6}$$

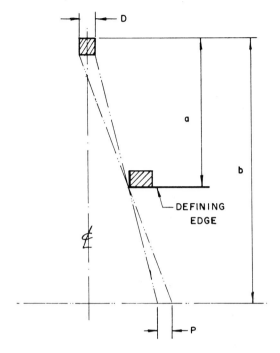

Fig. 4.13.  Geometrical penumbra. D, Source diameter; P, penumbra; *b*, source to surface distance; *a*, source to defining edge.

It can be seen that penumbra can be reduced by:

(1) *reducing source diameter:*   However, if the source is made small the radiation output will be reduced. This can partially be overcome by the use of high specific-activity cobalt.

(2) *reducing collimator-to-surface distance:*   This will destroy one of the important clinical advantages of a cobalt-60 beam; namely the fact that, when a high-energy gamma-ray beam enters the patient, the dose near the skin surface will be small, the maximum dose occurring at a depth below the skin. The proximity of the collimator to the skin surface will destroy this advantage as a result of increased electron scatter from the collimator. Clinical experience has shown that a distance of about 15 cm between the collimator and the skin surface preserves the *skin-sparing effect.*

(3) *increasing source-to-collimator distance:*   This will have the desirable effect of reducing the penumbra; however, because of the inverse square law, the activity of the source must be increased

to maintain a useable exposure rate. This is possible by the use of higher specific-activity material at increased cost.

### D. Support Structure

**1. Introduction.** The design of the cobalt source, its housing and collimator having been discussed, it is necessary to determine the manner in which the beam can be employed. The major objective is to apply a lethal dose to the tumor with as little damage as possible to surrounding healthy tissue. To achieve this it is necessary to have the capability of positioning the radiation beam so that it can enter the body at different locations to concentrate the radiation dose at the tumor site. The ideal situation would be to concentrate all the absorbed energy at the tumor site and have no absorption elsewhere. This would give the minimum integral dose for a given tumor dose.

In attempts to achieve the required dose distribution in the tumor volume the radiation may be combined in many different ways:

(1) *Opposed pairs.* The field is directed along the same axis from opposite sides of the patient.

(2) *Angled fields.* Two fields may be directed toward the tumor at a specified angle from the vertical.

(3) *Combination of fields.* Several fields may be directed toward the tumor center from different sides of the patient.

Radiation used in the ways described above is known as *fixed field therapy.* An extension of the combination of fields is to permit the movement of the radiation beam in such a way as to sweep out a circular arc centered at the tumor site. This technique is usually referred to as *moving beam* or *rotation therapy.* To allow the radiotherapist to accurately treat the patient it is essential that the beam of radiation does not deviate from its intended path. It is essential that all the structural components of the support structure be designed with utmost rigidity.

There have been many attempts to provide a satisfactory method of radiation beam movement. These included the rotation of the patient! Many techniques of rotation therapy have evolved; some are described in *The Physics of Radiology (8)*. Generally teletherapy units that have been developed for fixed-field therapy were improvements of the radium bomb and the supervoltage machines. Two basic types of machines are currently manufactured. They are *fixed-beam therapy units* or *vertical units* and the *rotational teletherapy unit.*

**2. Fixed-beam Teletherapy Unit.** This machine has been developed for treatments using single fields or combination of fields with the radiation beam remaining static during treatment. Such a unit is illustrated in Fig. 4.14. The unit normally incorporates three degrees of freedom for positioning the beam. One translational degree of freedom in the vertical direction to allow the source housing to move up or down from the floor. One or more rotational degrees of freedom in the horizontal plane that allow the source to be angularly positioned to direct the beam in the desired direction for treatment. Practical limits in the travel of the rotational motion must be incorporated if the primary shielding of the room is limited by economical or structural factors. This type of unit can be employed at any source-to-skin distance (SSD) within the limits of the vertical travel and patient position. Special rotational therapy modes can be considered by the use of a chair rotating about the vertical axis. Acceptance of this mode of treatment has been very slow; the reason is apparent when one considered the discomfort the patient would experience during his travels.

A typical "fixed beam" unit would consist of a source, a source housing collimator, and positioning mechanisms. The major function of a fixed beam unit is simple positioning of the beam for proper alignment with respect to the tumor site.

To facilitate the treatment set-up, the vertical drive mechanism should not allow the collimator center to deviate more than $\pm 0.5$ cm from the vertical axis. This can be readily achieved by the use of a ball screw drive and linear bearings riding on hardened steel shafts. To prevent the heavy source housing from coasting, the drive mechanism should be self-locking. This can be accomplished by the use of a drive mechanism incorporating a self-locking worm-gear. An alternative method would be the use of an electrically actuated brake mechanism which would be in the lock position when electrical power is removed.

**3. Rotational Teletherapy Unit.** To improve the effectiveness of radiotherapy by reducing the dose to the overlying tissue, the teletherapy system has evolved through many designs. Many treatment techniques have been developed, some using multifield cross-fire, opposed field, and eventually moving-field therapy. As it is more satisfactory to have the radiation beam move instead of the patient, the rotating teletherapy unit was developed *(11–13, 15)*. Such a unit is usually designed for 360° continuous rotation about a supine patient. The radiation beam focuses at the center of rotation of the machine during its motion.

With the moving-beam unit it was discovered that it was easier to

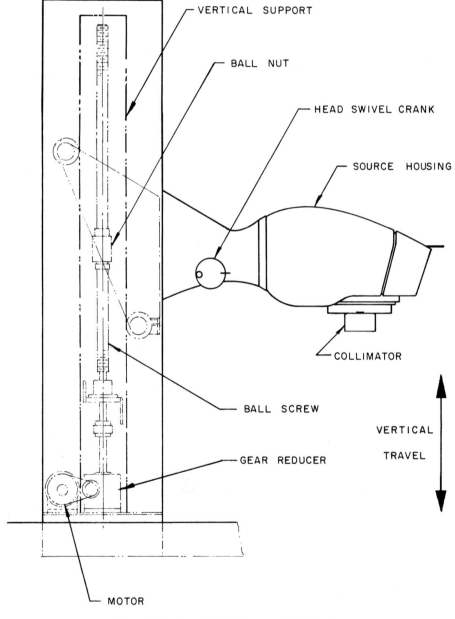

VERTICAL SUPPORT

BALL NUT

HEAD SWIVEL CRANK

SOURCE HOUSING

COLLIMATOR

BALL SCREW

VERTICAL

TRAVEL

GEAR REDUCER

MOTOR

FIG. 4.14.   A typical fixed-beam cobalt-60 unit.

position the beam relative to the patient, especially for multiportal treatments. With the patient located at the center of the unit in a fixed position all required beam directions for treatment are provided by a source moving on the surface of a sphere, the radius being the source-to-target distance. Once the tumor is located at the center of source movement, the beam direction can be changed by rotating the source housing-collimator assembly to a new angular position. This can be done by the remote actuation of the unit's rotation drive, thus increasing efficiency by eliminating the need for the operator to enter the treatment room. A typical rotational unit is illustrated in Fig. 4.15.

### E. Beam Stopper

In situations where the structural shielding of the therapy room is a limiting factor, a beam stopper is employed on the therapy unit to absorb the radiation transmitted through the patient during treatment. The moment of the source head of the unit about the axes of rotation must be balanced in some manner, and it is reasonable to assume that the beam stopper could be designed to perform this task as well as its job as a beam interceptor.

There are two approaches available for the design of a beam stopper; the first is a design which adheres to accepted practice as defined in NCRP Report No. 33 (19). Namely, the beam stopper must absorb all but 0.1 % of the primary beam and reduce by the same factor the scatter radiation from the patient through an angle of 30° from the central rays in all directions.

The second approach is the design of an optimum beam stopper. This beam stopper should reduce the transmitted radiation to a level that can be adequately handled by the limited room shielding as well as counterbalancing the movement of the source head. Figure 4.16 shows the reduction in dose rate for three different modes of therapy unit operations: no beam stopper, optimum beam stopper, and a beam stopper thicker than necessary. The data used to obtain these curves were obtained from beam stoppers which subtended a specific angle of the axis of rotation.

The practical width of the beam stopper is limited by the manner in which a patient must be positioned for various types of treatments as well as by the factors discussed above. Considering all these points, a good compromise is a beam stopper whose width subtends a solid angle of 60° at the isocenter of the therapy unit. The optimum beam stopper then will be of this width and of a sufficient thickness of a specific material to absorb 99 % of the primary beam (see Fig. 4.17).

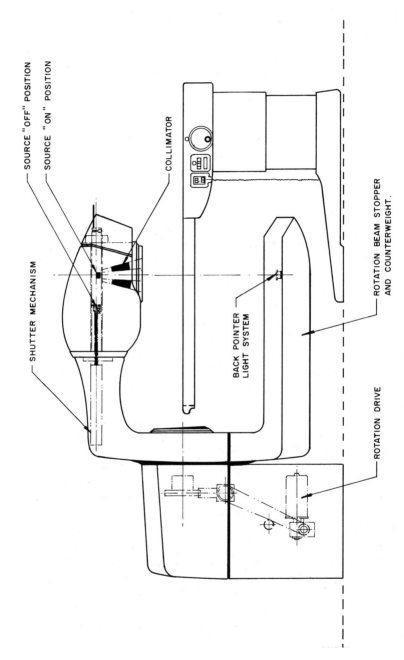

Fig. 4.15.   A typical cobalt-60 unit used for rotational therapy.

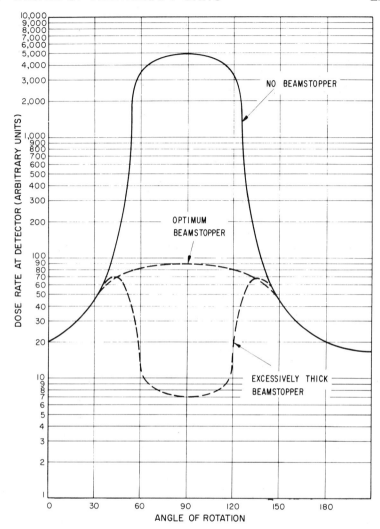

FIG. 4.16. Radiation incident upon detector versus angle of rotation.

The optimum distance of this beam stopper from the center of rotation of the unit will be that which exactly balances the unit. This distance can be found from a simple moment calculation.

Consider the simplified example of a beam stopper shaped as the section of a cylinder which subtends an angle of $60°$ at its center; the cylinder center is assumed to be the axis of rotation (Fig. 4.18a). Let $D$

be the distance from the axis of rotation to the face of the beam stopper and let $t$ be the thickness of the beam stopper. Divide the beam stopper into elemental volumes as shown in Fig. 4.18b. Let $\theta$ be the angle between an element and the horizontal. Let $M$ be the moment of the beam stopper about the axis of rotation. Then:

$$M = 2mg \int_0^{30} (D + t/2)\, \theta d\theta$$
$$= mg\,(D + t/2)$$

But the volume of the beam stopper is

$$V = \pi/6\, [(D + t/2)^2 - D^2]\, 2D \tan 30$$
$$= \frac{2\pi\, Dt}{3\sqrt{3}}\, (D + t/2)$$

also, $m = \rho V$ where $\rho$ is the density of the beam stopper and

$$M = \frac{2\pi\, Dt\, \rho g\, (D + t/2)^2}{3\sqrt{3}} \qquad (4.7)$$

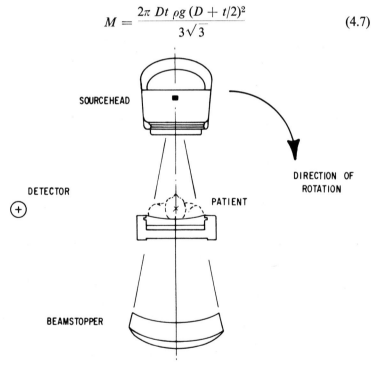

SOURCEHEAD

DIRECTION OF
ROTATION

DETECTOR

PATIENT

BEAMSTOPPER

FIG. 4.17.   Schematic representation of therapy unit and detector probe to produce radiation fields shown in Fig. 4.16.

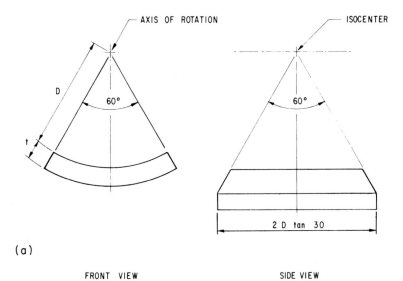

(a)

FRONT VIEW                    SIDE VIEW

FIG. 4.18a.  Simplified beam stopper.

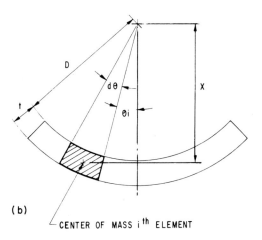

(b)

FIG. 4.18b.  Beam stopper moment calculations.

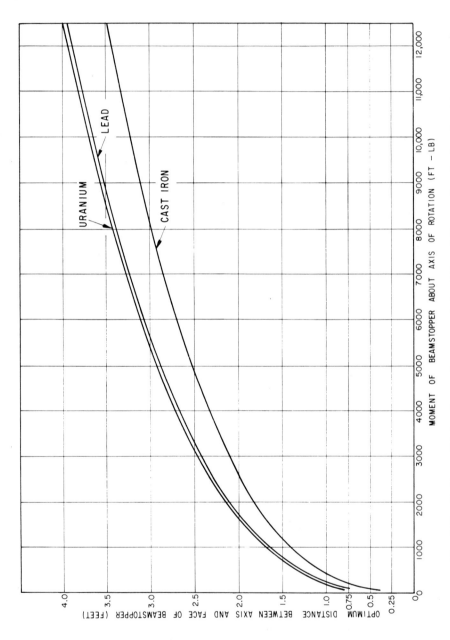

Fig. 4.19.   Optimum $D$ to produce a given moment about the axis for uranium, lead, and cast iron.

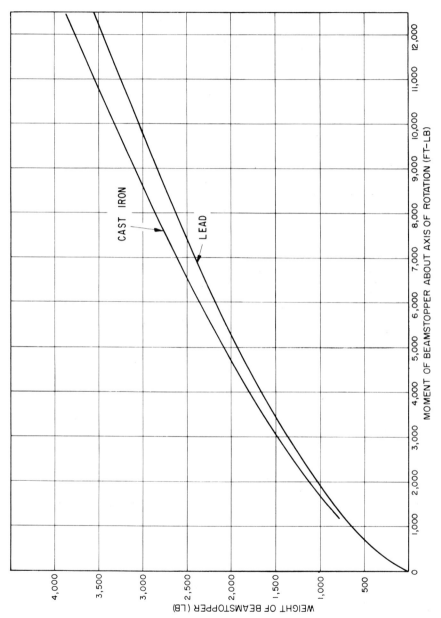

Fig. 4.20. Weight of beam stopper located at the optimum $D$ to produce a given moment about the axis.

TABLE 4.5

MOMENT EQUATION for VARIOUS BEAM-STOPPER MATERIALS

| Material | Density (pounds/ft³) | Optimum thickness (ft) | Moment equation (ft/pounds) |
|---|---|---|---|
| Iron | 491 | 0.500 | $M = 296.8gD(D + 0.25)^2$ |
| Lead | 698 | 0.262 | $M = 221.1gD(D + 0.131)^2$ |
| Uranium | 1177 | 0.154 | $M = 109.6gD(D + 0.077)^2$ |

Selection of a specific material gives us $\rho$ and $t$. The resulting moment equation for three possible beam-stopper materials is shown in Table 4.5.

Figure 4.19 shows optimum distance $D$ plotted against the moment for each of the materials in Table 4.5. Figure 4.20 shows the beam-stopper weight required to achieve a specific moment for cast iron and lead when the beam stopper is at the optimum distance $D$.

## REFERENCES

1.  M. Brucer, *Nucleonics,* **10**, 4, 40(1952).
2.  R. Robbins, *Nucleonics,* **10**, 4, 41(1952).
3.  C. B. Braestrup, *Nucleonics,* **10**, 4, 42(1952).
4.  M. Brucer, *Nucleonics,* **10**, 4, 43(1952).
5.  M. Friedman, M. Brucer, and E. Anderson, *Roentgens Rads and Riddles,* U.S. Atomic Energy Commission, 1959.
6.  Cancer Treatment, Technical Report Series No. 322, World Health Organization, Geneva, 1966.
7.  Planning of Radiotherapy Facilities, Technical Report Series No. 328, World Health Organization, Geneva, 1966.
8.  H. E. Johns and J. R. Cunningham, *The Physics of Radiology,* 3rd ed., Thomas, Springfield, Illinois, 1969.
9.  G. H. Fletcher, *Textbook of Radiotherapy,* Lea & Febiger, Philadelphia, 1966.
10. I. H. Smith, J. C. M. Fetterly, J. S. Lott, J. C. F. MacDonald, L. M. Myers, P. M. Pfalzner, and D. H. Thomson, *Cobalt-60 Teletherapy,* Harper, New York, 1964.
11. H. E. Johns and J. R. Cunningham, *Amer. J. Roentgenol,* **81**, 1, 2(1959).
12. D. T. Green and R. F. Errington, *Brit. J. Radiol.,* **25**, 309-313(1952).
13. C. B. Braestrup, D. T. Green, and J. L. Snarr, *Radiology* **61**, 614-624 (1953).
14. J. E. Richardson, H. D. Kerman, and M. Brucer, *Radiology* **63**, 25–36 (1954).
15. G. H. Fletcher et al., The Design of a Second Cobalt-60 Unit Based on the Experience Acquired with 1,000 Patients Treated with the First.
16. Classification of Sealed Radioactive Sources, American Institute of Chemical Engineers, New York.
17. F. Ellis and R. Oliver, *Brit. J. Radiol.,* **34**, 720-725(1961).
18. Radiation Protection: Protection against X-rays and Gamma-rays (Addendum), ICRP Publication 6, Pergamon Press, New York, 1967.
19. NCRP Report 33, National Council on Radiation Protection and Measurements, Washington, D.C.

# 5   DESIGN PROCEDURES FOR IRRADIATORS

*F. X. RIZZO, L. GALANTER, J. D. CLEMENT,\**
*AND B. MANOWITZ*

BROOKHAVEN NATIONAL LABORATORY
UPTON, LONG ISLAND, NEW YORK

---

\*Georgia Institute of Technology, Atlanta, Georgia.

# I.  INTRODUCTION

In recent years gamma radiation has emerged as a useful tool in industry as well as in research. In the radiation processing industry, gamma radiation is used for the destruction of bacteria in food and medical supplies, for the initiation of chemical reactions, and for the modification of properties of polymer materials. Some of the applications that have reached commercial use are food preservation, sterilization of medical products, polymerization of monomers in the chemical industry, production of wood–plastic and concrete–plastic combinations, and improvement of thermal resistance and other properties of plastic films.

In research, radiation has served for some time as a tool in biology, medicine, the physical sciences, and engineering. Some of the more glamorous research applications include the use of radiation in ecological and environmental studies, such as the treatment of solid and liquid wastes, and in medicine for blood irradiation for the control of leukemia and the study of the organ-implant rejection mechanism.

The increasing use of radiation has placed a demand upon electrical, mechanical, and nuclear engineers to perform dose distribution calculations as part of irradiator design.

The calculation of dose in an irradiator can range in complexity from the simple case of a point source in air to the very complicated case of a large-scale production irradiator. Although for the very complicated cases it is often necessary to use high-speed computers and the services of a competent radiation physicist, many of these calculations can be performed by the average engineer if he is provided with an understanding of the requirements and principles of irradiator design as well as a knowledge of the available calculational aids. In this chapter, irradiator design will be approached from an engineering point of view. It will be assumed throughout that the reader has a limited background in nuclear physics.

# II.  GENERAL IRRADIATOR DESIGN CONSIDERATIONS

A gamma irradiator system consists of

(1)   A radioactive source, such as $^{137}Cs$ or $^{60}Co$.

(2)  The target or product to be irradiated.
(3)  Means for conveying the target into and out of the radiation field.
(4)  Shielding.
(5)  Building, storage, and handling facilities.

The diversity of irradiator applications and consequent different design specifications lead to a limitless number of possible types of irradiators. Gamma irradiators can be classified in several different ways:

(1)  By irradiator geometry.
(2)  By application—experimental, research, demonstration, or production.
(3)  By mobility requirements—whether portable or stationary, shipboard or truck, etc.
(4)  By characterizing any or all of its components listed above (such as $^{137}$Cs source or wheat target).
(5)  By type of irradiation—batch, continuous, stop-dwell, or shuffle-dwell.
(6)  By radiation effect—biological, chemical, or physical.

An irradiator designer usually starts with a given set of parameters having to do with the amount of product to be treated, the treatment desired, and the dimensions of the unit product. From these he determines the amount of source activity required to effect the treatment and then decides upon a geometric configuration between source and target that will most efficiently or most economically satisfy the design requirements.

Parameters important for irradiator design are listed in Table 5.1 and are discussed below.

### A.  Target Parameters

MINIMUM AND MAXIMUM TOTAL DOSES. These parameters are usually specified by the user or customer, and therefore cannot be changed by the designer.

The minimum total dose is the lowest dose required for the treatment of the product. Typical minimum total doses are 8000–10,000 rads for insect sterilization; 15,000–25,000 rads for grain de-infestation; 75,000–500,000 rads for radiopasteurization of shellfish and other marine products; and 2.5–4.5 × 10$^6$ rads for sterilization of medical supplies and meat products.

The maximum total dose is the highest dose which the product may receive that does not represent an overdose or legal tainting of the product.

TABLE  5.1

SYMBOLS AND DEFINITIONS

| Symbol | Definitions | Units |
|---|---|---|
| 1. $D_{min}$ | Minimum total dose in target | Rads |
| 2. $D_{max}$ | Maximum total dose in target | Rads |
| 3. $U$ | Dose uniformity, $D_{max}/D_{min}$ | (Dimensionless) |
| 4. $w$ | Mass flow rate of target | lb/hr |
| 5. $Q$ | Capacity of irradiator, $w \times D_{min}$ | Rads-lb/hr |
| 6. $h_T$ | Target thickness | ft |
| 7. $H_T',L_T$ | Target height; target length | ft |
| 8. $\rho_T$ | Target density | lb/ft$^3$ |
| 9. $H_S',L_S$ | Source height; source length (extended source) | ft |
| 10. $S_g$ | Source specific activity (activity per unit mass) | Ci/g |
| 11. $S_a$ | Source activity per unit area | Ci/cm$^2$ |
| 12. $E_u$ | Source utilization efficiency | — |
| 13. $t_R$ | Total residence time in the irradiator | hr |
| 14. $V$ | Linear velocity of target package | ft/hr |

DOSE UNIFORMITY ($U$).   This is the ratio of the maximum allowable to the minimum allowable doses in the irradiator, where

$$U = D_{max}/D_{min}$$

Uniformity is a function of source-to-target geometry, target thickness, and the density and atomic number of the product. Since this parameter is usually stated in the irradiator specification, it also cannot be arbitrarily changed.

MASS FLOW RATE ($w$).   This parameter is also one which forms part of the customer's specifications. Typical mass flow rates are 100–2000 lb/hr in irradiators ranging from small research facilities to large production units.

IRRADIATOR CAPACITY ($Q$).   The irradiator capacity is given in units of power, usually rad-lb per hour or megarad-tons per hour, and is determined from the product of the mass flow rate and the minimum dose.

$$Q = w \times D_{min}$$

TARGET DIMENSIONS ($h_t$, $h_T$, $L_T$).   The maximum target thickness is controlled by the specifications for maximum dose uniformity and is therefore limited by target density, atomic number, and photon energy. These factors, in turn, affect the overall dose attenuation and absorbed dose variation within the target.

The target dimensions of length and height are somewhat arbitrary but are related to the specifications for mass flow rate and uniformity and to other parameters, such as source size and irradiator geometry (the type of irradiator selected for use).

In moving-target irradiators the relationships between the heights and lengths of the target and the source become increasingly important and affect the efficiency of the irradiator system. In final dose calculations these relationships must be optimized.

For example, in a moving-target irradiator, when the target length is short compared with the length of the source, the individual target or package length should be no larger than one-half the source length, otherwise the target travel can be varied only by rather large increments. Since there must be a void space into which the package will move, packages of small length result in a smaller void space and consequently a larger target volume and higher efficiency.

Frequently all three target dimensions will be set by the specification. This occurs when the product is already being marketed in a particular form and the manufacturer does not wish to change the packaging. Irradiators which are designed "around" package sizes are usually relatively costly and inefficient.

### B. Source Parameters

Although the dimension of source length is quite flexible for irradiators where the target moves parallel to the source axis, source height and thickness dimensions are more restricted. Usually the source height is governed by the target height as previously discussed and is some integral multiple of source element length for vertically stacked elements. Source element length is related to nuclear reactor specifications and ease of handling during encapsulating and shipping. Within reasonable limits (several inches to a foot), source length can be specified by the irradiator designer.

A range of source specific activities may be selected up to the practical maximum for the particular isotope. For reactor-produced sources the specific activity is related to neutron flux, isotopic abundance, activation cross section, half-life, and time in the reactor. For separated fission products, the specific activity is governed by isotopic abundance, fission yield, chemical purity, and half-life. The source strength per unit area for a fixed value of specific activity may be varied by adjusting the source thickness or by using more than one layer of source elements. Practical values for attainable specific activities range from 5 to about 500 Ci/g of cobalt metal for cobalt-60, and activities up to 25 Ci/g of cesium chloride for the separated isotope cesium-137.

## C.  *Efficiency*

The source utilization efficiency is related to many of the variables such as photon energy, source dimensions, source density, source-to-target geometry, target dimensions, and target density. Utilization efficiency is defined as the ratio of the power absorbed at the minimum dose point in the target divided by the total power emitted by the source, and is given by the relation

$$E_u = \frac{\text{energy absorbed in target at minimum dose point}}{\text{total electromagnetic energy emitted from source}}$$

Losses in efficiency may be classified separately according to their origin as follows:

(1)   Self-absorption in sources and cladding,
(2)   Absorption in nontarget material outside the source such as container walls and conveyor parts,
(3)   Energy escaping the system as unabsorbed radiation,
(4)   Excess energy absorbed in target material above the required minimum dose.

A quantitative relation for $E_u$ is as follows:

$$E_u = \frac{k_1 Q_{min}}{k_2 C}$$

where   $Q_{min}$ =   capacity, megarad-lb/hr at minimum dose
$C$   =   total source strength, curies
$k_1$   =   power absorption conversion factor: 1.26 watts per megarad-lb/hr
$k_2$   =   isotopic gamma power, = 0.0148 W/Ci for cobalt-60 and 0.00324 W/Ci for cesium-137.

In a typical irradiator design problem the customer will usually specify:

(1)   The mass flow rate in lb/hr.
(2)   The minimum allowable dose in rads.
(3)   The uniformity ratio.

(4) Other parameters such as the maximum residence time in the irradiator. (Residence time specifications are usually stated to prevent thawing and refreezing of frozen products and to prevent regrowth of bacteria in products that must be sterilized.) Another parameter which is sometimes stated is maximum temperature rise in the product.

The designer using these specifications must perform the following tasks.

(1) Select the irradiator geometry or type that is best suited for the product to be irradiated and that is consistent with the economic limitations placed upon him.

(2) Design of the unit package or target. (a) In designing the unit package, the maximum thickness of the package must be determined first. The thickness must be optimized taking into consideration the required dose uniformity, the nature of the product, and the expected dose distributions in the irradiator. Optimization of target thickness may require several separate dose calculations. (b) Once the target thickness has been optimized, the target length and height can be determined from the specification for the mass flow rate and assumption concerning conveyor velocity.

(3) The total source activity and the source specific activity then can be determined from the specification for minimum dose.

(4) The irradiator efficiency is then calculated.

(5) The parameters of source and target height and length, source activity, and irradiator efficiency must then be optimized through a series of trial and error calculations.

The procedure outlined in steps 1–5 is not necessarily the only one which is or can be used in irradiator design, but has been included as an example. It is the procedure that is generally followed for most systems.

The objectives of this chapter are to summarize the basic design principles and computational methods needed to perform these tasks. It is the authors' intention to provide a good reference on irradiator design rather than an all-inclusive design manual.

The subject will be introduced with a description of the simple, basic source design geometries and concepts used in research and processing. This will be followed by a discussion of the radiation physics and analytical methods used to calculate the dose in these simple systems. Complex irradiator concepts will then be descriptively introduced and will be followed by a discussion of computer methods, approximation techniques, and other computational aids used for these systems.

### III.   SOURCE GEOMETRIES

#### A.   Point Source Geometry

The simplest type of irradiator, from the point of view of dose calculation, is one in which the target material is exposed in a point source geometry. The point source can be used either in the narrow-beam or the broad-beam geometry.

**1.   Narrow-Beam Point Source Geometry.**   In Fig. 5.1, the narrow-beam geometry, the target is irradiated through a collimator that is usually made of lead or some other high density material. The purpose of the collimator is to create a beam of uncollided gamma rays. This is accomplished by eliminating from the beam all gamma rays that have undergone any kind of interaction before reaching the target. This is illustrated in Fig. 5.1. This geometry has very little practical application in industrial processing but is used quite often in research and in medical applications. Examples of irradiators using this geometry are medical teletherapy units, irradiators used for detector calibration, thickness gauging, and radiography.

The narrow beam geometry will be dealt with analytically in Section IV on dose calculation.

**2.   Broad-Beam Point Source Geometry.**   The difference between the narrow-beam and the broad-beam geometry is the absence of a collimator in the latter. When a target is irradiated without a collimator, the dose absorbed at the target point of interest is due not only to uncollided gamma rays but also includes a component deposited by gamma rays that may have undergone one or more interactions, where the resulting photon has

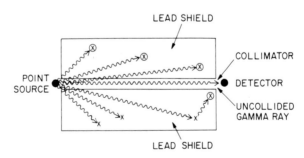

FIG. 5.1.   Narrow beam, point source geometry. ⊗, Gamma-ray absorption; X, scattering of gamma rays.

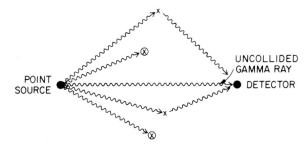

FIG. 5.2.   Broad-beam geometry; point source in infinite medium. ⊗, Gamma-ray absorption; X, scattering of gamma ray.

been Compton-scattered into the target point from the surrounding medium. This is illustrated in Fig. 5.2.

Examples of broad-beam geometries are a point source imbedded in an infinite target medium (Fig. 5.2) and a point source external to a semi-infinite or finite target (Fig. 5.3).

Although the point source geometry has relatively little practical application in research and industry as a source of radiation energy, the concept, both phenomenologically and mathematically, is an important one from several points of view. First, it is often possible to evaluate the effects of complicated source geometries by performing simple calculations based upon "point source" approximations. This can usually be done when the distance between a target point and the source is great compared with the dimensions of the source, resulting in the source

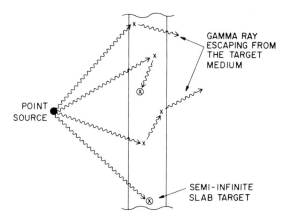

FIG. 5.3.   Point source irradiation of a semi-infinite slab target.

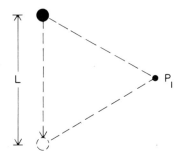

FIG. 5.4.   Line source generated from a moving point source.

approximating a point. Second, complicated source geometries can be generated by superimposing the effects of many point sources. This technique is often used in computer computations and is referred to as point kernel integration. Third, complicated irradiator concepts usually can be more easily understood if they are examined first in terms of the point source geometry.

### B.   Line Source Geometry

A uniform line source is the result of the superimposed effects of a series of point sources arranged in a straight line. The line source is also generated when a point source is moved at a uniform rate of speed in a straight line past a stationary target point. Similarly, the same result is obtained when the point source is stationary and the target point is moved. In both cases the line source generated is equal in length to the distance traveled by the point (see Figs. 5.4 and 5.5).

In practical irradiator design, the line source is particularly important because most high intensity gamma sources are manufactured in the form

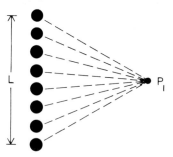

FIG. 5.5.   Line source resulting from the superposition of several point sources.

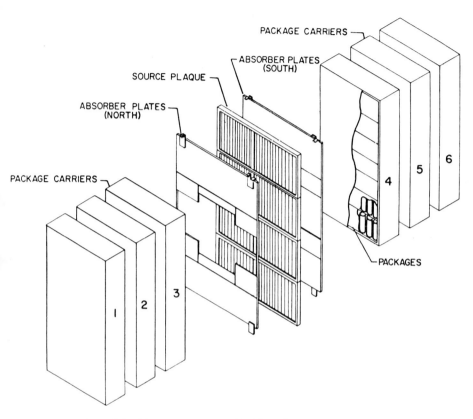

Fig. 5.6.   Plaque source assembled from line source elements.

of line source elements. Most practical extended source geometries are fabricated using the line source as the basic element (see Fig. 5.6).

There are only a limited number of practical applications in which the line source geometry as such is used in an irradiation system. Two examples of these are chemical gamma-ray reactors (see Fig. 5.7a, 5.7b) and extracorporeal blood irradiators (see Fig. 5.7c). In general, the line source geometry is likely to be used as an alternative whenever the point source geometry imposes limitations on an irradiator system insofar as curie content is concerned.

The number of source geometries possible using point or line source elements, or both, as building blocks is limitless. Among these are the disk source, the slab source, the truncated right circular cone source, the

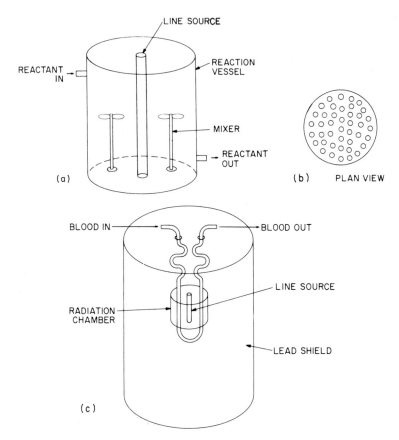

FIG. 5.7.   (a) Gamma-ray chemical reactor using a single line source.   (b) Chemical reactor using numerous line sources.   (c) Blood irradiator using a single line source.

cylindrical source, and the spherical source. Of these, only the slab source and the cylindrical source are commonly used in irradiator design; the others lead to rather complex design procedures and mechanical configurations.

### C.   Rectangular Source Geometry

Slab sources are usually assembled from line source elements as illustrated in Fig. 5.6. The rectangular slab source is the most commonly used geometry in large-scale production irradiation for the following reasons:

(1) It is best suited to the irradiation of targets having rectangular shapes such as plastic film, packaged products (food and medical supplies), wood and concrete plastic impregnated products. (2) It enables one to assemble extended sources containing large quantities of radioisotope in a reasonably efficient geometry. (3) It permits the use of source-dose shaping techniques, i.e., increasing the source strength and the dose rate in the vicinity of the low-dose regions of the target. This is usually referred to as *source overlap* and *augmentation*.

The slab source geometry is generated when a line source is moved past a stationary target point or when the line source is stationary and the target point is moved. In these cases the slab generated will be equal in height to the height of the line source and equal in length to the distance traveled by the line source or the target point. This is illustrated in Fig. 5.8.

### D. Cylindrical Source Geometry

The other source geometry that is used frequently in gamma irradiators is the cylindrical source. The cylindrical source geometry is generated when a line source is made to revolve around a stationary target point or when a target is rotated in front of a stationary line source.

Cylindrical source geometries are most often used when the requirements of the irradiation call for very good dose uniformities to be delivered to relatively small target volumes. In these cases irradiations are per-

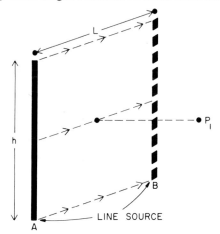

FIG. 5.8. Slab source generated from a moving line source.

formed inside the cylinder with the source material surrounding the target. Hollow cylindrical sources are also used to irradiate targets external to the source as in the case of the AECL Carrousel Irradiator (see Fig. 5.22) and in applications where line sources are desirable but limited in respect to source strength.

## IV.  GAMMA RADIATION FIELD CALCULATIONS

In Section III the basic source geometries encountered in irradiator design were described briefly. Before proceeding to incorporate these simple geometries into irradiator design concepts, attention will be turned to the analytical methods used to calculate the dose from these simple geometries with a few introductory remarks on gamma-ray interactions and narrow- and broad-beam attenuation.

### A.  Gamma-Ray Interactions

The theory of gamma-ray interactions and methods of calculating attenuation have been treated extensively in the literature (1–6), and tables of attenuation coefficients, buildup factors, and conversion factors, such as the conversion of radiation flux to dose rate, are available (1, 5, 6).

The three gamma-ray interaction mechanisms that need to be considered in gamma irradiator design are:

(1)  The photoelectric effect, characterized by the disappearance of the incident photon and the emission of an orbital electron;

(2)  Compton scattering, in which the photon imparts a portion of its energy to a free electron and is deviated in direction;

(3)  Pair production, which involves the transfer of all the energy of a photon to an electron–positron pair with the simultaneous disappearance of the photon.

The relative contribution of each of these mechanisms to the total dose received by any target material depends on the gamma-ray energy spectrum and on the composition of the absorbing material.

### B.  Attenuation of Gamma Radiation

**1.  Narrow-Beam Geometry.**  The absorption of a narrow beam of monoenergetic gamma radiation or attenuation occurs exponentially with absorber thickness because each photon is removed from the beam in a single interaction of any kind. Thus the number of photons removed $\Delta N$ is proportional to the thickness of the absorber $\Delta X$ and the number of incident photons $N$, and may be related by the following equation.

$$\Delta N = \mu N \, (\Delta X) \tag{5.1}$$

where $\mu$ is the proportionality constant known as the *total gamma absorption coefficient* (5). It is constant for monoenergetic gamma rays and in Eq. (5.1) is expressed in units of reciprocal length. If the path length is expressed in units of mass per unit area (g/cm²), the mass attenuation coefficient $\mu/\rho$ is used since the product of the coefficient and the thickness must be dimensionless. Integration of Eq. (5.1) yields the well-known Lambert law:

$$N/N_0 = e^{-\mu x} \tag{5.2}$$

The left-hand side of Eq. (5.2) may also be replaced by the ratio of energy flux density or intensity ($I$), or by the ratio of particle flux density. The equations are valid for narrow or collimated beams of monoenergetic photons (see Fig. 5.1). Photons are thus removed from the beam both by absorption processes and by scattering, and $\mu$ is the total absorption coefficient.

**2. Broad-Beam Geometry.** The situation described in the preceding paragraph represents a condition rarely encountered in practice. When extended sources and targets are involved and the scattering in shielding and target materials modifies the gamma-ray energy distribution significantly, the "narrow-beam" assumption clearly does not hold and more elaborate methods for calculating the radiation field must be employed. These methods must take into consideration the effect of scattering and *buildup*, the change in interaction mechanism as the radiation spectrum is degraded, and the effect of the finite dimensions of both source and absorber on the gamma-ray field.

### C. Simple Source Geometries

**1. Point Source.** The formulas used in calculating radiation flux from an extended source to a point in a target are derived by integration of the flux from a point source. This flux, or point kernel, may be extended to sources and targets of far greater complexity by integrations over source and target.

Consider an isotropic point source of photons in an infinite homogeneous medium emitting $S$ photons per second of energy $E_0$. The photon flux at any point may be expressed as

$$\phi = (S/4\pi r^2) e^{-\mu_0 r} \tag{5.3}$$

where $\mu_0$ is the total narrow-beam absorption cross section of the target for photons of energy $E_0$, and $r$ is the distance of the point from the source.

**2. Line Source.** The radiation flux at point $P_2$ at distance $a$ from the line of radiation may be expressed by the following equation:

$$\phi = (S_l/4\pi a) \left[ \int_0^{\theta_1} e^{-\mu_0 a \, \sec \theta} \, d\theta + \int_0^{\theta_2} e^{-\mu_0 a \, \sec \theta} \, d\theta \right] \tag{5.4}$$

At $P_1$ located on the perpendicular bisector of the line (see Fig. 5.9a)

$$\phi = (S_l/2\pi a) \int_0^{\theta_3} e^{-\mu_0 a \, \sec \theta} \, d\theta \tag{5.5}$$

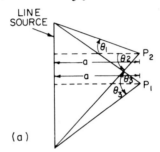

(a)

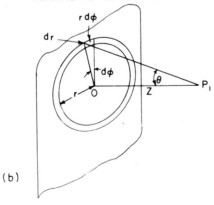

(b)

FIG. 5.9. Point source geometry.

The secant integral, $\int_0^\theta e^{-b \sec \theta} d\theta$, cannot be determined analytically. Various workers have evaluated it numerically and it has been tabulated ($1$, $16$).

3. **Plane Source.** The flux at a point $P_1$ at distance z from an infinite plane isotropic source emitting $S_a$ photons/cm² sec may be expressed by the following equation (see Fig. 5.9b):

$$\phi = S_a/2 \int_{\mu_0 z}^\infty (e^{-t}/t) dt \qquad (5.6)$$

The integral $\int_{\mu_0 z}^\infty (e^{-t}/t) dt$, where $t$ is a "dummy" variable of integration, is called the exponential integral $E_1 (\mu_0 z)$, and is quite useful in shielding calculations. Values of the $E_1$ function have been tabulated ($33$).

4. **Disk Source.** At $P_1$ on the center line of a disk of radius $R$, which is emitting $S_a$ photons per unit area per unit time, the uncollided flux is

$$\phi = S_a/2 [E_1 (b_1) - E_1 (b \sec \theta)] \qquad (5.7)$$

where $b_1 = \mu_0 z$ and $\theta = \tan^{-1} (R/z)$ (see Fig. 5.10).

5. **Slab Source.** The photon flux at $P_1$, a distance z in an infinite homogeneous target from a uniform isotropic slab source of thickness $h$, is given by the following equation (see Fig. 5.11):

$$\phi = (S_v/2\mu_s) [E_2(b_1) - E_2(b_1 + \mu_s h)] \qquad (5.8)$$

where $S_v$ = source strength per unit volume (photons/cm³ · sec), $\mu_s$ = linear absorption cross section of source (cm⁻¹), and $b_1 = \mu_0 z$, where $\mu_0$ is the linear absorption cross section of the target and

$$E_2(b_1) = b_1 \int_{b_1}^\infty (e^{-t}/t^2) dt \qquad (5.9)$$

For other source geometries such as cylindrical, trapezoidal, and spherical sources, the reader is referred to the standard shielding manuals of Rockwell ($12$), Goldstein ($10$), and references ($5$) and ($27$).

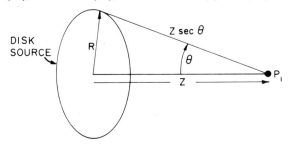

FIG. 5.10. Disk source geometry.

INFINITE SLAB SOURCE

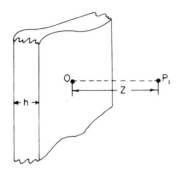

FIG. 5.11.    Slab source geometry.

**6.    Conversion of Radiation Flux to Dose Rate.**    To facilitate the conversion of gamma photon flux to radiation dose, Table 5.2 has been compiled. Values of energy absorption cross section, exposure dose in air, absorbed dose in air, and absorbed dose in water are listed for photon energies from 0.1 to 4 MeV based on a value of $W$, the energy required to create one ion pair in air, of 34.0 eV/ion pair and National Bureau of Standards energy absorption cross sections.

TABLE   5.2

ENERGY ABSORPTION CROSS SECTIONS AND RADIATION FLUX
TO DOSE RATE CONVERSION FACTORS

| Photon energy (MeV) | Linear energy absorption cross section (air), $(\text{cm}^{-1})$ $\mu_0$ | R/hr per MeV/cm²-sec, $D_r/\Phi$ | Absorbed dose[a] in air (rads/hr per MeV/cm²-sec), $D_{ab}/\Phi$ | Absorbed dose in $H_2O$, (rads/hr per MeV/cm²-sec) |
|---|---|---|---|---|
| 0.1 | $0.2994 \times 10^4$ | $0.1526 \times 10^{-5}$ | $0.1338 \times 10^{-5}$ | $0.1486 \times 10^{-5}$ |
| 0.2 | 0.3477 | 0.1772 | 0.1554 | 0.1726 |
| 0.4 | 0.3820 | 0.1947 | 0.1708 | 0.1896 |
| 0.5 | 0.3831 | 0.1953 | 0.1713 | 0.1902 |
| 0.6 | 0.3820 | 0.1947 | 0.1708 | 0.1896 |
| 0.663 | 0.3817 | 0.1945 | 0.1706 | 0.1895 |
| 0.8 | 0.3724 | 0.1903 | 0.1669 | 0.1854 |
| 1.0 | 0.3605 | 0.1838 | 0.1612 | 0.1790 |
| 1.25 | 0.3461 | 0.1764 | 0.1547 | 0.1716 |
| 1.5 | 0.3316 | 0.1690 | 0.1482 | 0.1646 |
| 2.0 | 0.3069 | 0.1564 | 0.1372 | 0.1523 |
| 3.0 | 0.2725 | 0.1389 | 0.1218 | 0.1353 |
| 4.0 | 0.2500 | 0.1274 | 0.1117 | 0.1241 |

[a] Based upon value of $W = 34.0$ eV per ion pair and density of $H_2O$ equal to unity.

**7. Buildup.** Buildup arises from the fact that in an actual medium scattering effects enhance the amount of radiation reaching a given target point. The buildup factor can also be defined as the ratio of the actual gamma-ray flux that would be calculated or measured accurately to that which would be calculated using simple exponential attenuation based on the total narrow-beam absorption coefficient. This definition results in a *number buildup factor*. However, it is more usual to use the absorbed dose buildup factor or *energy buildup factor*.

The *absorbed dose buildup factor* can be defined as the ratio of the actual dose rate that one could experimentally measure at a point in a medium to the dose rate due to uncollided flux at that point that one could calculate by using only simple exponential attenuation with the total absorption coefficient. The energy buildup factor is defined similarly.

Although a great deal is known about the interaction processes of gamma rays in matter, no completely satisfactory method of handling buildup has been found to date. A popular method, that of Taylor (*11*), expresses the buildup from a point isotropic source in an infinite homogeneous medium as a sum of two exponentials:

$$B = A_1 e^{-\alpha_1 \mu_0 t} + A_2 e^{-\alpha_2 \mu_0 t} \tag{5.10}$$

where $\mu_0$ = total absorption coefficient for the initial gamma energy, $E_0$; $B$ = the buildup at a depth $\mu_0 t$ mean free paths in the medium; $A_1 = 1 - A_2$; and $\alpha_1$ and $\alpha_2$ are functions of $E_0$.

In Table 5.3 the functions $A_1$, $\alpha_1$, and $\alpha_2$ are given for absorbed dose buildup in several different media. In Table 5.4 similar information is compiled for cesium-137 gamma-rays and a water target.

Readily available and reliable data on buildup are contained in the report by Goldstein and Wilkins (*9*), and others (*5, 10–15*). The results are based on calculations of the gamma-ray transport equation for point and plane sources in an infinite homogeneous medium using the moments method developed by Fano and Spencer (*23*). The important property of the buildup is that it is a function of photon energy, atomic number, and target depth. Since it is the result of the effect of multiple Compton scattering, it decreases with increase in incident energy and increases with penetration. At photon energies around 1 MeV the buildup decreases with increase in the atomic number of the target because of the shift in the absorption process in favor of the photoelectric effect. It is important to note that most data are available for only point or plane sources in infinite homogeneous targets.

TABLE  5.3

EXPONENTIAL APPROXIMATIONS TO ENERGY ABSORPTION BUILDUP FACTOR [a]

| | | POINT ISOTROPIC SOURCES — WATER TARGET | | |
|---|---|---|---|---|
| Substance | $E_0$(MeV) | $A$ | $-\alpha_1$ | $\alpha_2$ |
| Water | 1.0 | 13.5 | 0.100 | 0.010 |
| | 1.25 | 8.90 | 0.095 | 0.059 |
| | 2.0 | 8.1 | 0.068 | 0.0405 |
| | 3.0 | 5.6 | 0.059 | 0.073 |
| | 4.0 | 4.5 | 0.0555 | 0.11 |
| | 6.0 | 3.4 | 0.0525 | 0.156 |
| | 8.0 | 2.8 | 0.05 | 0.17 |
| | 10.0 | 2.5 | 0.0473 | 0.1719 |

$$B = Ae^{-\alpha_1(\mu_0 r)} + (1-A)\, e^{-\alpha_2\,(\mu_0 r)}$$

[a] Data obtained from Ref. (*10*), p. 378.

**8. Incorporation of Buildup into Equations for Uncollided Flux.** The methods of incorporating buildup into calculations of dose may be divided into two groups. In Group A for (1) a point source in an infinite medium or (2) an infinite plane isotropic source in an infinite medium, the appropriate buildup factors of Goldstein and Wilkins (*9*) may be incorporated directly by multiplying the uncollided dose rate at the required depth by the buildup at that point. Buildup factors have been tabulated for point sources, plane monodirectional sources, and plane angular sources in such media as air, iron, lead, tin, and uranium in USAEC Report NYO-3075 (*9*).

In Group B, where one requires the dose rate at a point from an extended source in a finite or infinite medium, the method requires the use

TABLE  5.4

EXPONENTIAL APPROXIMATION TO ENERGY ABSORPTION BUILDUP FACTOR [a]

| | POINT ISOTROPIC SOURCE — WATER TARGET | | |
|---|---|---|---|
| | ($^{137}$Cs source; $E_0 = 0.662$ MeV) | | |
| | Subscript | | |
| Parameter | 1 | 2 | 3 |
| $C$ | 3.50 | 3.00 | 0.50 |
| $\alpha$ | −0.308 | 0.231 | 1.824 |

$$B_a = C_1 e^{-\alpha_1\,(\mu_0 r)} + C_2 e^{-\alpha_2\,(\mu_0 r)} + C_3 e^{-\alpha_3\,(\mu_0 r)}$$

[a] Calculated at Brookhaven National Laboratory from data of Goldstein (*10*).

of the point source buildup factor in the mathematical expression of
the dose rate from a differential area of the source. The total effect of
buildup is thus obtained mathematically by integrating over the source
area. Because of the exponential attenuation of radiation, the use of
Taylor's method, where a sum of weighted exponentials is used to express
the buildup, does not result in a change in the mathematical function
within the integral. For example, for an infinite plane source, the uncollided radiation flux at some depth $b$ (in mean free paths) in the target
was given by Eq. (5.6) to be:

$$\phi = (S_a/2)\int_b^\infty (e^{-t}/t)dt = (S_a/2)E_1(b) \tag{5.6}$$

The uncollided dose rate may be obtained by multiplying the energy flux
by the appropriate conversion factor $K_1$. Thus,

$$D_{uncollided} = K_1 E_0(S_a/2)\int_b^\infty (e^{-t}/t)dt = K_1 E_0(S_a/2)E_1(b) \tag{5.11}$$

Since

$$B_{(E_0,\,b)} = A_1 e^{-\alpha_1 t} + (1-A_1)e^{-\alpha_2 t}$$

it may be shown that the total dose rate

$$D_{total} = K_1 E_0(S_a/2)\left[\int_{b(1+\alpha_1)}^\infty A_1(e^{-t}/t)dt\right.$$
$$+ \int_{b(1+\alpha_2)}^\infty (1-A_1)(e^{-t}/t)dt\left.\right] \tag{5.12}$$
$$= K_1 E_0(S_a/2)\left[A_1 E_1\,[b(1+\alpha_1)]\right.$$
$$+ (1-A_1)E_1\,[b(1+\alpha_2)]\left.\right] \tag{5.13}$$

Another method such as the use of linear buildup where $B = (1 + \alpha_3\mu t)$
would result in the following equation:

$$D_{total} = K_1 E_0(S_a/2)\left[E_1(b) + \alpha_3 e^{-b}\right] \tag{5.14}$$

## V.  PRACTICAL IRRADIATOR DESIGN

### A.  General Introductory Remarks

In Sections III and IV some of the basic source configurations and
methods of dose calculation used in the design of irradiators were discussed. In addition, examples of design concepts based upon these simple configurations were advanced. Most of these concepts were examples of simple, small-volume research-type irradiators for which dose

distribution calculations can be easily performed using the methods of Section IV.

Design calculations become increasingly difficult with increased source-to-target geometry complexity, which usually occurs with increased irradiator capacity. For most production-type irradiators one must resort to specialized computer programs and other calculational aids for design calculations. These aids will be discussed in Section VII.

In this section the reader will be introduced to the design concepts used for large-scale irradiation. This will be followed by discussions of the computational methods required to determine dose rates for these complex systems.

Since package irradiators with rectangular source and target geometries are the most widely used in production systems, this type irradiator will be used to a great extent to illustrate the general requirements, specifications, and complexities of large-volume, high-capacity irradiators and to introduce the reader to some of the design techniques and irradiator concepts commonly used in the design of all irradiator systems. At the end of this section other concepts and geometries will be illustrated and discussed.

## B.   Specific Design Considerations

Dose uniformity in an irradiator depends upon the target thickness, target density, and source-to-target geometry. The maximum target thickness is controlled by the specification for maximum allowable dose variation and is therefore limited by target density, atomic number, and photon energy. In any irradiator the uniformity is a composite effect depending upon the dose uniformity through the depth of the target and the lateral dose distributions in target planes parallel to the source (assuming here that the target is rectangular and that the source is a slab). Lateral dose distributions depend upon the source-to-target geometry. Since the designer usually strives to meet the uniformity specification with the thickest possible target package, he must minimize the lateral and depth dose distributions. Depth dose variations are minimized by employing two-sided irradiation of the product, by irradiating the target package equally from both sides through its depth, and through the use of multipass irradiation systems. Lateral dose distributions are minimized in several ways: (1) by introducing additional source material in the vicinity of the low dose target points (referred to as *source specific activity augmentation* or *enhancement*), (2) by allowing the source to overlap the target in the vicinity of the low dose regions (referred to as *source over-lap*), or (3) by allowing the target to move or sweep past the source at a uniform rate of speed or in a stop-dwell motion. The target motion assures the uniformity of the dose along any line in the target that is parallel to its direction of motion.

## C. Design Concepts

**1. Rectangular Slab, Package Irradiator Concepts.** There are many package irradiators in use today. Although each has unique characteristics, all use the simple ideas discussed in Section V.B to achieve uniformity, and on this basis they can be classed in three general categories: (1) stationary-type irradiator; (2) single-direction, multipass irradiator; (3) two-direction, multipass irradiator.

Each of these irradiator types utilizes the two-sided irradiation principle for minimizing depth dose distributions and at least one of the techniques discussed above for minimizing lateral dose distributions.

(a) STATIONARY-TYPE IRRADIATORS. The simplest type of large volme irradiator is the stationary irradiator. A simple, one-slab, two-position stationary irradiator is illustrated in Fig. 5.12. In this simple system there are only two packages in the irradiation chamber (one on each side of the source plaque) at any time. Two-sided irradiation is accomplished by moving the target package quickly into position number 1, with surface "A" facing the source, where it is allowed to remain for a predetermined period of time, then into position 2, where it remains for an equal period

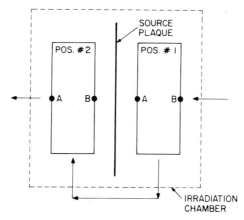

FIG. 5.12.   Single-slab, two-position stationary irradiator.

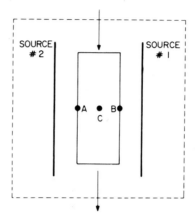

FIG. 5.13.   Two-slab, single-position stationary irradiator.

of time, and then out of the radiation chamber, completing one irradi-ation cycle. This is the simplest example of a two-sided irradiation, and all other irradiators, no matter how complicated, are in reality variations of this simple idea. Figures 5.13 to 5.16 are some of the simple variations of the stationary irradiator.

In the single-slab, multiposition, stationary-type irradiator, the one most commonly used (Fig. 5.14), there may be numerous target packages in the irradiation chamber at the same time. The direction of motion of of the packages as they are indexed up to and away from the source plaque is perpendicular to the plane of the source. This movement is usually referred to as "stop-dwell" motion. The advantages of multiposi-

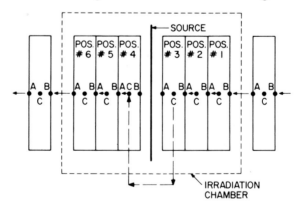

FIG. 5.14.   Single-slab, multiposition stationary irradiator.

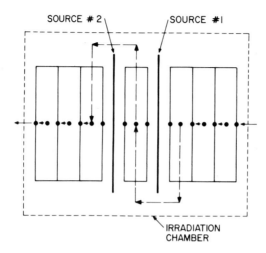

FIG. 5.15. Two-slab, multiposition stationary irradiator.

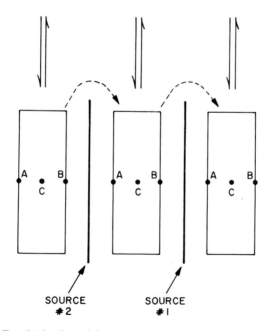

FIG. 5.16. Two-slab, three-position stationary irradiator.

tion irradiation are that it results in better depth dose uniformities and higher efficiencies than single-position irradiation. Lateral dose distributions are minimized in stationary irradiators by applying source overlap or augmentation or both.

Of the three modes of package irradiation, stationary irradiation is usually the least efficient and results in the greatest nonuniform lateral dose distribution, i.e., distributions in target planes that are parallel to the plane of the source plaque.

Examples of stationary-type irradiators are the five research irradiators that are located at the University of Washington, the University of Florida, the University of California at Davis, the Massachusetts Institute of Technology (see Fig. 5.16), and the University of Hawaii (see Fig. 5.13).

(b) SINGLE-DIRECTION, MULTIPASS IRRADIATOR. In this type, the target material is moved past the source plaque in a direction parallel to the plane of the source. In the single-slab, two-pass system (Fig. 5.17), a target package is introduced into the irradiation chamber at position "A," at one end of the chamber, and is moved horizontally past the source to the other end of the chamber (position "B") where it is then indexed to the other side of the source plaque (position "C"). It then traverses the irradiation chamber in the opposite direction to position "D," completing its two-sided irradiation. In moving past the source the target packages are butted and are moved either continuously, at a uniform rate of speed, or can be indexed from one target dwell position to another in a "stop-dwell" fashion. In the "stop-dwell" mode of operation each target package remains at each irradiator position for an equal time.

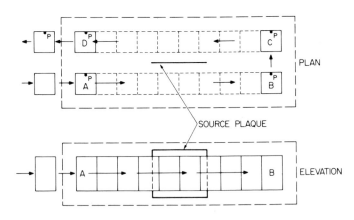

FIG. 5.17.    Single-slab, two-pass single-direction irradiator.

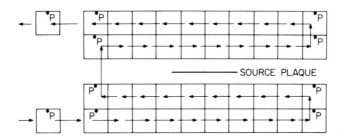

FIG. 5.18. Single-slab, multipass single-direction, stop-dwell irradiator.

The result of the horizontal motion of the target package is to eliminate or minimize dose variations in the horizontal direction. Dose variations in the vertical direction are minimized, as in stationary irradiators, either by source augmentation or overlap.

Figure 5.18 is a block diagram of a single-slab, four-pass, single-direction irradiator. The additional two passes, one on each side of the plaque, serve to minimize the lateral as well as the depth dose distributions.

This mode of irradiation usually results in efficiencies that are higher and lateral dose variations that are less severe than in stationary irradiators.

Examples of this type irradiator are the new BNL single-slab, two-pass irradiator, and the very versatile Hawaiian Development Irradiator, which can be operated as a single-direction, multipass system or as a modified quadrant irradiator.

(c) TWO-DIRECTION, MULTIPASS IRRADIATOR. The two-direction, multipass irradiator (Fig. 5.19) is, in principle, similar to the single direction systems discussed above, with the exception that the target material is moved vertically as well as horizontally as it undergoes its two-sided irradiation. Examples of this type irradiator are the simple quadrant irradiator (Fig. 5.19) and its various modifications (e.g., Figs. 5.20 and 5.21).

In Fig. 5.20, a complex two-direction, multiposition, multipass, shuffle-dwell motion irradiator is demonstrated. In this system there are twenty-five target positions on each pass and four passes (two on each side of the plaque). The arrows in the figure indicate a sequence of package movement arbitrarily selected for illustrative purposes because of its simplicity. In practice, the sequencing of the target packages will differ from one irradiator to another and will depend upon the design and the ingenuity of the conveyor system designer. The important fact is that each target

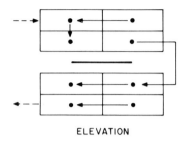

ELEVATION

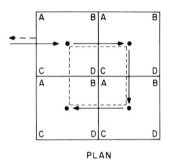

PLAN

Fig. 5.19.    Two-direction, multipass irradiator (simple quadrant irradiator).

package occupies each of the one hundred irradiation positions on each cycle through the irradiator.

In this type irradiator, the lateral dose distributions are essentially uniform or at a minimum in both the vertical and horizontal directions, and the efficiencies encountered are higher than in the other two types of irradiators.

Examples of this type of irradiator are the Marine Products Development Irradiator (Fig. 5.21) and the Mobile Gamma Irradiator (Fig. 5.19), the Irradco Meat Irradiator, the Hawaiian Development Irradiator, and the Medical Products Irradiator at Ethicon, Inc. (Fig. 5.20).

**2.   Other Irradiator Concepts.**   The three basic irradiator concepts presented in Section V.C.1 are illustrative of most of the gamma-ray irradiators in use today. Furthermore, most other possible arrangements of the source and target do not really represent serious departures from the concepts used in these systems.

One might, for instance, (1) change the source and/or the target geometry, (2) improve the method of conveying the target into, through, and

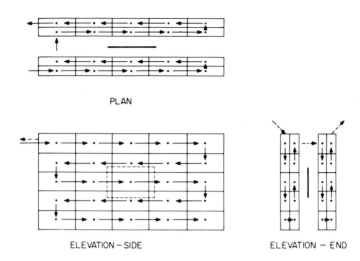

PLAN

ELEVATION – SIDE                    ELEVATION – END

FIG. 5.20. Two-direction, multipass, multiposition, shuffle-dwell irradiator.

out of the irradiation chamber, (3) introduce the concept of a moving line or point source of very high specific activity, (4) increase the number of source plaques and/or the number and location of target passes and positions, (5) introduce the concept of four-sided package irradiation, (6) use

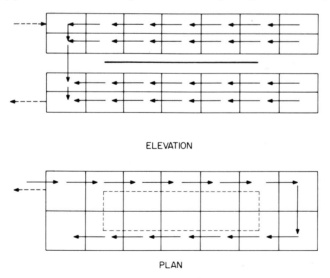

ELEVATION

PLAN

FIG. 5.21. Marine products development irradiator.

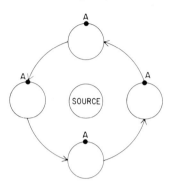

FIG. 5.22.    Carrousel irradiator concept.

an "infinite" array of target material (position target packages on all sides of the source), or (7) rotate the target in front of the source.

All of these ideas have been tried, and while many are useful design tools, some of them have been found to be impractical from several points of view:

(1) They may require very high specific activity source material that is usually not available or is too expensive (as in the case of the moving source concept).

(2) They may create unreasonable complications for the target conveyor and/or the source positioning mechanisms resulting in increased and sometimes prohibitive capital costs.

(3) They may result in unreasonable increases in the in-cell product in-

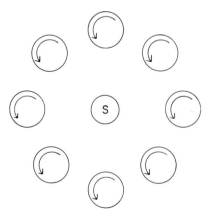

FIG. 5.23.    Cylindrical source, cylindrical target, turntable batch irradiator.

ventory giving rise to high risk (in case of breakdown) without the benefit of significant increase in efficiency.

The concepts that are described below are based upon the use of cylindrical sources and targets and four-sided package irradiation.

**3.  The Cylindrical Source Geometry.**  Figures 5.22 to 5.24 illustrate several possible cylindrical irradiator geometries. Figure 5.22 is a cylindrical source, cylindrical target irradiator concept, the essential feature of which is that the target undergoes a 360° revolution relative to the source on each irradiator pass without changing its orientation. The effect of this 360° irradiation is to minimize the radial or depth-dose distributions in the cylindrical target.

(a)

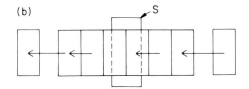

(b)

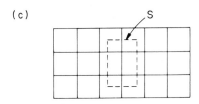

(c)

FIG. 5.24.  Rectangular target, carrousel-type irradiator. (a) Elevation; (b) single-direction, plan view; (c) two-direction, plan view.

This concept can be operated in a continuous or "stop-dwell" mode and can be used as a multipass system in the stationary, one-direction or two-direction modes as described above.

Although the cylindrical geometry is best suited for this concept, targets can be of any shape; and point, line, or slab sources can be used depending upon the source activity requirements. The simple concept, with little modification, can be used for batch irradiation, as shown in Fig. 5.23. This is a simple turntable-type irradiator with eight cylindrical targets arranged around a cylindrical source. All eight cylinders are brought into position in the irradiation chamber at the same time, the source is raised, and they are made to rotate about their axes until they receive the required total dose; they are then all removed. The effect on uniformity is the same as for the concept shown in Fig. 5.22. Again, the use of the cylindrical geometry here is not essential.

The carrousel type of irradiator in Fig. 5.24 is still another modification of this basic concept. In this system the target undergoes a four-sided irradiation. This system is similar to the concept used in Canada by Atomic Energy of Canada Limited.

The effect of the four-sided irradiation on dose uniformity is to minimize the depth dose variations as well as the distributions along target lines parallel to the directions of motion of the target. This results in the minimum dose regions lying along lines parallel to the axis of the cylindrical source at the center of the target. The dose variation along this line is minimized as in other irradiators by using source overlap and/or augmentation or by moving the target in the direction of the variation.

## D.  General Dose Distribution Patterns in Large Gamma-Ray Irradiators

**1.  Background Discussion.**    Irradiators of similar general design will possess individual differences depending upon the designer's goals and the use to which the irradiator is to be put. A qualitative discussion of the dose distribution patterns in large-scale gamma-ray irradiators serves mainly to illustrate what can be expected under ideal conditions. Nevertheless, even a general discussion may remove some of the common misconceptions concerning the complexity of irradiators and may clarify the recommended approach to the prediction of dose patterns.

Before proceeding, it might serve well at this point to discuss briefly the dose distribution requirements in radiation processing.

In food irradiation one is usually interested in the maximum and minimum absorbed doses in the product. U.S. Food and Drug Administration specifications are usually stated as the minimum total absorbed dose required to effect treatment of the product and the maximum total absorbed dose that still does not constitute an overdose or legal tainting of the product. Normally, maximum and minimum doses are also specified in medical product sterilization and chemical processing.

Although the situation does not arise very often in either research or processing, it may be necessary occasionally to know the average absorbed dose delivered to a product. When a processor requires that his product receive a near-uniform total dose, it is necessary to alter the source-to-target geometry, making the target small compared with the source. If the maximum and minimum doses are within 10% of one another, the average dose is relatively easy to determine. When there are large dose variations throughout the target, however, the average dose is not easily calculated and cannot be based upon the average of the doses at a few points. In the following discussion emphasis will be placed upon the determination of maximum and minimum doses.

The following paragraphs summarize some of the general ideas discussed at the beginning of this section on design principles.

—Most irradiators are designed to yield the lowest possible dose uniformity ratio $U$ ($U = D_{max}/D_{min}$).

—Uniformity is a composite effect depending upon the depth dose uniformity(distributions through the centerline of the target, perpendicular to the plane of the source), and the lateral dose uniformity (distributions in target planes parallel to the plane of the source).

—The depth dose uniformity is limited by target density, target thickness, and photon energy.

—Lateral dose distribution depends on the source-to-target geometry.

—Depth dose uniformities can be improved by irradiating the target from two or more sides and by using multipass irradiator systems.

—Lateral uniformities can be improved by source activity augmentation; by increasing the size of the source relative to the target and applying source overlap, i.e., by decreasing the size of the target or by increasing the size of the source; and by moving or sweeping the target past the source in the vertical and/or the horizontal directions.

Attention will now be turned to the dose distribution patterns in the basic irradiator types discussed above.

**2. Dose Distributions in Rectangular Slab Package Irradiators**

(a) STATIONARY-TYPE IRRADIATORS. In Section V.C.1 it was stated that greater lateral dose distributions are encountered in stationary irradiators

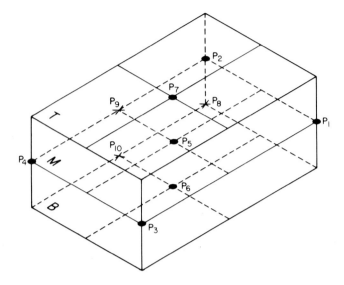

Fɪɢ. 5.25.   Typical stationary irradiator target.

than in the other two types and that the two techniques used to minimize lateral dose variations in these systems are source activity augmentation and source overlap. With both these techniques the designer raises the dose in the low dose regions of the target by increasing the total source activity in those regions.

To illustrate this, let us examine the irradiator packages shown in Figs. 5.25, 5.26, 5.27. In any two-sided stationary irradiation of a rectangular target, the minimum dose point would be expected to be in the midplane of the target; here the midplane is defined by points $P_1$, $P_2$, $P_3$, and $P_4$ (Fig. 5.25). This plane is parallel to the source and lies halfway between the front and back surfaces of the target. If the source used for the irra-

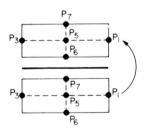

Fɪɢ. 5.26.   Stationary irradiator without source overlap.

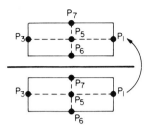

Fig. 5.27.  Stationary irradiator with source overlap.

diation is exactly the same size as the target, as in Fig. 5.26, the symmetrical points $P_1$, $P_2$, $P_3$, and $P_4$ in the corners of the package would be the minimum dose points for the entire target as well as for the midplane. The maximum dose would be found at points $P_6$ and $P_7$, at the center of the outside surfaces of the target. The point $P_5$ would be the maximum dose point in the midplane. If, now, the source were increased in size and allowed to overlap the four edges of the target, as in Fig. 5.27, the dose at points such as $P_1$ would be increased. The location of the minimum dose might no longer lie near the corners of the package but could begin to move along the line formed by point $P_1$ and point $P_5$. This, of course, is true only when the source-to-target spacing (the air gap) is very small (1 in. or less) and the source overlap is large (5 in. or more). For larger air gaps the location of the minimum point would not change although the dose at the minimum point would increase in value. Figure 5.28 illustrates this.

The plotted curves in Figs. 5.28 and 5.29 are dose distributions in a typical stationary irradiator target. In Fig. 5.28 the dose distribution is shown along the diagonals of the outside plane, going from the center point $P_6$ to point $P_8$ in the corner, and in the midplane going from $P_5$ to $P_2$. The cases of no source overlap and 5 in. overlap are shown. Figure 5.29 illustrates the same type of distribution, but in this case the distributions shown are from the center to the edges of the target (for the outside plane from the center point $P_6$ to points on the edge such as $P_{10}$, and for the midplane from the center point $P_5$ to the edge of that plane, such as point $P_9$ in Fig. 5.25).

From the above it may be seen that the maximum dose in any target plane parallel to the plane of the source is very likely to lie at the center of the plane. The dose decreases as the outside edges of the target are approached and falls to a minimum in the corner of the target. The maximum dose, therefore, is likely to be at the center of the outside planes and

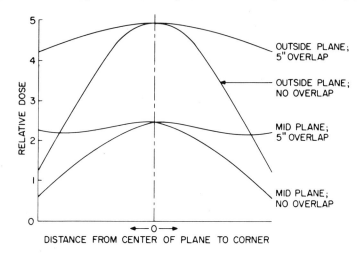

FIG. 5.28.   Dose distribution along diagonals from the center to the corners of the target.

the minimum is likely to occur at the corners of the midplane of the target. The effect of augmenting the activity of the source opposite the outside edges of the target is to minimize these lateral variations by raising the dose at the corner and near the edges of the target.

Figure 5.30 plots experimental correction factors for evaluating lateral dose distribution in the target midplanes. (The four-sided source overlap

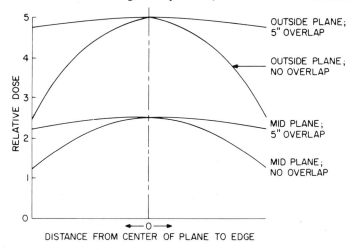

FIG. 5.29.   Dose distribution from center of target to center of edge of target.

curve represents data for stationary-type irradiators; the two-sided overlap is for one-direction, multipass irradiator types.) Data are presented for source-to-target air gaps of 1–6 in.

The correction factor $(F)$ in these curves, when multiplied by the dose at the center of the midplane ($P_5$ in Fig. 5.25), results in a good estimation of the true minimum dose in the middle plane when 5.0 in. of source overlap is used.

In Figs. 5.31 and 5.32 similar data are presented for 3.0-in. and 1.0–in. source overlap.

The use of these correction factors simplifies the task of evaluating the effects of source overlap. Reasonable interpolation and extrapolation of the data can be performed. The data can be used for target packages between 4 and 8 in. in thickness and for cesium-137 as well as cobalt-60 sources.

(b) SINGLE-DIRECTION, MULTIPASS IRRADIATORS. In this type of irradiator, the target is moved either vertically or horizontally past the source plaque in its transit through the irradiator. One would, therefore, not expect to encounter severe dose variations in the direction of motion of the target. The only distributions likely to exist in the direction of motion are those resulting, for example, from distortions of the radiation field near the metallic walls of the target carrier boxes.

If the direction of motion is horizontal, then the distribution in the vertical direction (perpendicular to the direction of motion) will resemble the dose distributions at the edges of targets shown in Fig. 5.29 for stationary irradiators. The effects of adding source overlap will also be the same as for stationary irradiators.

In single-direction irradiators, the maximum dose points are likely to be at the center of the outside planes and the minimum dose is likely to occur in the midplane at those edges of the target that are adjacent to the overlap portion of the source plaque.

The data in Figs. 5.30, 5.31, and 5.32 can be used to estimate the lateral dose distributions when source overlap is applied to the target. In this case the two-sided overlap data should be applied.

(c) TWO-DIRECTION, MULTIPASS IRRADIATORS. Since, in this type of irradiation, the target material is moved both horizontally and vertically past the source plaque, one does not expect to encounter any severe dose variations in either of these two directions. The only expected lateral dose variations will be those caused by the effect of transit dose and by distortions of the radiation field in the vicinity of absorbers located between the source and the target.

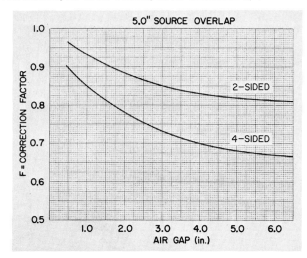

FIG. 5.30.   Correction factor vs. air gap for 5.0-in. source overlap.

The only general statements that can be made about the locations of the maximum and minimum doses are that the maximum dose point will be located on one of the outside surfaces and that the minimum dose point will occur somewhere in the midplane. In this type of irradiator the lateral dose variations rarely can be reduced to less than 5% and are usually between 5 and 10%.

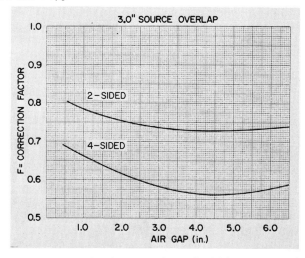

FIG. 5.31.   Correction factor vs. air gap for 3.0-in. source overlap.

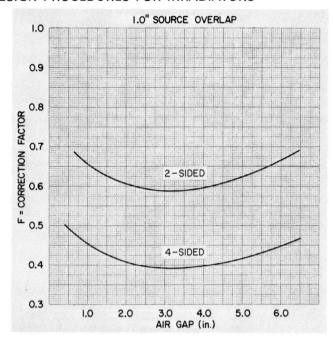

FIG. 5.32. Correction factor vs. air gap for 1.0-in. source overlap.

**3. Cylindrical Geometry Irradiators.** In the carrousel type of irradiators shown in Fig. 5.24 the maximum dose should occur at the center of the four vertical outside surfaces of the rectangular target. The minimum dose should lie inside of a small "line" or volume element along the center of the target as illustrated in Fig. 5.33. To evaluate the lateral dose distributions and the effect of source overlap the criteria and data used for the three rectangular geometry irradiators can be used.

### E. Summary

All irradiators in use to date for thick target irradiation use the two- or four-sided irradiation principle to improve the depth-dose uniformity. This is true of all bulk irradiators regardless of type (stationary and one- and two-direction, multipass types). Consequently, the following general statements are applicable to most bulk irradiator systems regardless of type or any other geometrical or mechanical considerations.

The maximum absorbed dose point or points will always occur in one of the outside planes or surfaces of the target which, during some phase of

MINIMUM DOSE REGION

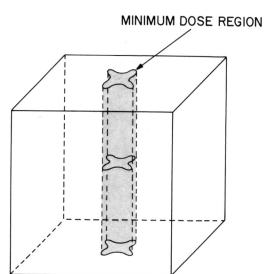

FIG. 5.33. Minimum dose region in carrousel irradiator target.

the radiation cycle, are oriented parallel to the plane of the source. Other points in other planes may exist with doses nearly equal to points in the outside planes, but none will be higher than the highest dose points in the outside planes.

When the target is irradiated equally from two sides, the minimum absorbed dose point or points will always occur in the middle plane of the target (relative to depth), i.e., in the case of four-sided irradiation the minimum dose will lie along the central line of the target, i.e, the line that is parallel to the source and perpendicular to the direction of motion of the target.

These statements are true in most cases if the target is thick and is subjected to two- or four-sided irradiation. They are true even in the following situations.

—When the target is not homogeneous in composition.

—When the source activity or material is not uniformly distributed.

An exception may arise in the case of two-sided irradiation, when the target is not irradiated equally from both sides and the doses on the outside surfaces differ by more than 10–15%. However, irradiators are nearly always designed to deliver equal doses to the outside planes. An equivalent exception can be made for four-sided irradiation.

The task of calculating the maximum and minimum dose points in any bulk irradiator target thus requires only that one calculate doses in the midplane and outside planes of the target.

## VI. CALCULATION OF DOSE IN COMPLEX IRRADIATOR SYSTEMS

### A. *A Simple Calculational Model for Irradiator Calculations*

Up to this point the techniques discussed have dealt with radiation field calculations in simple geometries. The calculation of dose in very complex irradiator systems however, presents problems that in many cases require the use of specialized computer programs, computational aids, and approximation methods. To better understand some of the difficulties involved in these calculations it is helpful to examine a typical irradiator design concept. The single-slab, two-pass, single-direction irradiator with source overlap in Fig. 5.34 can be used as an example. For illustrative purposes let us also assume that this irradiator is a cobalt-60, stop-dwell system with a heterogeneous target consisting of regularly arranged cans of food with ten target lengths along the conveyor.

If one were to attempt to calculate the dose in this geometric configuration, dealing with each physical dimension rigorously, it would soon

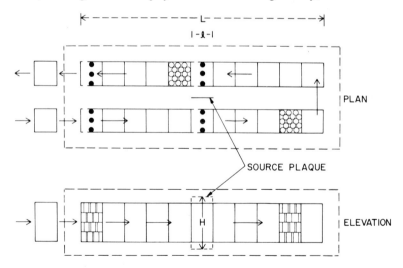

FIG. 5.34. Single-slab, two-pass single-direction irradiator with source overlap and heterogeneous target.

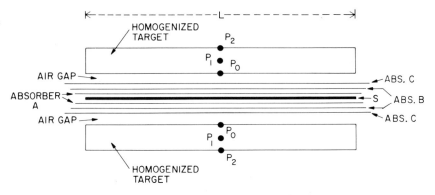

FIG. 5.35.   Calculational model.

become apparent that the computation could not be easily performed even using a high-speed computer.

It is evident that this concept must be modified, using approximation methods, to a form which is simpler but yet equivalent insofar as dose calculation is concerned.

The relatively simple calculational model shown in Fig. 5.35 is an equivalent system for calculating the maximum and minimum doses in the complicated irradiator shown in Fig. 5.34. In progressing from the real system to the calculational model it was necessary to make several assumptions and approximations which are discussed below.

**1.   Source Approximations.**    (a)    STATIC EQUIVALENT SYSTEM (SES). The designer must account for the fact that the target is irradiated from twenty different lateral positions during each irradiator cycle (in this illustration).   It is also necessary sometimes to account for the dose accumulated during transit time, which is the time it takes the package to enter and leave the irradiation chamber, to go from one irradiator position to another, and to go from one side of the source plaque to the other. The transit dose can be neglected only in those cases where it is a negligible part of the total accumulated dose. In the calculational model in Fig. 5.35 the effect of transit dose has been neglected and the source target system in Fig. 5.34 has been replaced with a static equivalent system to account for the multilateral position irradiation of the target.

A static equivalent system is a static representation of the irradiator geometry that yields results exactly equal to the results that would be obtained from the equivalent dynamic system. Static systems are generated by interchanging the source and target motions in the system. For example, if a target is moved in steps past a small source, the same dose will be accumulated if the target were kept stationary and the source made to move over the same path. Likewise, the same dose would be accumulated if the target were stationary and was irradiated with a large stationary source equal in length to the distance moved by the target in the real system.

The use of an SES here permits the calculation of the dose using a static source of height $H$, the height of the real source, and length $L$, the length of the target array in the real system (see Fig. 5.34).

It should be noted that the relatively simple SES generated in this example resulted from selecting the length of the real source, $l$, in the dynamic system, equal to that of the target carrier boxes in the real system. If these two lengths were not equal, the SES generated in a stop-dwell system of this type would be considerably more complicated. In most preliminary calculations, however, this assumption can usually be made without loss of accuracy.

More complete and detailed discussions of static equivalent systems can be found in Section VI. B, Refs. (*1*) and (*34*).

When an SES is used, it is necessary only to calculate the dose along the centerline of the target at points such as $P_0$, $P_1$, and $P_2$ in Fig. 5.35. The doses at these points are equivalent to the doses that would be accumulated in the real system when the target is indexed from one position to another. If there is symmetry in the irradiator, then the maximum and minimum doses ($D_{max}$ and $D_{min}$) could be found from the SES for stationary irradiators (see the discussion on static systems in Section VI. B) where:

$$D_{max} = D_0 + D_2$$

where $D_0$ is the dose at point $P_0$,..., etc. and $D_{min} = 2D_1$.

The doses found in this manner are centerline doses and as such are not the true maximum and minimum doses in the irradiator. The effects of lateral dose distributions and those of source overlap and boundary leakage must be taken into consideration. This is done by making corrections to the centerline doses based upon the computational aids which are discussed below.

(b) SOURCE SELF-ABSORPTION. In the calculational model self-absorption in the source is accounted for by assuming that the source is a hypothetically thin plane of source material attenuated by a cobalt metal absorber, semi-infinite in extent and equal in thickness to one-half the total thickness of the source. This is referred to as absorber "A" in

Fig. 5.35. (The source is "S".) This assumption has been found to be adequate for most irradiator calculations.

**2. Other Absorber Approximations.** Because the rectangular geometry is easy to handle mathematically, all absorbers in the computational model are represented by semiinfinite slabs of material with absorbers of similar material combined into single absorbers with thickness equal to the sum of the thicknesses of all the similar materials. For example, the stainless steel source cladding is represented by a semi-infinite slab of steel equal in thickness to the combined thicknesses of the first and second encapsulations. This is absorber "B" in the model. Absorber "B" in Fig. 5.35 should also incorporate any other stainless steel absorbers that may be present in the irradiator and located between the source and the target. Likewise, absorber "C" in the model can represent all of the aluminum present between the source and target.

**3. Other Assumptions.** In constructing the calculational model the following absorber and scattering effects can be assumed to be negligible:

(a)    The absorption and scattering effects in all air spaces. The effect of an air gap can be considered purely a geometrical one. In the model the thickness of the air gap is found by subtracting the space occupied by the source and other absorbers located between the source and the target from the total distance between the source and target on each side of the source plaque.

(b)    The attenuation in those absorbers that are positioned in planes perpendicular to the plane of the source. This includes similarly placed absorbers in the source, the conveyor carrier boxes and frames and supports located between the source and target. It does not include absorbers associated with the target material itself, such as food cans.

(c).    Differences in scattering effects resulting from absorber position. It can be assumed that all absorbers, positioned parallel to the plane of the source and located between the source and the target, have the same attenuation and buildup effects regardless of where they are located. For example, two 0.001-in. absorbers, one located on the top of the source and the other on the bottom of the target, can be treated as a single 0.002-in. absorber located anywhere between the source and the target.

**4. Heterogeneous Targets.** In the calculational model the heterogeneous target was replaced with a homogeneous one with a calculated "effective" density.

It is important when homogenizing the target that it be done on the basis of the unit cell of the product (see Fig. 5.36). When the effective density of the product is calculated simply by considering the inside volume

SQUARE ARRAY, CLOSE PACKED

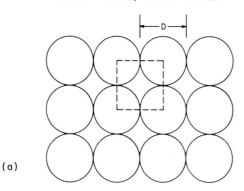

(a)

STAGGERED ARRAY, CLOSE PACKED          OPEN STAGGERED ARRAY

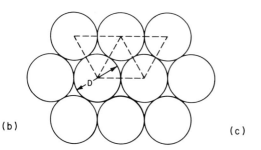

(b)

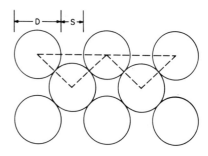

(c)

FIG. 5.36.  (a) Square array, close packed;  (b) staggered array, close packed;
(c) open staggered array.

of the conveyor carrier box and the mass of product in the carrier, serious
overestimations of the dose and of irradiator efficiency can result. Better
agreement between computation and experiment is obtained, however,
when the effective density is based upon the density of the unit cell formed
by the particular array of cans being used. Equations (5.15), (5.16), and
(5.17) are the recommended forms for calculating effective density for the
three different square and staggered arrays of food cans shown in Fig.
5.36.

Square array:

Effective density $= W/D^2h$                (5.15)

Staggered array, close packed:

Effective density $= 2W/(D^2h\sqrt{3})$        (5.16)

Open staggered array:

Effective density $= 2W/(D+S) h (3D^2-2DS-S^2)^{1/2}$    (5.17)

where $W =$ the total weight of the individual food can, including the weight of product and of the metal can, in grams; $D =$ diameter of the can, in cm; $S =$ spacing betweeen cans, in cm; and $h =$ height of individual food can, in cm.

A limitation of this method of target homogenizing occurs in the case of thin heterogeneous targets irradiated in multipass systems (for example, single rows of 3-in. diameter food cans in a four-pass irradiator). When dose calculations are performed using calculated effective densities, the results do not agree with experimental measurements for the system. Better agreement is obtained if, for example, in this case, the array is represented by a 3-in. thick homogeneous slab target with a density equal to the density of the product itself, neglecting the air spaces and the weight of the metal can.

The justification for using the homogenized target technique in irradiator calculations is illustrated in Fig. 5.37, which shows the result of experimental studies of the lateral and depth dose distributions inside food cans arranged in heterogeneous arrays. The study indicates that, when square or close-packed and open-staggered arrays of food cans are irradiated in large multipass continuous or stop-dwell irradiators, where the source itself or the source generated is extended (not a point or line), there are no lateral dose distributions that can be attributed to void spaces between the cans. The only distributions found (Fig. 5.37b and c) are those that would be predicted on the basis of the external spatial relationship of the target and the source.

It is also found that the minimum dose in the depth dose distribution always occurs at the centerplane of the target array, as would be predicted for a homogeneous target, and not near the center of a can.

**5. Source Overlap and Augmentation.**    As was stated previously, the effect of source overlap upon the minimum dose point may be neglected in the calculational model and taken into account as a correction to the centerline doses when the calculation is completed. It should be noted, however, that the overlap portion of the source must be included in the size of the source plaque in calculating the centerline doses.

Source augmentation may also be neglected in the calculational model as it is presented here. The effects of source augmentation and methods of calculating it will be discussed below.

**6. Boundary Effects.**    The finite nature of the target gives rise to gamma-ray "leakage" or "escape" at the target-air interfaces and other

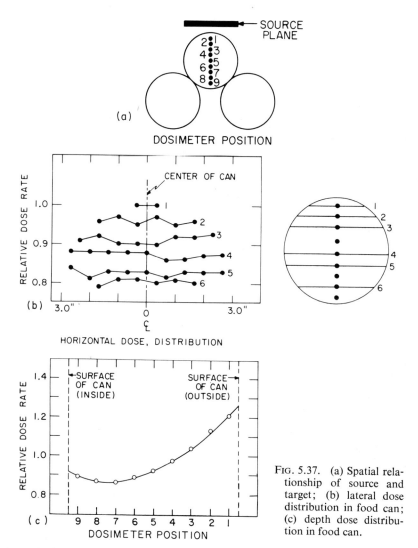

FIG. 5.37.  (a) Spatial relationship of source and target; (b) lateral dose distribution in food can; (c) depth dose distribution in food can.

boundaries. This usually results in overestimation of the dose at these points when the dose calculation is performed using infinite medium buildup factors, as is usually the case.

The effects of boundary leakage can be neglected in the calculational model. In most efficiently designed irradiators this effect is indeed negligible because of the presence of reflecting or scattering material in the vicinity of the target. When boundary effects are not negligible they must be accounted for as "after-the-fact" corrections (except when Monte Carlo calculations are used). These corrections will also be discussed below.

## B.    Computational Aids in Gamma Irradiator Design

In Section VI.A considerable space was devoted (1) to developing a calculational model for complex gamma irradiators, (2) to elaborating on the simplifications that may be made with the geometry, and (3) to listing the approximations that can be made.

The need for a simplified calculational model arises from the fact that actual irradiator geometries defy rigorous calculation using the usual computer techniques. Furthermore, the use of the calculational model together with other approximation methods and computational aids makes it possible to evaluate accurately and quickly dose distributions in irradiators without using high-speed computers. (It is recommended, however, that for the most accurate results computers be used whenever they are available.)

In this section computer programs as well as other computational aids and approximation techniques available for dose calculations will be listed and described.

**1.    Computer Programs.**    Rigorous solution of gamma photon energy transport is quite complicated for finite source target geometries. In fact, techniques such as the method of moments lend themselves only to simple and idealized geometries such as a point isotropic source, or a plane monodirectional source in an infinite medium. Monte Carlo methods (5) offer a means of solution but require unreasonably large amounts of computer time and storage and become quite complex for multiboundary systems.

The method used most often in those computer codes written specifically for or adaptable to irradiator calculations is that of "point kernel" integration.

Two such computer code series are the FUDGE series developed at Brookhaven National Laboratory and the QAD series developed at Los Alamos National Laboratory.

(a)    FUDGE SERIES COMPUTER CODES.    The FUDGE series codes were written at Brookhaven National Laboratory specifically for plane source gamma irradiator dose calculations. The codes use a calculation method indirectly based on a point kernel integration over a source area by means of Gauss quadrature techniques rather than point-by-point integration. The available FUDGE series programs are listed below:

(1) FUDGE-3. This computer code calculates the specific dose rate due to uncollided flux from any finite plane isotropic gamma source in an infinite homogeneous water target at any point in the target. This program is unpublished, but a FORTRAN listing is available from Brookhaven National Laboratory.

(2) FUDGE 3A. This code calculates the specific dose rate distribution from any finite plane isotropic gamma source in an infinite homogeneous target at any point in the target, based on a modified 12-point Gauss quadrature integration over the source plane. Buildup due to multiple scattering may be included as the sum of up to three exponentials. FORTRAN listing can be found in Ref. (1), together with the required input data and input format.

(3) FUDGE 4. This code handles problems involving several absorbers and air gaps. The program is basically identical to FUDGE 3A; however, it sums up the total absorber thickness to a point in the target from the source plane and calculates a fictitious mean free path or linear absorption coefficient based on the total linear distance. This calculation is performed for all depths of interest in the target. For FORTRAN listing and other information see Ref. (1).

(4) FUDGE 4A. This code is a substantially modified and updated version of FUDGE 4, with increased accuracy, efficiency, and applicability. This new version was written in FORTRAN IV for use with the CDC 6600 computer at Brookhaven National Laboratory. For listings and other information see Ref. (17a).

(5) GIRD. This program is essentially a FUDGE series program written specifically to calculate directly the dose in the "shuffle-dwell" type irradiator (two-direction, multipass type irradiator). The code can also be used to calculate the dose from source plaques with nonuniformly distributed source activity, such as is used in source activity augmentation techniques. Listings and all pertinent information can be found in Ref. (17b).

(b) QAD SERIES CODES. As mentioned above, there are numerous computer codes that perform a numerical summation of the contribution to the dose rate of the individual kernels. The codes differ in details in the way the input describes the boundary between regions, the source spatial distribution, and especially in the way that the buildup is treated.

The QAD code (*7,8*), which is a point kernel code developed by the Los Alamos Scientific Laboratory, is a good example of this technique since versions of the programs are readily available in FORTRAN IV. In the QAD program the gamma-ray source is represented by a number of point isotropic sources, and the line of sight distance is computed from each source point to the predetermined and input detector point. The attenuation is calculated from the path length through the attenuating regions and the characteristics of the shielding materials. On the basis of this attenuation the energy transferred along the line of sight and the appropriate buildup factor (*7*) to account for the scattered radiation are then calculated. For a source emitting a range of gamma-ray energies, the point kernel, including the buildup, is summed over the source volume for each source point and the source energy spectrum.

There are several versions of QAD:

(1)   QAD-IV, the general-purpose basic QAD prototype that estimates the uncollided gamma-ray flux, dose rate, and energy deposition at specified detector points (and also the fast-neutron dose).

(2)   QAD-P5, which incorporates a technique for interpolating the results of neutron calculations, has additional source description routines, and has an increased number of output options.

(3)   QAD-HD, which evaluates the heat deposition and temperature rise of the propellant and the dose to a crew during nuclear rocket reactor operation.

(4)   QAD-P-5, another version of QAD-P5, which includes a built-in library of gamma-ray attenuation coefficients, buildup factor coefficients, neutron removal cross sections, and neutron moments-method spectra coefficients.

(5)   QAD-INT, which calculates gamma-ray heating rates within a source region or in a semi-infinite region surrounding the source zone, as well as unscattered and built-up fluxes and dose rates.

(6)   QAD-V, which permits heating calculations with a two-dimensional integration scheme.

(7)   QAD-8, which is an expanded version of QAD-P5 with a simplified input format and a more detailed output format that includes a data library of many of the required input parameters.

The use of a point kernel code such as QAD is probably the most straightforward approach to computing gamma-ray fields.

(c)   NUMERICAL SUMMATION OF LINE SOURCES USING THE QAD CODE. Another method especially useful for finite slabs [see Ref. (*18*)] which can be readily programed for a digital computer involves the integration of the point kernel analytically to obtain the results for a line source. The slab is subdivided into $N$ equivalent lines and the contribution to the dose due to each line source is numerically summed.

The model is very flexible allowing as input the source plane length and height, and the number of equivalent lines one chooses to use in the approximation. $N$ is selected to be large enough so that the change in the value of the computed dose rate is negligible as $N$ is increased further.

**2. Other Computational Aids and Approximation Techniques.** When high-speed computers are not available, the dose in an irradiator can be evaluated using (1) the computational model developed in Section VI.A; (2) static equivalent systems; (3) approximation techniques for estimating lateral dose distributions, effects of source overlap and augmentation and boundary corrections; and (4) computational aids for evaluating centerline depth dose distributions.

(a) TARGET MOTION AND STATIC EQUIVALENT SYSTEMS. Static equivalent systems (SES) were discussed in Section VI.A. There the SES for the one-direction stop-dwell irradiator was used along with that for the stationary type of irradiator to set up the simplified calculational model for irradiator calculations. In this section the SES models for some other types of irradiators will be illustrated.

(1) Static Equivalent Systems (SES). Target motion in an irradiator system can complicate the problem of dose calculation unless SES are used. The use of SES is discussed in detail in Ref. ($1$).

To illustrate how these systems are used, simplified SES for the three basic types of rectangular source irradiators are presented here.

(b) GENERALIZED SES FOR STATIONARY-TYPE IRRADIATORS. Figure 5.38 is the SES for a stationary irradiator. This model is intended for the calculation of the dose along the centerline of the source plaque with the following assumptions: (1) that the transit dose can be neglected; (2) that lateral distributions can be estimated from centerline doses; (3) that each target package occupies every irradiator position in sequence during each irradiator cycle; (4) that each irradiator position is filled at all times; and (5) that adjacent target packages are butted or touching. In the equivalent dynamic system (Fig. 5.14) target points $A$ and $B$ are located at the center of the outside surfaces of the target packages and point $C$ is located at the center of the midplane of the unit package. In the static system (Fig. 5.38), points $P_0$ through $P_6$ and $P'_0$ through $P'_6$ are fixed locations in the irradiator on either side of the source plaque.

If there is symmetry in the irradiator and if each target carrier resides

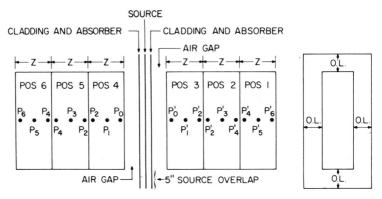

FIG. 5.38.    Static equivalent system for stationary-type irradiator.

for an equal period of time at each irradiator position during each pass through the irradiator, the dose received by outside target points $A$ and $B$ of the dynamic system can be expressed in terms of static doses and can be represented by the general equation:

$$D_B = D_A + D_0 + D_n + 2(D_{n-2} + D_{n-4} + \ldots + D_2)$$

where $D_B = D_A = D_{max}$,
$\quad n$ = total number of passes in the irradiator, and
$\quad D_n$ = the total dose at point $P_n$.
Likewise,

$$D_C = D_{min} = 2(D_{n-1} + D_{n-3} + D_{n-5} \ldots + D_1)$$

The general equation for the depth of the target points ($P_i$), where $i = 0 \rightarrow n$, is

$$\text{Depth of } P_i = i(z/2),$$

where $z$ is the thickness of the unit target package.

(c)  SINGLE-DIRECTION MULTIPASS IRRADIATORS.    These systems can be either of the stop-dwell or continuous motion type. In both these systems the technique used involves the use of two SES forms. The first reduces the dynamic system to the SES for stationary irradiators described above, and the second, the SES for stationary irradiators, is used to calculate the dose.

(1)  Single-Direction Stop-Dwell Irradiator.    A typical single direction, stop-dwell irradiator is shown in Fig. 5.39. In this irradiator the length of the irradiation chamber is "$L$" ("$L$" is also the total length of the target

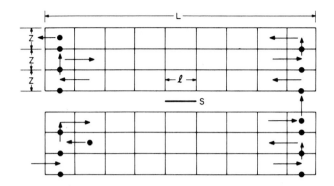

FIG. 5.39. Typical single-direction-type irradiator.

array in each pass) and the thickness of the unit package is $z$. As was pointed out in Section VI.A, when the source is equal in length to the length of the unit package $l$, the dynamic system can be replaced with the simple static system shown in Fig. 5.40. In the static system the real source has been replaced with one whose height is the same as that of the real source but whose length is equal to the length $L$ of the irradiator. The target points which are of interest are $P_0$ through $P_6$ on both sides of the source plaque. The line formed by these points is perpendicular to the center of the source plaque.

*(2) Continuous Motion, Single-Direction Irradiators.* The static equivalent system for the continuous motion, single-direction irradiator is the

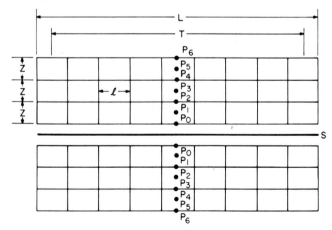

FIG. 5.40. Static equivalent system for single-direction-type irradiator.

same as the one shown for the stop-dwell system. In both systems the real
source plaque is replaced by one which is of the same height and whose
length is equal to the length of the irradiation chamber $L$. In both cases

$$L = T + l,$$

where $T$ is the total distance traveled by the target and $l$ is the length of
the unit target package and of the source.

In this system the relationship between the target size and the source
size is not significant as it is in the stop-dwell system.

An important limitation on this system is that the length of the static
equivalent source $L$ must be no less than six to seven times the length of
the real source. When this ratio becomes as low as 6:1 the error between
the actual dose in the dynamic system and the dose calculated using the
static system begins to become significant (1% or more).

The dose in the static system and the dose in the real or dynamic system
are related in the following way. The centerline dose rate in the static system, when multiplied by the total target residence time in the real irradiator, is equal to the integrated dose accumulated at a point in the target
package in traversing the distance $T$ in the real system. This relationship
is valid if the following conditions are satisfied: The heights of the real

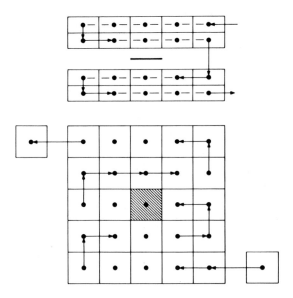

Fig. 5.41.   Typical two-direction-type irradiator.

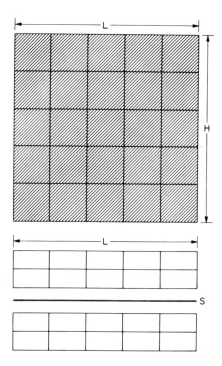

FIG. 5.42.  Static equivalent system for two-direction-type irradiator.

and the static equivalent sources must be equal; both sources must contain the same total number of curies.

The relationship and conditions should be studied carefully and the
reader should be certain that they are thoroughly understood before
they are applied.

*(3)  Two-Direction, Multipass Irradiator.*  Although it is possible for
a two-direction irradiator to be either of the continuous or stop-dwell
type, the continuous motion type is not a practical design and will not
be considered here.

The SES for the two-direction, stop-dwell system is found in a manner
similar to its single-direction counterpart.

The irradiator shown in Fig. 5.41 is a typical multipass, multiposition,
two-direction, stop-dwell motion system. In this system there are twenty-
five target positions on each source pass and four passes. This system can
be replaced by the static system illustrated in Fig. 5.42.

As in the case of the single-direction irradiators, if the target and source
motions are interchanged, a source plaque is generated that is equal in

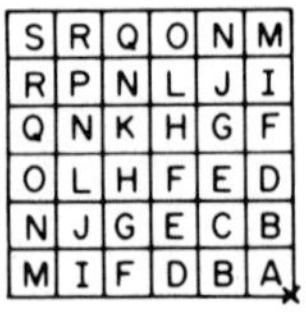

| S | R | Q | O | N | M |
|---|---|---|---|---|---|
| R | P | N | L | J | I |
| Q | N | K | H | G | F |
| O | L | H | F | E | D |
| N | J | G | E | C | B |
| M | I | F | D | B | A |

FIG. 5.43.    Square source element.

size to the target array shown in the dynamic system (Fig. 5.41). The length of the static equivalent source is $L$ and its height is $H$.

As in the case of the one-direction irradiators, this static equivalent system is used with the SES for stationary irradiators to find the center-line doses. When the source and target sizes are not equal, the resulting static equivalent systems are complicated.

In the calculational model in Fig. 5.35, the effects of transit dose have been neglected, as they can be in most irradiator calculations. In those cases where the transit dose is not a negligible entity and must be calculated, the static equivalent system method can be applied in a separate but similar calculation. In transit dose calculations, the transit motion must be considered a continuous one, and while the SES is the same as for the stop-dwell systems demonstrated above, the dose cannot be found simply from superimposed dose rates, but must take the total residence time in the irradiator into consideration, as stated above. For detailed discussions see Refs. (*1*) and (*34*).

### C.    Aids for Calculating Centerline Depth Dose Distributions

**1.    Plane Source Superposition Method.**    The source superposition method was designed to provide a simple and accurate technique for synthesizing dose distributions for hypothetically thin plane sources imbedded in an infinite homogeneous water medium. The data are tabulated as the specific dose rate contribution at a point in the medium from a small source element as it is placed at various grid positions in a plane through-

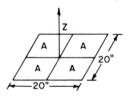

FIG. 5.44.    Square source geometry: central position.

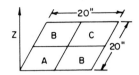

FIG. 5.45.   Square source geometry: corner position.

out the medium. By summing up or superimposing the contributions from the source element in its various positions it is possible to generate dose distribution information for plane sources of any size and shape at any point in the medium.

In Fig. 5.43, a 10 × 10-in. source element is shown in numerous positions, lettered A through S. The source positions are arranged symmetrically about the point X, which is located at the corner of source position A. The dose rate at X from any combination of these source positions can be obtained by simply summing up their contributions to the dose rate at point X.

For example, the specific dose rate along the central axis of a 20 × 20-in. plane source at a distance $z$ from the plane is four times the contribution at point X from source position A at distance $z$ (see Fig. 5.44). Likewise, the specific dose rates at the corner and the edge of a 20 × 20-in. plane source would be found by adding the contributions from the following positions:

Corner dose = A + (2 × B) + C      (Fig. 5.45)
Edge dose   = 2(A + B)      (Fig. 5.46)

In Table 5.5 the specific rates from 10 × 10-in. source elements in positions A through S in an infinite water medium at distances from the source plane ranging from 1 to 12 in. are tabulated for cobalt-60 sources. The target-to-source distance is the perpendicular distance to the plane from the point X as shown in Fig. 5.43 to 5.46. Superposition tables are available for cesium-137 as well as cobalt-60 and for 10 × 10-in., 5 × 5-in., 2.5 × 2.5-in., and 1 × 1-in. plane source elements. These are tabulated in Ref. (1).

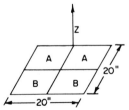

FIG. 5.46.   Square source geometry: edge position.

TABLE
DOSE RATE FROM $10 \times 10$-IN. PLANE

| | | | | Specific dose rate, | |
| $d^a$ | $A^b$ | B | C | D | E |
|---|---|---|---|---|---|
| 1 | $4.558 \times 10^4$ | $2.207 \times 10^3$ | $5.954 \times 10^2$ | $2.528 \times 10^2$ | $1.170 \times 10^2$ |
| 2 | 3.117 | 2.145 | 5.69 | 2.508 | 1.135 |
| 3 | 2.296 | 2.048 | 5.500 | 2.500 | 1.099 |
| 4 | 1.744 | 1.930 | 5.312 | 2.400 | 1.064 |
| 5 | 1.347 | 1.790 | 5.050 | 2.295 | 1.029 |
| 6 | 1.052 | 1.640 | 4.720 | 2.169 | $9.932 \times 10$ |
| 7 | $8.272 \times 10^3$ | 1.494 | 4.400 | 1.940 | 9.579 |
| 8 | 6.540 | 1.324 | 4.130 | 1.880 | 9.225 |
| 9 | 5.200 | 1.176 | 3.750 | 1.810 | 8.871 |
| 10 | 4.149 | 1.033 | 3.450 | 1.709 | 8.518 |
| 11 | 3.320 | $9.05 \times 10^2$ | 3.090 | 1.570 | 8.165 |
| 12 | 2.667 | 7.855 | 2.810 | 1.428 | 7.800 |
| | K | L | M | N | O |
| 1 | 6.800 | 5.350 | 3.530 | 2.870 | 2.000 |
| 2 | 6.705 | 5.209 | 3.486 | 2.836 | 1.980 |
| 3 | 6.609 | 5.068 | 3.443 | 2.803 | 1.960 |
| 4 | 6.514 | 4.927 | 3.399 | 2.769 | 1.940 |
| 5 | 6.418 | 4.786 | 3.356 | 2.736 | 1.920 |
| 6 | 6.323 | 4.646 | 3.312 | 2.702 | 1.900 |
| 7 | 6.227 | 4.505 | 3.268 | 2.668 | 1.880 |
| 8 | 6.132 | 4.364 | 3.225 | 2.635 | 1.860 |
| 9 | 6.036 | 4.223 | 3.181 | 2.601 | 1.840 |
| 10 | 5.941 | 4.082 | 3.137 | 2.567 | 1.820 |
| 11 | 5.846 | 3.941 | 3.094 | 2.534 | 1.800 |
| 12 | 5.750 | 3.800 | 3.050 | 2.500 | 1.780 |

$^a d$=distance from target point to source plane, inches.

The superposition method is usually used in irradiator calculations along with scale modeling techniques, which will be discussed below.

**2. Disk Source Approximation.** In some cases it is possible to use a disk source approximation when plane source dose distribution information is needed. With this method one can obtain information similar to that obtained from the plane source superposition method described above.

When calculating the dose from a plane rectangular source, the technique usually involves the calculation of the dose from a disk source of equal area. The approximation is most useful for centerline points of square or nearly square plane sources but can be used for other plaque shapes by superpositioning doses from several plaques. The disk source calculation is described in detail in Ref. (*12*) as well as in Section IV.C.4.

5.5
COBALT-60 SOURCE AT VARIOUS PLANE POSITIONS

rads/hr per Ci/cm²

| F | G | H | I | J |
|---|---|---|---|---|
| $4.250 \times 10$ | $2.850 \times 10$ | $1.500 \times 10$ | $1.120 \times 10$ | 8.650 |
| 4.150 | 2.793 | 1.475 | 1.102 | 8.523 |
| 4.050 | 2.736 | 1.449 | 1.085 | 8.396 |
| 3.950 | 2.678 | 1.424 | 1.067 | 8.268 |
| 3.850 | 2.621 | 1.398 | 1.049 | 8.141 |
| 3.750 | 2.564 | 1.373 | 1.031 | 8.014 |
| 3.650 | 2.506 | 1.347 | 1.014 | 7.886 |
| 3.550 | 2.449 | 1.322 | $9.959 \times 10^0$ | 7.759 |
| 3.450 | 2.392 | 1.296 | 9.782 | 7.632 |
| 3.350 | 2.335 | 1.271 | 9.605 | 7.505 |
| 3.250 | 2.277 | 1.246 | 9.427 | 7.377 |
| 3.150 | 2.220 | 1.220 | 9.250 | 7.250 |

| P | Q | R | S |
|---|---|---|---|
| 1.420 | 1.180 | $6.500 \times 10^{-1}$ | $3.450 \times 10^{-1}$ |
| 1.406 | 1.169 | 6.441 | 3.405 |
| 1.391 | 1.158 | 6.382 | 3.359 |
| 1.376 | 1.147 | 6.323 | 3.314 |
| 1.362 | 1.136 | 6.264 | 3.268 |
| 1.347 | 1.255 | 6.205 | 3.223 |
| 1.333 | 1.115 | 6.146 | 3.177 |
| 1.318 | 1.104 | 6.086 | 3.132 |
| 1.304 | 1.093 | 6.027 | 3.086 |
| 1.289 | 1.082 | 5.968 | 3.041 |
| 1.275 | 1.071 | 5.909 | 3.000 |
| 1.260 | 1.060 | 5.850 | 2.950 |

[b]Positions A to S refer to source positions as shown in Fig. 5.43.

**3. Tabulated Dose Distribution Data.** In Refs. (*30*) and (*31*) tabulated dose distribution "look-up" data have been made available for use in gamma irradiator design calculations.

The first of these reports is entitled "Tabulated Dose Distribution Data for Gamma Irradiator Design" (BNL 50147). The data presented in the tables are centerline depth dose distributions in semi-infinite homogeneous media over a range of densities (0.1–1.3 g/cc) from both cobalt-60 and cesium-137 square source plaques of various sizes (from 10 × 10-in. to 120 × 120-in.). The targets are assumed to be bounded only at the front surface by the source, air gap, and absorbers. The calculation also assumes that the target material is present on both sides of the plaque. The thickness of the sources and of the absorbers between the source and the target

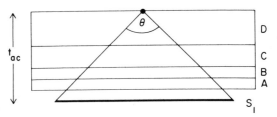

FIG. 5.47.   Scaling geometry.

are treated as constants (0.036-in. stainless steel, 0.25-in. aluminum, and 0.060-in. cobalt metal or 0.25-in. cesium chloride), and the air gap was varied (0 to 7.0-in.).

The second report is entitled "Tabulated Dose Uniformity Ratio and Minimum Dose Data for Gamma Irradiator Design" (BNL 50145). The data in the tables are calculated values of the centerline uniformity ratios and the minimum doses in 2, 4, and 6-pass irradiators using target thicknesses from 2 to 12 in. The calculation was performed for irradiator parameters identical to those used in BNL 50147 (30).

**4.  Scale Modeling Techniques.**   It is often convenient to use scale modeling techniques with the plane superposition method or the disk source approximation to evaluate dose rates for material densities other than 1.0 g/cc or for points in a target with interposed absorbing material and air gaps. Briefly, modeling depends upon transferring from material of one density to material of another density while maintaining constant total attenuation, multiple scattering and solid angle, assuming that the mass absorption cross sections of both materials are the same or reasonably similar.

The basis for this procedure has been explained by various workers such as Dove (28) and Johnson (29). A detailed discussion of this subject can also be found in Ref. (1). The principles are best illustrated by an example. In the cross-sectional view shown in Fig. 5.47 plane angles are considered rather than the actual solid angle for reasons of simplicity.

Figure 5.47 shows the cross section of an actual system consisting of of absorbers A and B, air gap C, and target D. Figure 5.48 shows an arrangement that preserves the angle and in which the total attenuation is preserved, but the absorbers A and B and the air gap C have been replaced with their water equivalents.

The water equivalent distance $t_{we}$ is

$$t_{we} = \frac{\Sigma \mu t}{\mu_w} = \frac{\mu_A t_A + \mu_B t_B + \mu_C t_C + \mu_D t_D}{\mu_w}$$

A scale factor $(SF)$ is found from the actual distance $t_{ac}$ in the real system and the water equivalent distance $t_{we}$ and is equal to

$$SF = t_{we}/t_{ac}$$

The size of the source in the scaled model is found by multiplying each dimension of the real plaque by the scale factor.

The dose in the real system is equivalent to and can be calculated from the scaled model case of a plane source imbedded in an infinite homogeneous water medium provided the model source has the same activity per unit area as the real source. The use of scale modeling techniques can simplify dose calculations for complicated heterogeneous target systems using the disk source approximation and high-speed computers, and makes possible the use of "look-up data," such as the superposition method.

**5. Boundary Corrections.** The accurate calculation of dose distributions in a finite target depends on the knowledge of the buildup at or near the boundaries of the target. Currently the information available is inadequate for the accurate handling of all finite medium problems. The data at hand are primarily applicable to either point source or plane monodirectional sources and are limited to the case of one boundary. For a more complete discussion of finite buildup factors and dose distributions near and at the interface between two media of different densities, the reader is referred to Berger and Doggett (22), Galanter and Rizzo (15), and Ref. (1).

As previously stated, in most irradiators boundary effects are not considered a serious problem because of the presence of scattering medium in the vicinity of the target.

**6. Effects of Source Overlap and Source Activity Augmentation.** The effects of source overlap are adequately accounted for by using the plotted experimental data in Figs. 5.30, 5.31, and 5.32 in Section V.D of this chapter and the criteria cited for lateral distributions in the three basic types of irradiators.

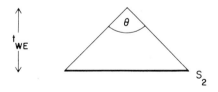

FIG. 5.48. Equivalent geometry.

Source activity augmentation problems can be solved with either the GIRD, FUDGE series computer codes or by using the plane source superposition method.

## VII.   HEAT GENERATION

It can be stated that the major consideration regarding heat absorption concerns the irradiator source rather than the target. Much larger radiation fluxes exist within the source and the source absorption coefficient is much higher than the target; therefore, temperature rises within the source will be much more significant than rises within the target.

Methods used to calculate the fraction of gamma energy absorbed in sources are described in (*32*). To this one must add the beta energy that may be considered totally absorbed within the source. The computer code QAD (*7,8*) can be used to calculate the gamma-ray heating in the target. The reader is also referred to standard textbooks on heat transfer such as Jakob (*35*).

Heat losses within targets and sources must also be known or calculated to obtain the net heating rate in order to calculate true temperature rises. For high specific activities and high heating rates source temperature rises may be significantly large to require forced cooling.

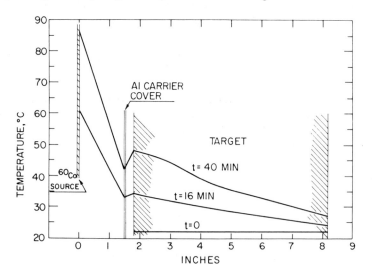

FIG. 5.49.   Thermal gradient in a phenolic target.

Some typical measurements made for a noninsulated phenolic target irradiated by a 35 × 30-in. vertical plaque of cobalt-60 in still air, where the average source specific activity was 54 Ci/g, are shown in Fig. 5.49. Figure 5.49 depicts the thermal gradient through the source and target after 0, 16, and 40 min of irradiation time. The dose rate at the target frontal face was approximately $12.0 \times 10^6$ rads/hr. The curve shows that the temperature rise at the front face was 26 °C above room temperature after 40 min. The accumulated dose at that point was $8.0 \times 10^6$ rad.

## VIII.   ILLUSTRATIVE EXAMPLE

### A.   Design Requirements

1.   The target to be a food product with an effective density of 0.7 g/cc.
2.   The throughput to be 290 lb/hr.
3.   The minimum dose to be 2.5 megarads.
4.   Uniformity ratio to be 1.20
5.   Maximum residence time in the irradiator to be 21 hr.
6.   The unit package to be rectangular in shape. The size of the package unspecified.
7.   Source material: cobalt-60.

### B.   Design Tasks

**1.   To Select an Irradiator Geometry.**   On the basis of the uniformity ratio requirement of 1.20, which is a difficult one to meet, the irradiator most suited would be the two-direction, multipass type, since this system is capable of delivering lowest uniformity ratios with highest efficiencies. For the purpose of this illustration the four-pass, two-direction type of system shown in Figs. 5.20 and 5.41 will be used. This system has a 5 × 5-unit package array on each of the four passes.

**2.   Design of the Unit Package.**   (a) OPTIMIZE THE TARGET THICK-NESS.   This is accomplished quickly and easily by using the data for uniformity ratios in Ref. (30). For this purpose centerline dose distribution data for a very large (infinite) plaque should be used since in two-directional systems very large plaques are generated.

On page 61 of Ref. (30) centerline uniformity data are tabulated for a 120 × 120-in. cobalt-60 plaque, using a 0.7 g/cc target in a four-pass irradiator with a source to target air gap of 3.0 in. These data are reproduced in the following:

| Target thickness (in.) | Uniformity ratio |
|:---:|:---:|
| 2 | 1.031 |
| 4 | 1.093 |
| 6 | 1.177 |
| 8 | 1.283 |
| 10 | 1.412 |
| 12 | 1.564 |

For best results, these data could be plotted as uniformity ratio ($U$) vs. target thickness ($z$). For purposes of brevity in this illustration this will not be done, but it will be assumed that the 4 in. thick target with a center-line uniformity of 1.093 is the optimum. This would allow between 5 and 10% for lateral dose variations in the target. [Note: If the reference data in (30) are not used, several lengthy irradiator calculations would have to be performed.]

(b) DETERMINE THE LENGTH AND WIDTH (OR THE CROSS-SECTIONAL AREA) OF THE UNIT PACKAGE. These are found from (1) the target thickness which was found above, (2) the throughput of the irradiator, (3) the number of dwell positions in the irradiator (100, 25 on each pass), and (4) the maximum residence time in the irradiator (21 hr).

If a target package must occupy 100 irradiator positions in 21 hr (1260 min), then the maximum time it could spend at each position is 12.6 min, or 12 min if time is allowed for target transit from position to position. This implies that one target carrier must leave the irradiator every 12 min (5 carriers per hour).

If the throughput is 290 lb/hr, then each target carrier contains approximately 58.0 lb of product and has a volume of 1.33 ft$^3$. Since the target thickness is set at 4.0 in. (or 0.33 ft), then the cross-sectional area is 4.0 ft$^2$. For convenience in this illustration the unit package size will therefore be set at 2 × 2 × 0.33 ft (or 24 × 24 × 4 in.).

3. **Determination of the Total Source Activity Required.** To do this it is first necessary to perform a dose calculation in the irradiator selected for use here. This is best done using one of the computer programs referred to in Section VI.B. However, it can also be done using the computer aids that have been discussed.

The statement of the dose calculation problem is as follows:

a. **Irradiator Parameters**
(1) Source: cobalt-60
(2) Source plaque (active size): 24 × 24 in. (This size was selected

to be the same as the target size to simplify the problem).
(3) Cobalt metal thickness: 0.06 in.
(4) Source-to-target air gap: 3.0 in.
(5) Source cladding: doubly encapsulated in stainless steel ($\rho = 7.8$ g/cc); total thickness of the stainless steel, 0.036 in.
(6) Target: food products ($\rho = 0.7$ g/cc).
(7) Unit target dimensions: $24 \times 24 \times 4$ in, thick.
(8) Other absorbers between the source and target planes: 0.25 in. of aluminum ($\rho = 2.7$ g/cc). This includes the metal in the carrier boxes as well as any other aluminum absorbers present.
(9) Irradiator geometry: The two-direction, four pass, shuffle-dwell irradiator in Fig. 5.41. This irradiator has a $5 \times 5$ target array with the source located at the center of the array.

b. **Procedure:** Calculate the maximum and minimum doses in this system.

Before the calculation can proceed, a static equivalent system and a simplified calculational model must be set up in the manner described in Sections VI.A and VI.B.

The static equivalent system calculational model is the one shown in Fig. 5.41. It consists of a $120 \times 120$-in. stationary plane source and a stationary target consisting of 4 semi-infinite slab targets (2 on each side of the plane), each 4.0 in. thick with a material density of 0.7 g/cc.

Between the plane source and the target, on each side of the source there are three semi-infinite plane absorbers and a 3.0-in. air gap. The three absorbers are (1) a 0.03-in. cobalt metal absorber (one-half the thickness of the source), (2) a 0.036-in. stainless steel absorber, and (3) a 0.25-in. aluminum absorber.

The centerline maximum and minimum doses for this irradiator can be obtained quickly from the tabulated data in either Refs. (30) or (31).

If the dose distribution data in Ref. (31) are used, the dose rates can be found on page 35, tabulated under cobalt-60, $120 \times 120$ in, slab source, $Z = 4$ in., and air gap is 3.0 in.

*Note:* The absorber thicknesses used in calculating the doses for that report are the same as those selected in this illustrative example.

The maximum dose

$$D_{max} = D_0 + D_4 + 2D_2$$

and the minimum dose

$$D_{min} = 2(D_3 + D_1)$$

The depths of target points are (in inches):

$$P_0 = 0$$
$$P_1 = 2.0$$
$$P_2 = 4.0$$
$$P_3 = 6.0$$
$$P_4 = 8.0$$

The centerline specific dose rates from Ref. (*31*) are (in rads/hr/Ci/cm²):

$$D_0 = 19.65 \times 10^4$$
$$D_1 = 12.99 \times 10^4$$
$$D_2 = 9.38 \times 10^4$$
$$D_3 = 7.02 \times 10^4$$
$$D_4 = 5.36 \times 10^4$$

and

$$D_{max} = (19.65 + 5.36 + 2 \times 9.38)\ 10^4\ \text{rads/hr/Ci/cm}^3$$
$$= 43.77 \times 10^4\ \text{rads/hr/Ci/cm}^3$$
$$D_{min} = 2(7.02 + 12.99) \times 10^4\ \text{rads/hr/Ci/cm}^3$$
$$= 40.02 \times 10^4\ \text{rads/hr/Ci/cm}^2$$
$$U_c = \text{Centerline uniformity ratio} = 1.094$$

These are total centerline specific dose rates and the time is in terms of dwell time (the time the target spends at each dwell position).

Again in this case the total centerline minimum specific dose rate and the uniformity ratio can be found directly from Ref. (*30*). From that report:

$$U = 1.093$$
$$D_{min} = 40.03 \times 10^4\ \text{rads/hr/Ci/cm}^2$$

To this point the doses calculated were centerline doses. While the maximum dose is a true one, the minimum dose is not. From the criteria stated in Section V.D, the minimum dose must be reduced by 5–10%. The value selected will depend upon how successful the mechanical designer is in eliminating unnecessary absorbers near the target and upon the final physical dimensions of the source plaque and the target boxes. For purposes of this illustration 7.5% variation in the midplane of the target will be selected.

Reducing the minimum dose by 7.5%:

$$D_{min} = 40.02 \times 0.925 \times 10^4$$
$$= 37.02 \times 10^4\ \text{rads/hr/Ci/cm}^2$$

$$D_{max} = 43.77 \times 10^4 \text{ rads/hr/Ci/cm}^2$$
$$U = 43.77/37.02 = 1.18$$

From the throughput of 290 lb/hr (5 carrier boxes per hour) and the minimum dose requirement of 2.5 megarads, the total source strength required in the irradiator can be calculated.

*Before proceeding it is important to note that the source strength requirements cannot be based on the large static equivalent plaque size (in this case 120 × 120 in.). It must be based upon the real plaque size of 24 × 24 in.*

If a throughput rate of one box per hour at a minimum dose of $37.02 \times 10^4$ rads requires a plaque activity of 1 Ci/cm² (total curies = 3716), then a throughput rate of 5 boxes per hour, with a minimum dose of 2.5 megarads will require:

$$\text{Total activity} = \frac{5 \times 2.5 \times 10^6 \text{ rads} \times 3716 \text{ Ci}}{37.02 \times 10^4 \text{ rads}}$$
$$= 1.25 \times 10^5 \text{ Ci}$$

or a surface activity of the source plaque:

$$S_a = 33.6 \text{ Ci/cm}^2$$

The specific activity of the required cobalt is:

$$S_g = \frac{\text{Total activity (Ci)}}{\text{Weight of cobalt metal (g)}} = \frac{1.25 \times 10^5 \text{ (Ci)}}{5.93 \times 10^3 \text{ (g)}} = 211 \text{ Ci/g}$$

c. **Utilization Efficiency** (see Section V.B)

$$E_u = \frac{1.26 \text{ (watts/megarads - lb/hr)} \times 2.5 \text{ megarads} \times 290 \text{ lb}}{0.0148 \text{ (watts/Ci)} \times 1.25 \times 10^5 \text{ (Ci)}}$$
$$= 0.490 \text{ or } 49.0\%$$

d. The parameters of source and target height and length, source activity, and irradiator efficiency must at this point be optimized through a series of trial and error calculations. This will not be undertaken in this illustrative example; however, in practice, it is best to use a high-speed computer for this purpose.

## REFERENCES

*1.* B. Manowitz, R. H. Bretton, L. Galanter, and F. X. Rizzo, "Computational Methods of Gamma Irradiator Design," U.S. AEC Rept. BNL 889 (T-361), December 1964.

2.   W. Heitler, *Quantum Theory of Radiation,* 3rd Ed., Oxford University Press, 1954.
3.   R. D. Evans, *The Atomic Nucleus,* McGraw-Hill, New York, 1955.
4.   H.A. Bethe and T. Ashkin, in *Experimental Nuclear Physics* (E. Segré, ed.), Vol. 1, John Wiley and Sons, Inc., 1953.
5.   R.G. Jaeger (Editor-in-Chief), *Engineering Compendium on Radiation Shielding,* Vol. 1, Shielding Fundamentals and Methods, Springer Verlag, 1968.
6.   "Reactor Physics Constants," U.S. AEC Rept. ANL-5800, 2nd Ed. July 1963.
7.   R. E. Malenfant, "QAD: A Series of Point Kernel General Purpose Shielding Programs," Los Alamos Scientific Laboratory Report LA 3537, April 1967.
8.   G. P. Lahti, "QAD-HD Point Kernel Radiation Shielding Program to Evaluate Propellant Heating and Dose to Crew," National Aeronautics and Space Administration Report NASA-TM-X-1397, April 1967.
9.   H. Goldstein and J. E. Wilkins, "Calculations of the Penetration of Gamma Rays," U.S. AEC Rept. NYO-3075, 1954.
10.  H. Goldstein, *Fundamental Aspects of Reactor Shielding,* Addison-Wesley, 1959.
11.  J. J. Taylor, Westinghouse Report WAPD-RM-217, 1954.
12.  T. Rockwell, Ed., *Reactor Shielding Design Manual,* McGraw-Hill, New York, 1956.
13.  J. H. Hubbell, *J. Res. Nat. Bur. Stand.* **67C** (1963.)
14.  B. J. Price, C. C. Horton, and K. T. Spinney, *Radiation Shielding,* Pergamon Press, 1957.
15.  L. Galanter and F. X. Rizzo, *Trans. Am. Nucl. Soc.* **4,** 261 (1962).
16.  A. Foderaro and F. E. Obenshain, "Fluxes from Regular Geometric Sources" WAPD-TN-508, 1955.
17a. L. Galanter and K. Krishnamurthy, "FUDGE 4A, A Computer Program for Gamma Dose Rate Distribution from Rectangular Sources," U.S. AEC Rept. BNL 50126 (T-503), 1968.
17b. L. Galanter, S. Rosen. F. X. Rizzo, and L. Barziak, "GIRD-A Computer Program for Design of Shuffle-Dwell Gamma Irradiators," U.S. AEC Rept. BNL 50148 (T-519), 1969.
18.  B. Manowitz, O. A. Kuhl, L. Galanter, R. H. Bretton, and S. Zwickler, "Experimental Parameter Study of Large-Scale $Co^{60}$, $Na^{24m}$ and $Cs^{137}$ Slab Irradiators," Large Radiation Sources in Industry **I**, 68. *Proc. Conf. Application of Large Radiation Sources in Industry, Warsaw, Sept. 1959;* Int. Atomic Energy Agency, Vienna, 1960.
19.  M. G. Brown, "The Canadian Approach to Medical Product Sterilization Plants," AECL Report 2264, 1965.
20.  S. Jefferson, *Massive Radiation Techniques,* John Wiley & Sons, Inc., New York, 1963.
21.  A. Oltmann and O. A. Kuhl, "Gamma Radiation Source and Irradiator Design," U.S. AEC Rept. BNL 9281, 1965.
22.  M. J. Berger and J. Doggett, *J. Res. Nat. Bur. Stand.,* **56,** 89C (1956).
23.  L. V. Spencer and U. Fano, *Phys. Rev.,* **81,** 464L (1951).
24.  A. Oltmann and O. A. Kuhl, "Fabrication of BNL Standard Cobalt-60 Source," U.S. AEC Rept. BNL 845 (T-334), Feb. 1964.
25.  O. A. Kuhl, A. Oltmann, and J. Wagner, "Report on the Mark II Standard Cobalt Radiation Source, Bonded Type, U.S. AEC Rept. BNL 986 (T-418), Apr. 1966.
26.  B. Manowitz, "Elements of Gamma Irradiator Design," in *Radiation Preservation of Foods.* American Chemical Society, Washington, D.C., 1967.

27.  A. V. Bibergal, V. I. Sinitsyn, and N. I. Leshchinskii, *Gamma Irradiation Facilities*, 1965 (Translated from the Russian, available from U.S. Dept. of Commerce, USAEC Report AEC-tr-6469, 1965).
28.  D. B. Dove, J.P.A. Rideout, and G. S. Murray, *Intern. J. Appl. Radiation Isotopes* **9**, 27-33 (1960).
29.  S.A.E. Johansson, *Nucl. Sci. Eng.* **14**, 196-201 (1962).
30.  F. X. Rizzo, L. Galanter, and K. Krishnamurthy, "Tabulated Dose Distribution Data for Gamma Irradiator Design," U.S. AEC Rept. BNL 50147, 1969.
31.  F. X. Rizzo, L. Galanter, and K. Krishnamurthy, "Tabulated Dose Uniformity and Minimum Dose Data for Gamma Irradiator Design," U.S. AEC Rept. BNL 50145, 1969.
32.  L. Galanter and O. A. Kuhl, "Theoretical Calculations of Self-Absorption in Gamma Radiation Sources," *Trans. Am. Nucl. Soc.,* **9**, 97 (1966).
33.  *Tables of Sine, Cosine and Exponential Integrals,* NBS WPA, 1940.
34.  F. X. Rizzo, "Irradiator Design Calculational Techniques Based on Centerline Depth Dose Distributions," U.S. AEC Rept. BNL 50146, 1969.
35.  M. Jakob, *Heat Transfer,* Vols. I and II, John Wiley, New York, 1962.

# 6  GAMMA IRRADIATION SYSTEMS

*JOHN C. BRADBURNE, JR.*

LOCKHEED-GEORGIA CO.
DAWSONVILLE, GEORGIA

A gamma irradiation system used for industrial processing consists of the following major components: (1) the radioactive source assembly with its positioning and shielded storage equipment, (2) the irradiator, and (3) the product conveyor mechanism.

The radioactive source assembly consists of the encapsulated radioisotope and the framework used to rigidly position the encapsulated sources in a predetermined array. Encapsulation of the sources is required to preclude the spread of radioactive contamination throughout the irradiation facility and possibly into the product being irradiated.

The source assembly positioning and shielded storage equipment is employed to move, in a positive manner, the radioactive source assembly from a shielded storage container into a fixed position for irradiating the product and for return to the storage container. The shielded storage container is of course necessary to provide safe entry into the irradiation facility for maintenance, inspections, etc. A highly reliable, fail-safe source assembly positioning device is a critical requirement for the irradiation system.

The irradiator consists primarily of the shielding material required to adequately shield the surrounding area when the source is out of the shielded storage container within the irradiation facility structure. The facility structure can also assist in providing environmentally controlled conditions necessary to support the irradiation process such as special inert gas blankets, humidity controls, etc.

Finally, the product conveyor mechanism is the device used to move the product to be irradiated into the irradiation facility structure from a loading station, exterior to the facility. The conveyor then moves the product past the radioactive source assembly, usually on a continuous basis, after which the product is moved again to the exterior of the irradiation facility structure and to an unloading station. Figure 6.1 shows a typical irradiation facility which is used for irradiating prepackaged products. The major components as they have just been described are illustrated in this figure.

Before an irradiation system is constructed it must first be analyzed for its economic feasibility. This analysis is based not only on the initial cost, or capital investment, required for basic construction of the system but on continuing cost requirements which will be incurred during the operation of the system. In fact, operational costs can be a prime factor relating to economic feasibility or economic disaster in most systems of this type. For example, high capital expense incurred for highly automated equipment can greatly reduce annual system operating costs; however, there obviously must be a point of diminishing returns and hence arises the necessity of exacting economic analyses to be considered.

The information presented in this chapter can be used to develop an engineering analysis of an irradiation processing application so that the economic factors relating to the process can be determined. Basic data are presented which are applicable to package irradiation systems, bulk solid irradiation systems, and liquid irradiation systems.

## I. PLANT COST DETERMINATIONS

A process using ionizing radiation will require a determinable quantity of energy to affect the product. This means that energy emitted from a radioisotope must be absorbed within a given product to be processed by radiation and by this absorption the desired radiation-induced effect is produced in the product. Therefore, the initial factor to be investigated is the source of energy, the radioisotope source.

Economic analyses of irradiators involve optimization of the overall

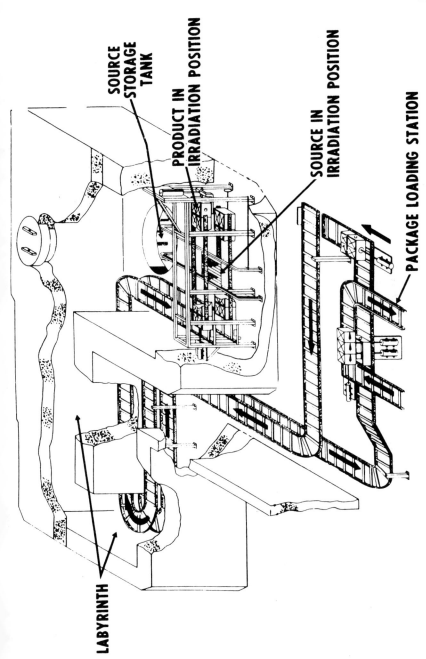

FIG. 6.1.  Hawaii Development Irradiator. *Purpose*: semicommercial scale processing of tropical fruits for large-scale shipping, storage, distribution, test marketing, and economic studies. *Type*: fixed facility; pool storage for source. *Source*: 250,000 Ci of $^{60}$Co. *Capacity*: 4,000 lb/hr at 75,000 rad.

process system. For the purpose of economic analysis, a process irradiation system can be considered to consist of four major parts: (1) the radiation source; (2) the product, or target, holder and conveyor system; (3) the radiation shield including the source shield; (4) the building, associated storage facilities, and handling equipment. (In the case of mobile irradiators, this may be the truck-bed and portable power equipment.)

For economic acceptability the complete process irradiation system must satisfy competitive economic factors while meeting radiation application criteria. The four factors are independent technical regimes; however, the initial analysis of the candidate radiation application will begin with source optimization. The result of this initial analysis will dictate design considerations for the other three process irradiation system parts.

### A.  The Radiation Source

A very simple illustration of the important factors to be considered in determining source requirements can be found in the equation for calculating dose rate from a point source in a given medium. This equation is (1):

$$D = \frac{kS_0 B e^{-\mu x}}{4\pi R^2} \tag{6.1}$$

where $D$ = dose rate in millirad/hr, $S_0$ = source strength in MeV/sec, $B$ = dose buildup factor, $\mu$ = total gamma-ray attenuation coefficient in cm$^{-1}$, $x$ = shield or product thickness between source and dose point, $k$ = conversion factor from gamma flux (photons/sec) to dose rate (mR/hr), and $R$ = distance between dose point and source. Figure 6.2 explains these relationships. Equation (6.1) clearly relates the distinction between the

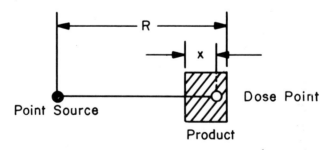

FIG. 6.2.   Dose–source diagram.

total energy emitted by a source of radiation and the dose absorbed within a product. In fact, considering only this equation it could be assumed that an irradiation processing plant would make use of the most energetic gamma rays available to accomplish the processing. The energy of the gamma rays must be chosen to be in a range that is most efficiently absorbed in the material of the target and in its volume thickness. Applications calling for low-energy radiation or involving very thin target materials could possibly be candidates for machine irradiators (see Chapter 7). The choice of gamma rays is also limited to those emitted by radioisotope sources which are available in sufficient quantities to assure an adequate and economic supply. There are now only two gamma-ray emitting radioisotopes that can be considered as practical processing sources. These are cesium-137 and cobalt-60.

To make a preliminary evaluation of source requirements there are three factors that must be known about the radioactive isotopes. These are cost, annual radioactive decay (an exponential function), and radiation energy. The values for these factors are presented in Table 6.1. Since one disintegration of cobalt-60 yields 2.50 MeV (1.17 + 1.33) of gamma-ray energy as compared to only 0.662 MeV for cesium-137, nominally 3.79 Ci of cesium-137 are required to emit the same total energy as 1 Ci of cobalt-60, assuming negligible self-absorption in the source.

From Table 6.1 the cost of doubly encapsulated cobalt is \$0.58/Ci at 1969 prices as available from commercial suppliers. The radioisotope is a capital asset and must be depreciated like any other piece of equipment in the processing plant. A ten-year depreciation period is normally used in the United States. The cobalt source will be decaying while it is in use and must be replenished to maintain an economical processing capability.

TABLE 6.1

COBALT-60 AND CESIUM-137 COST DATA[a]

| | Annual radioactive decay (%) | Radiation energy (MeV) | Doubly encapsulated source cost (1969) (\$/Ci for quantities over 200,000 curies) |
|---|---|---|---|
| Cobalt-60 | 12.6 | 1.17 + 1.33 | 0.58 (Specific activity at 30 Ci/g) |
| Cesium-137 | 2.34 | 0.662 | 0.93 (4000 Ci source as CsCl-27Ci/g) |

[a]The prices per curie for cesium and cobalt shown in this table are subject to negotiation with commercial suppliers in the case of cobalt and subject to U.S. AEC pricing policy decisions in the case of cesium.

The dose rate will decrease 12.6% in a year due to radioactive decay which means that the amount of product which can be processed in that year would also be reduced 12.6%. Therefore, assuming the ten-year depreciation period and a 12.6% replenishment for decay, the annual cost for a cobalt-60 source will be

$$(0.126 + 0.10) (\$0.58) = \$0.131/Ci\text{-}yr$$

The same analysis can be made for cesium-137. For a high-level cesium source, the annual cost per curie would be as follows:

$$(0.0234 + 0.10) (\$0.93) = \$0.115/Ci\text{-}yr$$

There are three primary types of radiation processes. These are package, bulk solid and bulk liquid processes. There are other applications, but the large majority of applications will fit one of these three categories. For optimum source utilization the sources will be arranged as either a planar source plaque or as a line source for the three types of processes. The plaque source will be used in a package process and sometimes in a bulk solid process. The line source will be used in a bulk liquid process and sometimes in a bulk solid process where the product would travel along a spiral or annular path around the source. Each disintegration, each photon, has a cost and that is the importance of the source efficiency relationships developed in the previous chapter. The source cost is significant and is usually the sole determining factor as to economic feasibility of the process.

Initial design calculations for source requirements are based on the dose rate required to process a unit weight of product per unit time. The source arrangement can be satisfactorily analyzed to determine what percentage of the radiation is lost due to leakage, to self-absorption in the source holder, and to escape from the product without being absorbed. The ratio of energy absorbed in the product to energy emitted from the source is called *source efficiency* (see Section II).

The source plaque should be arranged for maximum efficiency. As shown in Chapter 5 the most efficient array will be to "overlap" the plaque with the product to assure maximum absorption in the product of the emitted radiation from the plaque. The plaque will be arranged for maximum dose rate uniformity over the frontal area of the plaque in the case of a planar array and for a maximum dose rate uniformity over the vertical axis in the case of a line source array.

Figure 6.3 presents relative dose rate in rad/hr/Ci in a plane normal to

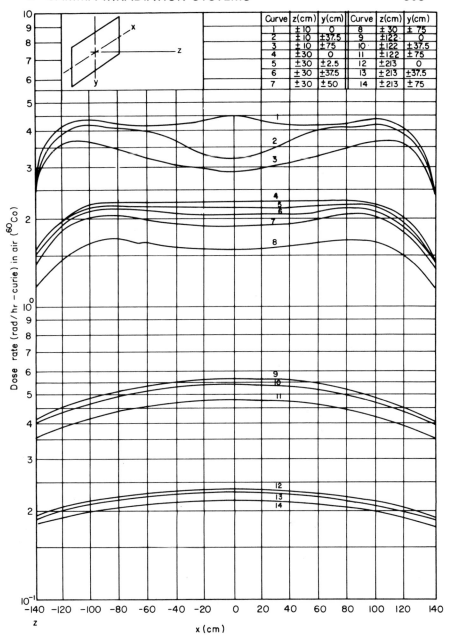

| Curve | z(cm) | y(cm) | Curve | z(cm) | y(cm) |
|-------|-------|-------|-------|-------|-------|
| 1 | ±10 | 0 | 8 | ±30 | ±75 |
| 2 | ±10 | ±37.5 | 9 | ±122 | 0 |
| 3 | ±10 | ±75 | 10 | ±122 | ±37.5 |
| 4 | ±30 | 0 | 11 | ±122 | ±75 |
| 5 | ±30 | ±2.5 | 12 | ±213 | 0 |
| 6 | ±30 | ±37.5 | 13 | ±213 | ±37.5 |
| 7 | ±30 | ±50 | 14 | ±213 | ±75 |

FIG. 6.3.   Planar source plaque dose rates.

the frontal area of the plaque at several distances from the plaque,* for a typical rectangular cobalt source array which has been arranged for optimum uniformity over a 4 ft by 8 ft frontal area on either face of the plaque. Figure 6.4 presents relative dose rates in rad/hr Ci radially around a simple line source which has been arranged for optimum uniformity over an approximate length of 60 in.† Figures 6.3 and 6.4 are examples of the two most common source arrays which will be used in irradiation facilities and, although they are explicit examples, the arrangement of source material in the plaques for several requirements can be satisfied with the general arrangements shown, as described in the next paragraph. The major precaution in arranging the source material in any given plaque is to minimize gamma-ray absorption in the plaque's structural material and in the source materials themselves.

Now that specific source plaque examples have been illustrated it is possible to develop some simple approximations which the reader will be able to use to derive approximate source strength requirements. The plaque source shown in Fig. 6.3 can be averaged over a frontal area as shown in Fig. 6.5 and should be a valid estimate as long as $l$ is never less than 4 ft, $h$ is never less than 2 ft and $l$ is always approximately $2h$. The line source shown in Fig. 6.4 can be averaged vertically as shown in Fig. 6.6. This assumption should be valid for values of $l$ between 2 and 5 ft. Data shown in Figs. 6.3 and 6.4 are expressed in rad/hr/Ci in air. Since these figures show dose rate per curie in air, corrections will have to be made for actual applications to determine the dose delivered to the target material. An approximation of these corrections can be made from the equation (4)

$$I_x = BI_0 e^{-\mu x} \tag{6.2}$$

where $I_x$ = intensity of monoenergetic beam of photons after passing through the target, $B$ = dose buildup factor, $I_0$ = intensity of monoenergetic beam without target, $\mu$ = linear absorption coefficient, and $x$ = target thickness.

The numbers shown in Figs. 6.5 and 6.6 are the relative source strengths in each plaque expressed in curies. They represent the fraction of the whole source strength to be located at that position in the plaque. (It is

---

*Note: Self-shielding in the source plaque structure has been taken into account.

†Note: If volume-integrated dose rates per curie are investigated for line sources, it will make no difference whether the source plaque is shaped or not. The volume-integrated dose rate per curie for the plaque shown in Fig. 6.4 is 1.12 rad/hr/Ci for $^{60}$Co, and 0.241 rad/hr/Ci for $^{137}$Cs.

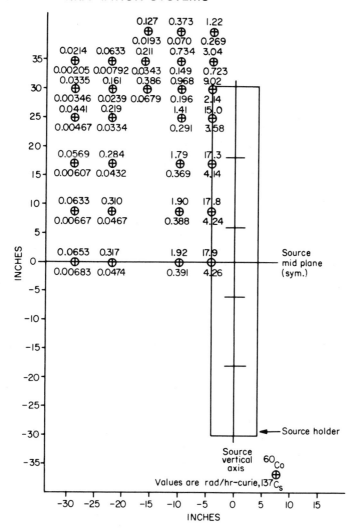

FIG. 6.4.  Line source dose rates.

customary to normalize relative activities in this way so that their sum equals unity.) These source distributions have been developed under the assumptions stated in the text so that the specific activity is immaterial for Fig. 6.5 (the source can even be a point source) or for Fig. 6.6 as long as the values are integrated over the whole volume.

The data presented thus far are sufficient to enable the reader to develop

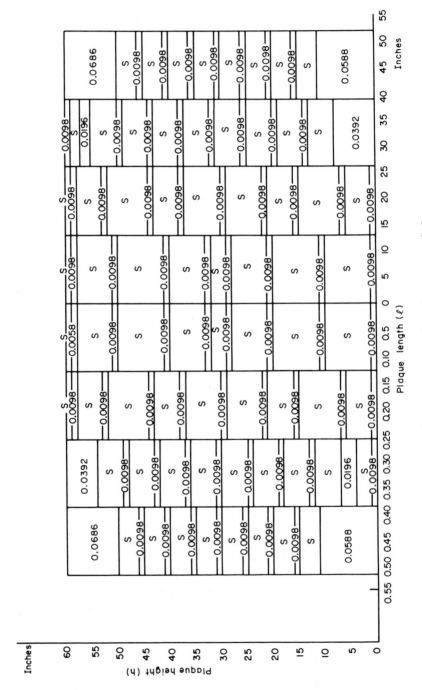

Fig. 6.5. Relative source strengths—planar source. S, Spacer.

Inches

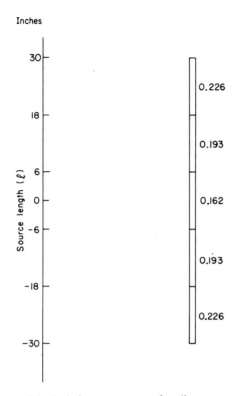

FIG. 6.6.   Relative source strengths—line source.

reasonably accurate approximations of radioisotope quantity and cost for a given radiation application.

*Example 1:*

Determine the cost of cobalt-60 required to achieve a dose rate of $4 \times 10^5$ rad/hr at a depth of 30 cm in a material which is placed on either side of a planar source plaque having a frontal area of 4 ft by 8 ft. Assume a buildup factor $B$ of 4.0 and a linear absorption coefficient $\mu$ of 0.1 cm$^{-1}$ for the target material.

From Fig. 6.3 the dose rate in air from a planar source plaque 4 ft by 8 ft at 30 cm from the plaque is fairly uniform along the $y$ axis of the plaque. Therefore, it can be assumed that the frontal dose rate per curie in air is about 2.0 rad/hr. The dose rate per curie in the target at a depth of 30 cm, assuming no gap between the plaque and the edge of the target material nearest the plaque, will be $4.0 \times 2.0 \times e^{-0.1 \times 30}$ or 0.39 rad/hr/ Ci [see Eq. (6.2)]. Then the total quantity of cobalt-60 required is $4.5 \times 10^5/0.39$ or approximately $10^6$ Ci.

From Table 6.1 the cost of $^{60}$Co is shown to be $0.58/Ci. Therefore, the cost of the cobalt will be $0.58 \times 10^6$ or $580,000.

## B. Conveyor Systems

The particular irradiation facility to support a given radiation application will depend on four primary factors. These are:

(1) Physical state of the target material.
(2) Whether the target material is to be handled in bulk form or in package form.
(3) Necessary environmental conditions for the target material (considering chemical properties, etc.).
(4) Product throughput.

Factors 1 and 2 are interrelated to some extent in that the physical state of the target material will in most cases determine how the material can be handled during irradiation. However, in some applications the target material must be prepackaged to maintain the advantageous effects induced by irradiation of the material. An obvious example here is the use of radiation to produce partial or complete biological sterilization in the irradiated product. Factor 3 must be considered in applications that require attention to toxicity of the target material or its radiation-induced by-products; volatility of the target material or its radiation induced by-products; biological stability of the target material during preirradiation periods, irradiation periods, and postirradiation periods; and exclusion of infection or reinfestation during postirradiation periods. Factor 4 is the predominant economic determinant and must be accurately evaluated to assure maximum utilization of the radioisotope source and an optimum output of irradiated product.

Once these four factors have been carefully considered and the irradiation parameters related to these factors have been defined, the type of irradiation facility can be selected. There are three basic types of irradiation facilities. These are: (1) package irradiation facility, (2) bulk solid irradiation facility, and (3) bulk liquid irradiation facility. (These are in no way exclusive as far as irradiation facilities are concerned since other types such as continuous loop irradiators, batch irradiators, etc., may also be required. The three basic types listed do, however, satisfy the large majority of existing and potential irradiation applications and should provide the reader with an ample background to analyze other facility concepts as the needs present themselves.)

The designer should strive to use either the bulk solid or bulk liquid irradiation concept wherever possible as these concepts most readily lend themselves to a line source which tends to yield higher source efficiencies. This is due to:

(1) Elimination of void space between product containers and absence of container materials to absorb radiation, i.e., better target homogeneity.
(2) Simplified product conveyor systems (hydraulic or pneumatic versus mechanical).
(3) Virtual elimination of manual handling.
(4) Minimum leakage of radiation from the ends of the source plaque that is not absorbed in the product.

The package irradiation facility in general represents the most expensive of the three basic facilities discussed. This is due to:

(1) Complexity and attendant costs of the conveyor system.
(2) Expensive capital and maintenance costs of the conveyor system.
(3) Manual handling requirements of the packaged target material in some cases.
(4) Complexity and attendant costs of the planar source plaque storage and lift mechanism.
(5) Large size of the irradiation chamber which results in increased costs for shielding.

Mention should be made of batch irradiators at this point since there are several of these facilities in operation today. The batch irradiator serves a useful purpose in that it can and usually does serve a multipurpose use. For example, the source and/or conveyor system can be arranged to irradiate large packages of product for a given period of time. When this requirement is fulfilled a changeover can be made in the facility to accommodate smaller packages of another product at different dose rate and/or dose rate uniformity requirements. This approach is advantageous to the facility user to allow maximum facility use time and consequently a better return on capital investment; however, this type of facility is now being used primarily to process research and development quantities of materials or limited production quantities of some materials. As markets for irradiation-processed materials develop and increase, the batch irradiator will prove to be less economical for production applications. The several batch irradiation facilities in existence today represent sufficient capacity to handle research and development demands for several years to come and, therefore, should not be considered as a potential design problem in the near future. Table 6.2 presents comparative capital costs and capital cost estimates for several existing and studied irradiation

TABLE 6.2

CAPITAL COST COMPARISONS FOR IRRADIATION FACILITIES

| Plant | Investment | Cost |
|---|---|---|
| 1. Proposed fish irradiation plant (package concept) (2) | Radioactive source | $130,000 |
| | Land | 15,000 |
| | Building | 65,000 |
| | Miscellaneous equipment | 74,500 |
| | Conveyors | 30,000 |
| | Engineering, etc. | 55,400 |
| | Contingencies | 28,000 |
| | Total investment | $397,900 |
| 2. Bulk grain irradiation(2) (bulk flow concept) | Radioactive source | $35,000 |
| | Land | 15,000 |
| | Building | 50,000 |
| | Miscellaneous equipment | 60,000 |
| | Conveyors | 25,000 |
| | Engineering, etc. | 40,000 |
| | Contingencies | 20,000 |
| | Total investment | $245,000 |
| 3. Meat sterilization facility (study) (3) (package concept) | Radioactive source | $1,295,200 |
| | Land | 15,000 |
| | Building | 135,000 |
| | Miscellaneous equipment | 35,000 |
| | Conveyors | 50,000 |
| | Engineering, etc. | 22,000 |
| | Contingencies | 25,000 |
| | Total investment | $1,577,200 |
| 4. Chemical irradiation facility (estimate) (bulk flow concept) | Radioactive source | $30,000 |
| | Land | 15,000 |
| | Building | 70,000 |
| | Miscellaneous equipment | 50,000 |
| | Conveyors | 25,000 |
| | Engineering, etc. | 30,000 |
| | Contingencies | 20,000 |
| | Total investment | $240,000 |

facilities to better illustrate the higher cost requirements for package irradiation facilities when compared to bulk solid or bulk liquid (continuous flow) irradiation facilities.

When selecting a material conveyor system or combination of systems for a particular irradiation application there are six prime considerations. These include:

(1) The conveyor system should be designed for at least an 8,400-hr annual duty cycle without major maintenance and preferably without any maintenance since facility down-time usually carries a high cost.*

(2) Materials such as hydrocarbons, fluorocarbons, etc. may degrade under the high-level gamma-radiation environment within the irradiation cell. This necessitates the selection of noncorrosive all-metal components in the conveyor mechanism including metal-to-metal bearings free of organic lubricants. In addition, serious consideration must be given to possible ozone corrosion and toxicity within the cell.

(3) All electrical controls such as switches and wiring should be located outside the irradiation cell to preclude costly maintenance situations (shutting down the process) since the wiring insulation and plastic switch components usually will not endure the gamma-radiation environment or high ozone levels.

(4) The target material must be positively contained in the conveyor system while being irradiated to assure proper integrated doses as well as the desired dose rate uniformity.

(5) The conveyor system should be arranged so as to preclude mechanical interference with the plaque storage and lift mechanism. In no case should it be possible to interfere with the return of the radioisotope source to its shielded storage position under normal or emergency conditions.

(6) A conveyor system should be selected which will minimize or eliminate manual handling operations during conveyor loading and/or unloading operations to reduce labor costs and ensure maximum throughput.

There are several types and combinations of conveyor systems that are adaptable to handling the target material in package form. Some of the

---

*The 8400-hr duty cycle is predicated on 350 days of operation, 24 hr per day with 14 days down-time for annual maintenance and source replenishment if required.

TABLE 6.3

Conveyor Systems in Existing Irradiation Facilities

| Facility | Conveyor system(s) |
| --- | --- |
| 1. Bulk grain irradiator | Gravity feed, vibratory conveyors |
| 2. Mobile gamma irradiator | Hydraulic cylinder actuators, gravity feed roller conveyors |
| 3. U.S. Army Natick Laboratory Food irradiator | Continuous monorail conveyor |
| 4. Experimental food irradiator Wageningen, Holland (I.T.A.L.) | Belt conveyor |

more common types include: (1) continuous monorail conveyors, (2) hydraulic cylinder actuators, (3) pneumatic cylinder actuators, (4) in-line screw actuators, (5) belt conveyors, and (6) vibratory conveyors. Existing irradiation facilities employ one or more of these conveyor systems and in some cases couple these mechanisms with gravity feed. Examples are shown in Table 6.3.

There are numerous considerations pertaining to the selection of a type or combination of types of conveyor systems to be employed in a given package irradiation application, including product density, packaging material, number of passes by the source plaque, irradiation position dwell time, and others. Each case must be considered on an individual basis and evaluated in light of the six prime factors for conveyor system selection. The final selection of the conveyor should satisfy these six factors as they are applicable and should represent the lowest reasonable capital investment.

To guide the reader in making preliminary economic determinations regarding package conveyor systems, Table 6.4 has been developed. This table lists approximate installed costs per foot of linear motion for the six more common types of conveyors including their control systems.

A bulk solid conveyor system or a liquid conveyor system will be less complicated and consequently less expensive. In fact, in most cases a gravity flow-through concept for both bulk and liquid irradiation applications will satisfy the conveyor system requirements. Careful consideration must be given to hydraulic parameters for the target material during detail design so that proper baffling and adequate hydraulic diameters can be selected with minimum danger of plugging or blocking the flow. However, for the purpose of initial economic considerations, the reader need only generally consider the criteria and select a suitable conveyor mecha-

TABLE 6.4

APPROXIMATE INSTALLED COST PER FOOT OF LINEAR MOTION
SYSTEMS FOR PACKAGE CONVEYOR

| Conveyor system | Cost per foot of linear motion ($) |
|---|---|
| (1) Continuous monorail | 80 |
| (2) Belt | 45 |
| (3) Hydraulic cylinder actuators[a] | 400 |
| (4) Pneumatic cylinder actuators[a] | 400 |
| (5) Power roller | 45 |
| (6) Gravity roller | 20 |

[a]These conveyors have travel limits of approximately 5 ft per cylinder due to hydraulic and pneumatic efficiencies.

nism to move the target material through the irradiator. Table 6.5 has been developed to assist the reader in determining capital cost requirements for several types of conveyors including their control systems.

There is the possibility that a pilot mock-up of some part of the irradiation process will be required before the final plant design can be initiated. This, of course, has an effect on the plant economics since additional funds must be allocated to perform the pilot studies. The probable area where the requirement for a pilot process may arise is in the case of a bulk solid or liquid irradiation application. It is conceivable that the bulk solid or liquid to be irradiated, such as wheat flour or polyethylene oxide, cannot be compared to known media in order to determine hydraulic characteristics. Therefore, a mock-up of the irradiation chamber should be prepared to study flow characteristics of the target material to assure that the desired dose uniformity in the material can be achieved. In addition, material velocities within the irradiation chamber should be studied to

TABLE 6.5

APPROXIMATE BULK SOLID AND LIQUID CONVEYOR SYSTEM COSTS
PER FOOT OF LINEAR MOTION

| Conveyor system | Cost per foot of linear motion ($) |
|---|---|
| (1) Screw conveyor | 375 |
| (2) Vibratory conveyor | 300 |
| (3) Belt conveyor | 345 |
| (4) Air conveyor | 150 |
| (5) Fluid pumping conveyor[a] | 300 |

[a]Note: This conveyor cost is highly sensitive to pumping requirements. The cost shown in the table is based on 20 h.p. pumping requirements.

optimize product flow rates and therefore select the final radioisotope
source strength to deliver the desired integrated dose to the product.

Package irradiation concepts will not usually require a pilot mock-up of
the process. Instead, the reader will be confronted with the challenge of
selecting a conveyor mechanism or combination of conveyors to properly
move the target material through the irradiation chamber at a rate that
will satisfy plant throughput requirements. Table 6.6 shows typical total
industrial costs for piloting a bulk solid flow process and a liquid flow
process at 1969 rates. These costs include all materials and labor required
to erect the pilot equipment, perform the tests, reduce the data, and report
the findings.

TABLE 6.6

APPROXIMATE DEVELOPMENT COSTS FOR PILOTING BULK SOLID AND LIQUID FLOW
PROCESS CONCEPTS

| Task | Cost ($) |
|---|---|
| (1)  Pilot equipment | 5,000 |
| (2)  Pilot runs | 3,000 |
| (3)  Data reduction, analysis and reporting | 2,000 |
| Total approximate costs | 10,000 |

## C.  Shielding

The cost of shielding the irradiation chamber and source storage well
in a radiation processing system will represent a significant capital cost
factor. Considerable experience in facility study, design, and construction
has led to a sizeable reduction in the choices of shielding materials in recent years. These materials are ordinary concrete, lead, and earth. There
will obviously be other materials used in construction, such as steel and
aluminum or even water, but they will not serve as primary shielding media and, therefore, they need not be considered as such except where required during the detail design phase of the overall plant design program.
The potential radioisotopes to be used in a radiation processing application have been previously narrowed to either cobalt-60 or cesium-137.
Nomograms for both of these radioactive isotopes in ordinary concrete,
lead, and earth for infinite line sources have been prepared to assist the
reader in selecting the desired shielding thickness of the chosen shield ma-

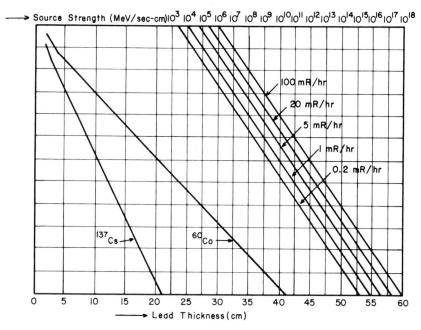

FIG. 6.7.   Cobalt-60 and cesium-137 nomogram for lead shields.

terial *(1)*. These nomograms are presented in Fig. 6.7 through 6.9.*
Table 6.7 presents typical costs for preparing the three different shields
for selected thicknesses.

   Radioisotope source plaque storage and handling mechanisms must be
considered in determining preliminary economic evaluations of radiation
applications. Water-filled pool storage of source plaques has been widely
used in existing irradiation facilities because of the flexibility in altering
the source array for the irradiation of various products. This approach is
more costly than dry storage due to the requirement for water purification
systems to maintain large volumes of water at optimum conductivity, pH,

---

   *Note:   To use the nomograms the source strength in MeV/sec must first be
determined. The source strength must then be corrected for attenuation in air for the
distance from the plaque to the inner edge of the shield by using Fig. 6.3 since these
dose rates are in free air. The allowable dose rate at the outer surface of the shield is then
selected on the nomogram and the intersection of the source strength with that curve
is traced on the nomogram. From this intersection, move horizontally to the left until
the isotope curve is intersected and then read the shield thickness on the nomogram.
A more accurate calculation will be required during final design but these nomograms
should provide a basis for analyzing facility shield costs.

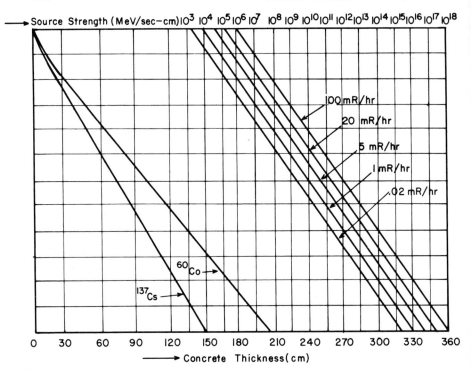

FIG. 6.8. Cobalt-60 and cesium-137, nomogram for concrete shields. Concrete density, 2.3 g/cm³.

and temperature so as to protect the source cladding material from undue chemical degradation.

Dry storage of the source plaque is now considered to be satisfactory and has been proven to be more economical. This concept allows for use of the primary shield structure as storage space thereby minimizing capital costs for the storage well. The source plaque conveyor mechanism

TABLE 6.7

Approximate Shield Costs for Irradiation Facilities

| | Type of shield | Installed cost ($) |
|---|---|---|
| (1) | Ordinary concrete (includes forming, reinforcing and finishing) | 0.05/pound |
| (2) | Earth (includes excavation, drainage, grading, compacting, and stabilization) | 100/yd³ |
| (3) | Lead (includes steel encasements) | 1.00/pound |

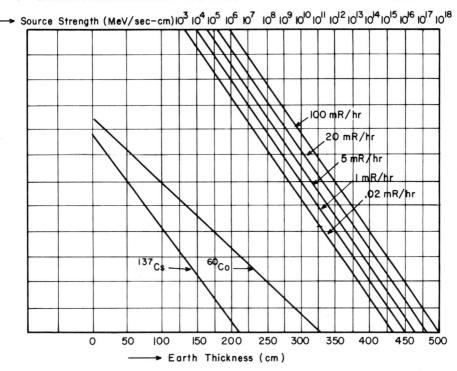

Fig. 6.9. Cobalt-60 and cesium-137, nomogram for earth shield. Earth density, 1.5 g/cm³.

thereby becomes the most significant cost factor in this area. Representative costs are presented in Table 6.8 for both planar and line source plaques conveyor mechanisms. These costs include a dry storage well in the primary shield. Figure 6.10 shows this source storage concept for a horizontal arrangement. Note the rotating shield plug.

TABLE 6.8

SOURCE PLAQUE DRY STORAGE AND CONVEYOR MECHANISM APPROXIMATE COSTS

| Type of mechanism | Installed cost ($) |
|---|---|
| (1) Line source storage and conveyor mechanism | |
|     A. Up to 10 kCi $^{60}$Co | 10,000 |
|     B. Up to 100 kCi $^{60}$Co | 15,000 |
|     C. Up to 1000 kCi $^{60}$Co | 22,000 |
| (2) Planar source storage and conveyor mechanism | |
|     A. Up to 100 kCi $^{60}$Co | 15,000 |
|     B. Up to 1000 kCi $^{60}$Co | 28,000 |
|     C. Above 1000 kCi $^{60}$Co | 50,000 |

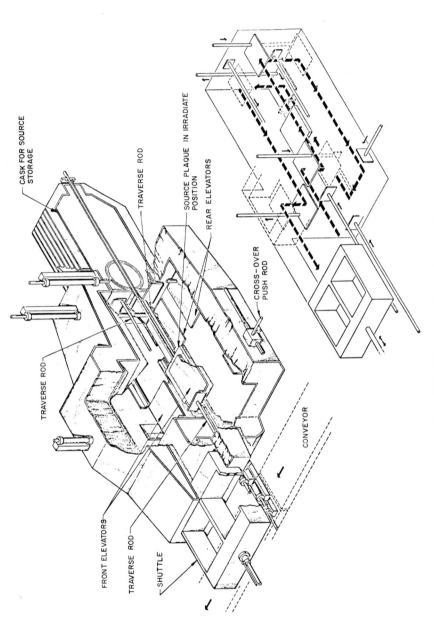

CASK FOR SOURCE STORAGE

TRAVERSE ROD

SOURCE PLAQUE IN IRRADIATE POSITION

REAR ELEVATORS

CROSS-OVER PUSH ROD

TRAVERSE ROD

CONVEYOR

FRONT ELEVATORS

TRAVERSE ROD

SHUTTLE

Fig. 6.10.   Dry source plaque storage wells

### D. System Costs

The final cost factors to be considered in a processing plant can be grouped as miscellaneous costs. These include: (1) miscellaneous equipment, (2) annual maintenance costs, (3) annual operating costs (not including source replacement), (4) interest on capital investment, (5) local taxes and insurance, (6) architect and engineering services. Table 6.9 has been prepared to define these six miscellaneous cost areas for the three basic processing plant concepts. The costs given in Table 6.9 represent the following considerations for each of these miscellaneous areas.

*1. Miscellaneous equipment:* (a) building utilities, (b) radiation detectors and safety interlock systems, (c) radioisotope source shipping and replenishing cask and associated tools, and (d) plaque and product dosimetry equipment.

*2. Annual maintenance costs:* (a) mechanical system and electrical system preventive maintenance, (b) emergency maintenance allowance.

*3. Annual operating costs:* (a) operating personnel direct cost and overhead, (b) supervisory personnel direct cost and overhead, (c) service personnel direct cost and overhead, (d) operating supplies.

TABLE 6.9

APPROXIMATE MISCELLANEOUS COSTS FOR IRRADIATION PROCESSING FACILITIES

| Item | Annual cost ($) |
|---|---|
| (1) Building utilities | 1% of plant cost |
| (2) Radiation detectors and safety interlock systems (nonrecurring) | $5,000 |
| (3) Radioisotope source shipping cask and tools (nonrecurring) | $20,000 |
| (4) Plaque and product dosimetry equipment (nonrecurring) | $2,000 |
| (5) Preventive maintenance | 5% of plant cost |
| (6) Emergency maintenance allowance | $3,000 |
| (7) Operating personnel: direct cost and overhead | $4.00/hr/man required + $4.00/hr/man overhead |
| (8) Supervisory personnel: direct cost and overhead | $5.50/hr/man required + $ 5.50/hr/man overhead |
| (9) Service personnel: direct cost and overhead | $3.00/hr/man required + $3.00/hr/man overhead |
| (10) Operating supplies | 1/2% of plant cost |
| (11) Approximate interest on capital investment | 8%/yr |
| (12) Local taxes and insurance | 2% of plant cost |
| (13) Engineering costs (nonrecurring) | 10% of plant cost |

*4.  Interest on capital investment:* This is an annual charge for use of capital and will vary from year to year depending on prime interest rates.

*5.  Local taxes and insurance:* This is assumed to be 2% of the capital cost. However, this percentage will vary for different locations.

*6.  Architect and engineering services:* This category makes allowance for the cost of plant design and supervision of construction to assure compliance to the design specifications.

The reader now has sufficient data to construct a preliminary cost analysis for a facility to accomplish a particular radiation process. It can be seen that the facility concept must be at least partially developed to properly analyze the economics of a radiation application and if the economics appear marginal, a more detailed concept must be developed to better define the economic analysis. The approach to detailed economic determinations is presented in the following sections.

Figures 6.11, 6.12, and 6.13 are artists' concepts of package, bulk solid, and liquid irradiation facilities which are presented to exemplify the facility concepts discussed in this section.

## II.  ANALYSIS OF PLANT ECONOMICS

The factors presented in Section I present guidelines for approximate economic analysis of radiation processes. This section will develop the economics for a given plant.

The most important parameter to be defined is product throughput. Section I developed a method for determining dose rate per curie for given source plaque arrays and established a method for correcting those dose rates to a given point. These data can be used to determine source efficiency. Source efficiency is defined as

$$E_U = \frac{\text{useful photon absorption in product}}{\text{total photon emission from source}}$$

Integrated exposures to the target material will range from 5,000 to 5,000,000 rads depending on the desired induced effect in the target. Some examples of induced effects and the required integrated exposures to achieve these effects are shown in Table 6.10.

To determine product, or target, throughput in a plant it is necessary to know: (1) the required integrated exposure, (2) the quantity of product to be processed in a given time, and (3) the plant duty cycle. It has been previously discussed that the optimum plant duty cycle is 8400 hr. The

TABLE 6.10

REQUIRED DOSES FOR VARIOUS IRRADIATION PROCESSES

| General applications | Radiation dose (rads) |
|---|---|
| (1) Insects | |
|     De-infestation dose | $7 \times 10^3 - 6 \times 10^5$ |
| (2) Bacteria | |
|     Pasteurization dose | $9 \times 10^4 - 9 \times 10^5$ |
|     Sterilization dose | $1.5 \times 10^6 - 7.5 \times 10^6$ |
| (3) Virus inactivation | $1 \times 10^6 - 9 \times 10^6$ |
| (4) Seeds | |
|     Growth stimulation | $0.75 \times 10^2 - 1 \times 10^3$ |
|     Inhibition | $6.5 \times 10^3 - 3.5 \times 10^4$ |
|     Mutations | $4.5 \times 10^4 - 1 \times 10^6$ |
| (5) Fruits | $5 \times 10^4 - 7.5 \times 10^5$ |
|     Extended storage and shelf life | |
| (6) Vegetables | |
|     Extended storage and shelf life | $7.5 \times 10^3 - 7 \times 10^4$ |
| (7) Chemistry | |
|     Polymerization | $1 \times 10^5 - 9 \times 10^6$ |
|     Crosslinking | $1 \times 10^6 - 1 \times 10^8$ |

| Specific applications | Dose (megarads) |
|---|---|
| (1) Fish (pasteurization) | 0.15 |
| (2) Clams (pasteurization) | 0.45 |
| (3) Shrimp (pasteurization) | 0.16 |
| (4) Ham (sterilization) | 4.5 |
| (5) Mangos (extended storage and shelf life) | 0.025 |
| (6) Strawberries (extended storage and shelf life) | 0.2 |
| (7) Oranges (extended storage and shelf life) | 0.2 |
| (8) Beef (sterilization) | 4.5 |
| (9) Shrimp (sterilization) | 4.5–5.6 |
| (10) Chicken (sterilization) | 4.5–5.6 |
| (11) Pork (sterilization) | 4.5–5.6 |
| (12) Bacon (sterilization) | 4.5–5.6 |
| (13) Pharmaceuticals and medical supplies (sterilization) | 2.5 |
| (14) Flour (deinfestation) | 0.015 |
| (15) Polyethylene film (crosslinking) | 20 |
| (16) Methyl methacrylate-purified (polymerization) | $1.0^a$ |
| (17) Vinyl acetate-purified (polymerization) | $0.2^a$ |
| (18) Styrene-purified (polymerization) | $1.0^a$ |

[a]These radiation doses may be varied significantly by alterations in dose rates and atmosphere.

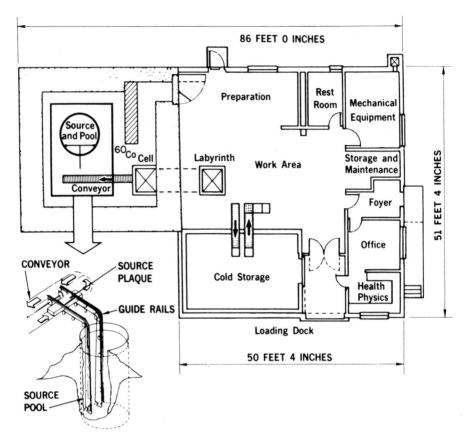

FIG. 6.11. Marine Products Development Irradiator. *Purpose:* semicommercial sea-
food irradiation. *Type:* fixed facility; four-pass quadrant irradiation, pool storage
for source. *Source:* 250,000 Ci of $^{60}$Co. *Capacity:* 2,000 lb/hr at 250,000, rads. *Facility cost:* $600,000 exclusive of source.

integrated exposure to achieve the desired effect in the product will have
been previously specified. This specification will include exposure tolerances and dose rate effect consideration. For a commercial process, the
required quantity of product will be determined by the existing and
projected market or by the projected market only.

Since many of the existing and potential radiation applications are in
the integrated exposure range of from 200,000 to 5,000,000 rads, the integrated exposure can be conveniently expressed as rads $\times 10^6$ or megarads.
The quantity of product to be irradiated will usually be expressed in

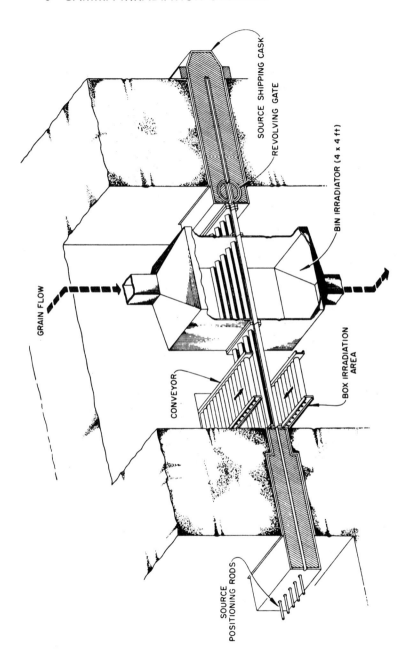

FIG. 6.12.  Bulk Grain Irradiator.  *Purpose:* de-infestation of bulk grain or packaged products.  *Type:* fixed grid of $^{60}$Co strips; two irradiation positions, one for bulk grain and one for packages.  *Source:* 250,000 Ci of $^{60}$Co.  *Capacity:* 5,000 lb/hr bulk or 2,800 lb/hr packaged product, either at 25,000 rads.  *Facility cost:* $200,000, exclusive of source.

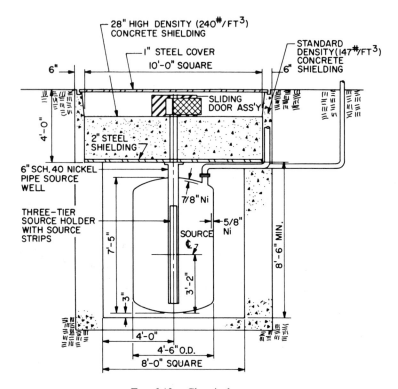

FIG. 6.13.   Chemical reactor.

pounds and will usually be in large enough quantities to be conveniently expressed in tons. The plant duty cycle has been defined as 8400 hr and can be more conveniently expressed in calendar days. Therefore, product throughput can now be defined in terms of units of megarad-tons/day.

### A.   Package Irradiation Plant

Assume that an annual market of approximately 6,700 tons of radiation sterilized beef now exists. From Table 6.10 it can be seen that the required integrated exposure to sterilize beef is 4.5 megarads. If the plant duty cycle is 350 days/year then the required plant throughput becomes:

$$\frac{4.5 \text{ megarads} \times 6,700 \text{ tons}}{350 \text{ days}} = 86.2 \text{ megarad-tons/day}$$

As discussed in Section I it may be necessary to consider environmental controls (temperature) for the target material. In developing the case for radiation sterilized beef it has been determined through extensive research that beef must be irradiated at liquid nitrogen temperatures to preclude undesirable flavor changes. To minimize liquid nitrogen consumption the maximum dwell time or irradiation time for a twenty-pound package of beef should be approximately one hour.

Since the plant throughput is to be 86.2 megarad tons/day a total of approximately 1,915 twenty-pound packages of beef will be irradiated in a 24-hr day. Assuming a one-hour dwell time per package the product thickness on either side of a planar source plaque can be determined by using Fig. 6.3 and correcting the dose rate with Eq. (6.2).

It has been shown in Section I and in Chapter 5 that a line source would be the most reasonable source array considering source efficiency relationships. However, the conveyor mechanism for transporting liquid nitrogen cooled packages of meat around a line source would be economically unfeasible both from the standpoint of conveyor costs and source efficiency. Therefore, a proper trade-off between source arrangement and conveyor system is made in this case and a planar source plaque is selected. The conveyor system best suited for the sterilized beef application is a monorail system. This is due to the following factors: (1) minimum void spaces between the product packages, (2) reasonable costs of monorail conveyor system (see Table 6.4), (3) minimum maintenance requirements, and (4) ease of manual loading and unloading of packages. (Note: manual handling is required since liquid nitrogen envelope must be supplied.) Once a conveyor system, a source plaque shape, and a product throughput have been selected it is possible to develop a finite irradiator concept.

The size of a twenty-pound package of beef will be 24 in. by 24 in. by 10 in. The product thickness on either side of the plaque will be taken as 50 in. and the package dwell time as one hour. Therefore, the maximum plaque dimensions can be 48 in. by 96 in. with five passes on either side of the source. The integrated dose to the target on one side of the plaque must be 2.25 megarads thus requiring approximately 950,000 Ci of cobalt-60 in the plaque to achieve a total integrated dose to the target of 4.5 megarads.

At this point cesium-137 should be considered as an alternative source. In Section I it was determined that the annual cost of cobalt-60 was $0.131 per curie as compared to $0.115 per curie for cesium-137. However 3.79 Ci of cesium-137 are required for every curie of cobalt-60 to produce equivalent exposure thereby producing an effective cost of $0.436 per curie for cesium-137. This eliminates cesium for this application as it requires an annual cost of $415,000 for the cesium as compared to $124,000 for the cobalt.

The total product thickness on either side of the plaque will be 50 in., and a single package will make five passes on either side of the plaque. Figure 6.14 shows a representative multipass system of this type. These findings can now be used to: (1) calculate the internal volume and size of the irradiation facility; and (2) determine the total length of the conveyor system within and outside the irradiation facility. The internal volume of the facility will be approximately 1080 ft³ based on internal dimensions of 5 ft by 12 ft by 18 ft.*

Using the data presented in Figs. 6.7, 6.8, and 6.9, the thickness of concrete, lead, and earth required to adequately shield the source plaque can be determined. It has already been shown that cesium-137 cannot be considered for this case due to the great difference in capital investment for the two sources when such large quantities of radioisotopes are required. Therefore, only shield thicknesses for cobalt-60 need be considered and evaluated for relative cost even though cesium-137 might result in some savings in shield thickness. For a 950,000 Ci source plaque the shield thickness would be 12.5 in. for lead, 67 in. for concrete, and 98.5 in. for earth fill.†

It can be seen immediately that such large quantities of lead would be much higher in cost as compared to either concrete or earth leaving the latter two as the shield materials to be considered. However, considerable savings may be achieved if the storage volume were below ground level and/or if a composite shield were considered involving a lead shield as an inner shell to save space followed by a concrete structure, or a double-wall concrete shell with dry earth fill. Finally, savings can be achieved with a concrete building partially below ground having earth graded against the walls and some earth covering the roof with grass planted in the earth to preclude erosion. In all these cases moisture-proof construction becomes essential. To consider earth as a potential shield material, the topography and geology of the proposed facility site should be known. For example, it would be unwise to use earth shielding on a perfectly flat site unless a below-grade structure were to be considered and it would be

---

*Allowance is made for monorail supports and clearances, source plaque structure, and product carrier maneuvering.

†This assumes a line source strength of $1.46 \times 10^{13}$ MeV/sec-cm.

unwise to consider a below-grade structure if ground water levels were high enough to create persistent moisture problems within the facility. These factors not only cause problems in design and construction, but also have considerable effect on the nuclear safety aspects of the facility which could complicate and impede nuclear licensing of the facility.

For the purpose of the beef sterilization facility, it will be assumed that a topographically flat site exists with no ground water levels that could cause moisture problems. A concrete structure would consist of approximately 270 yards of concrete assuming internal facility dimensions of 5 ft by 12 ft by 18 ft and a concrete shield wall thickness of 5.6 ft. Therefore, from Table 6.6, the shield cost can be determined to be $54,000. An excavated earth shield roof for the facility would bear a cost of $31,000 as determined from Table 6.6. Additional shield costs for providing a labyrinth at the entry/exit point to the irradiation facility will be incurred (see Fig. 6.15) since the labyrinth is required to adequately shield the entry/exit portal. These additional costs will be $6,250 for the concrete structure assuming 50 ft of additional shield wall and ceiling is required at a reduced average thickness of 1.5 ft. (This reduced thickness is due to increased scatter and $1/r^2$ attenuation of the gamma-rays.) The earth shield will require additional costs of approximately $3,600 for the labyrinth using the same assumptions as for the concrete structure.

Under the assumptions given for this particular case the shield costs can now be compared. The excavated earth shield represents a savings of $26,650 over the concrete shield and should be used for this application.

The total length of the conveyor system will be essentially the same for either facility shield concept. This length can be determined by calculating the total distance traveled on both sides of the source plaque and adding to that distance the length of conveyor required for entry into and exit from the facility. Therefore, the total length of monorail conveyor required for the facility plus loading and unloading lengths will be approximately 160 ft. Referring to Table 6.4 the conveyor cost is found to be $12,800.

The next factor to be considered in the economic analysis is the source plaque conveyor mechanism and storage well. Since a planar source plaque has been selected this cost factor can be determined from Table 6.7. For the proposed facility a capital cost of $28,000 will be incurred.

The process techniques involved in beef sterilization by radiation have been thoroughly investigated thereby eliminating the need for piloting this package irradiation concept. It was previously mentioned that refrigeration of the beef during irradiation was necessary to ensure an acceptable

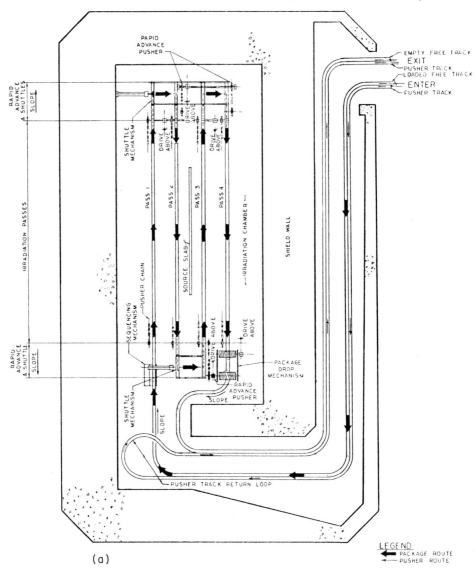

(a)

<u>OVERHEAD CONVEYOR</u>
<u>PLAN</u>
BOTTOM OF RAIL ELEV.+8-4"

FIG. 6.14a.   Overhead conveyer plan.

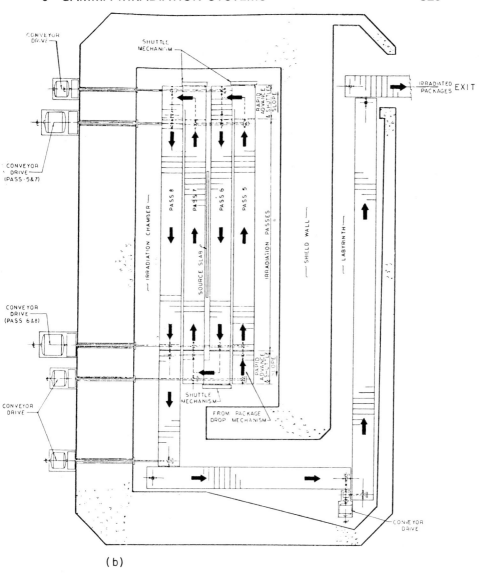

(b)

FLOOR  CONVEYOR
PLAN
TOP OF CONVEYOR ELEV=1'-3"

FIG. 6.14b.  Floor conveyor plan.

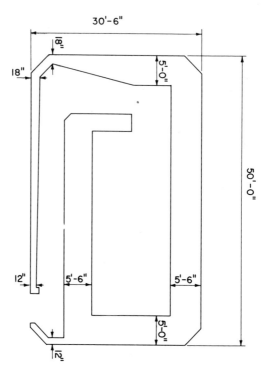

FIG. 6.15.   Labyrinth shield (entrance maze).

end result in the sterilized product and that liquid nitrogen was proved to be the best refrigerant. Based on extensive experimental work at the U.S. Army Natick Laboratory, the refrigerant costs have been determined to be $0.023 per pound of product or $308,000 per year. This cost includes the total capital cost, return on investment, and nitrogen supply at 1.5 cents per pound. It can be calculated (4) from the equation

$$P = \frac{\$84,000}{X} + 0.0164 \qquad (6.3)$$

where $P$ is the cost in dollars per pound and $X$ is the annual throughput in pounds; 0.0164 is a constant covering depreciation on capital costs, etc.

The final economic factors can now be considered for the beef irradiation facility. Table 6.9 can be used to apply dollar amounts to the six miscellaneous cost areas defined in Section I. These costs will be as follows:

(1) Miscellaneous equipment        $27,000
(2) Annual maintenance costs        17,300 (includes 1/2 man year)
(3) Annual operating costs         185,489 (includes 9 operators
                                           and 1 supervisor)
(4) Interest on capital investment  51,500 (Capital investment in-
                                           cludes full, initial cost
                                           for source of $550,000)
(5) Local taxes and insurance        4,380
(6) Architect and engineering
    services                        21,934

All economic factors have now been determined for the irradiation processing facility to sterilize 6,700 tons of beef per year. Since meat proces-
sors will be interested in the cost per pound of processing by this technique the cost factors must be summed and presented in this manner
(Table 6.11).

TABLE 6.11
SUMMARY OF IRRADIATOR COSTS

| Item | Total cost/year[a] | Cost/pound/year |
|------|-------------------:|----------------:|
| (1) Cobalt-60 source | $124,000 | $0.009250 |
| (2) Shield | 3,460 | 0.000259 |
| (3) Conveyor system | 1,280 | 0.000096 |
| (4) Source plaque conveyor system and storage well | 2,800 | 0.000209 |
| (5) Refrigeration costs | 308,000 | 0.023000 |
| (6) Miscellaneous equipment | 2,700 | 0.000202 |
| (7) Annual maintenance costs | 17,300 | 0.001292 |
| (8) Annual operation costs | 185,989 | 0.013800 |
| (9) Interest on capital investment | 51,500 | 0.003840 |
| (10) Local taxes and insurance | 4,380 | 0.000327 |
| (11) Architect and engineering services | 2,193 | 0.000163 |
| Total | $703,092 | $0.052437 |

[a]Capital costs are written off over ten-year period. Source costs include replacement
and shipping costs.

## B.  Bulk Solid Irradiation Plant*

For the case of a bulk solid irradiation facility, a complete comparison
will be made between a planar source plaque and a line source plaque.
This analysis will be based on a complex requirement to irradiate a chemical which will be called Polymer A. The effects of irradiation will enhance

*Any process details presented here are representative and do not relate to any actual
plant. They are presented here to illustrate design procedure only.

the mechanical properties of Polymer A at a point within a total chemical process thereby making this irradiation facility one unit within the complete chemical processing facility. The concept employing the planar plaque will be called Facility Concept A and the concept employing the line source will be called Facility Concept B.

Polymer A will be assumed to have characteristics like polyethylene and has several unique characteristics which must be considered to assure safe and reliable processing.

The unique characteristics of Polymer A to be considered are:

(1)   good hydraulic characteristics due to small particle size (approximately 25 microns);

(2)   explosive characteristics of an atmosphere saturated with Polymer A.

(3)   maintenance of chemical purity of Polymer A, and

(4)   maximum Polymer A temperature limited to 50°C.

Throughput requirements for the facilities will be 2,000,000 pounds per year at an integrated exposure of $0.4 \times 10^6$ rads. The annual duty cycle will be 7,000 hr and the maximum to minimum dose ratio is 1.4.

It should be noted that the planar source plaque in this evaluation has been modified significantly from the plaque shown in Fig. 6.3. This is not meant to cause confusion for the reader but to optimize the uniformity over a smaller frontal area than the 4 ft × 8 ft plaque shown in Fig. 6.3 and, thereby, develop a more exacting economic analysis. This alteration in the design of the source plaque will illustrate methods which must be employed on final facility design and evaluation. A comparative analysis using the source data presented in Section I will show the accuracy of these data.

Computer calculations have also been performed to determine shield structure thicknesses. Here again a comparison of the shield data given in Section I with the computer-developed data for this specific case will show very good agreement. Greater detailed attention will be given to all aspects of this problem to exemplify the detailed consideration for the reader making an accurate economic and design analysis of a potential radiation processing facility.

It will be assumed that due to geological conditions an excavated earth shield is not acceptable, thereby necessitating an above ground concrete structure. A lead shield will not be economically feasible due to the large size of the facility.

The product conveyor system used for Facility Concept A can be the most economical system shown in Table 6.5 which is the belt conveyor and gravity flow combined. This concept is for a bin-type irradiator, utilizing highly reliable and economical belt and gravity feed systems and a shaped, planar irradiation source.

Facility Concept B is for an irradiator employing a mixing technique to greatly enhance irradiation source efficiency. Here again highly economical and reliable belt conveyors are used. In addition, a ribbon conveying-mixing system is employed which, when coupled with a shaped-line source array, results in more efficient use of the gamma energy being emitted from the source.

**1. Facility Concept A: Summary.** Arrangement and details for this concept are shown in Fig. 6.16. The system will be housed in a shielding structure of concrete equipped with carbon steel liners for all equipment and service penetrations. All materials in contact with Polymer A will be stainless steel, chrome-plated carbon steel, and aluminum. An exhaust fan will be provided to clear the irradiation bin of dust during filling of the system prior to startup to preclude the possibility of explosion and to minimize ozone. The process system will be completely sealed. Storage and discharge bins, conveyor belts, chutes, and the irradiation bin will be stainless steel construction. All drive units and bearings will be located outside the sealed system for ease of maintenance and prevention of radiation damage.

The radiation source will be normally positioned in seven 2-in. diameter tubes which penetrate the irradiation bin. These sources can be retracted into the building wall storage area by means of a manually operated rod to allow personnel access to the irradiation room.

System operation will be accomplished from an operating room adjacent to the irradiation facility. An instrument rack in the operating room will contain all the necessary controls and indicators for normal operation of the facility.

Material flow in the system will be accomplished by a combination of gravity and powered belt conveyor. Polymer from the input hopper located on top of the shielding building will flow onto the input belt conveyor through a gate and will be moved into the irradiation bin. Flow through the irradiation bin will be by gravity and outflow will be on a second powered belt conveyor. The output conveyor will dump the irradiated polymer into a second bin.

A synchronized driving system for the input and output conveyors will give accurate control of polymer flow through the irradiator.

**2. Facility Concept B: Summary.** Arrangement and details for this concept are shown in Fig. 6.17. The system will be housed in a shielding structure of concrete equipped with carbon steel liners for all equipment and service penetrations. All materials in contact with Polymer A will be stainless steel, chrome-plated carbon steel, and aluminum. The process

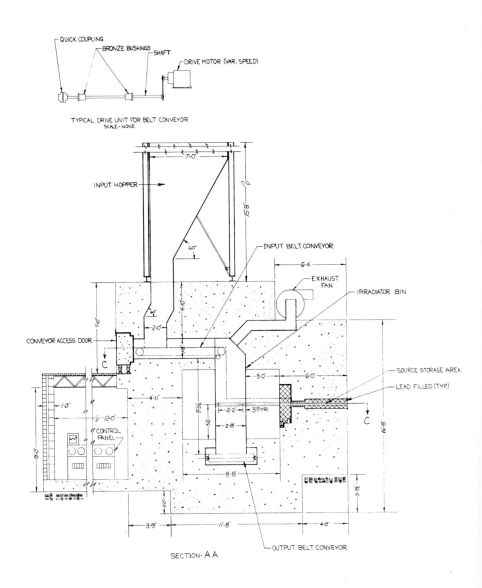

FIG. 6.16a.   Facility Concept A—vertical section.

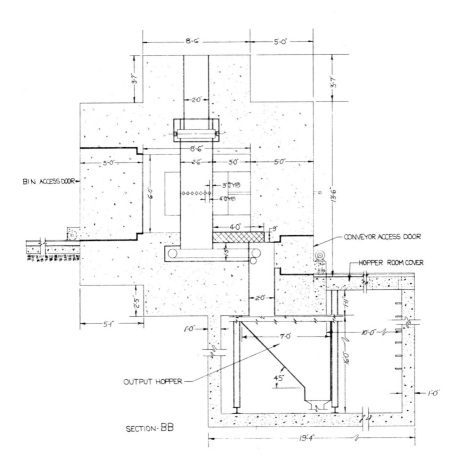

FIG. 6.16b.   Facility Concept A—elevation.

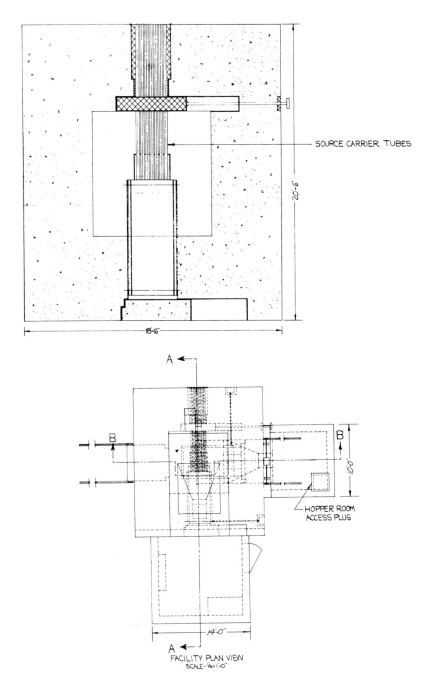

SOURCE CARRIER TUBES

HOPPER ROOM ACCESS PLUG

A

B

B

A

FACILITY PLAN VIEW
SCALE-¼"=1'-0"

20'-6"

18'-6"

10'-0"

14'-0"

Fig. 6.16c.   Facility Concept A—details of source and hopper.

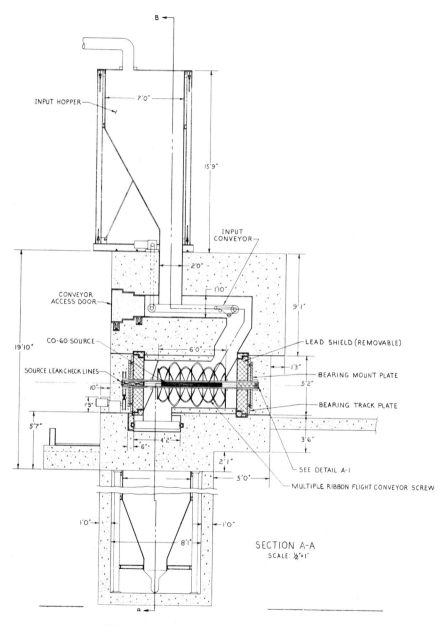

FIG. 6.17a.  Facility Concept B—vertical section.

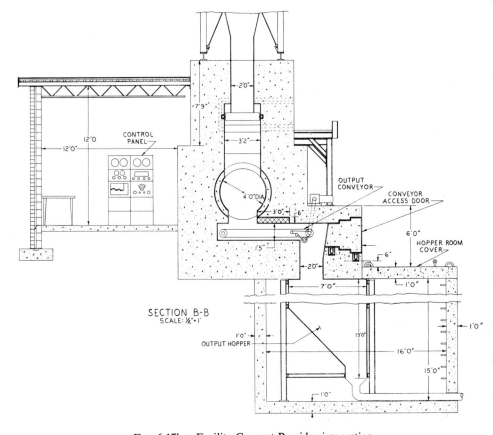

FIG. 6.17b.   Facility Concept B—side view section.

system will be completely sealed. Storage and discharge bins, conveyor belts, chutes, and the irradiation bin will be of stainless steel construction. The ribbon conveyor-mixer will be high strength aluminum construction. All drive units and bearings will be sufficiently shielded to preclude radiation damage and will be easily accessible for routine maintenance.

The radiation source will be positioned within the drive shaft for the ribbon conveyor-mixer. The source holder will contain a total of eighteen source strips arranged in five tiers and the source holder will be locked in a second aluminum tube within the drive shaft. Storage of the source within a shielded container in this facility will not be required.

System operation will be accomplished from an operating room adjacent to the irradiation facility. An instrument rack within the operating

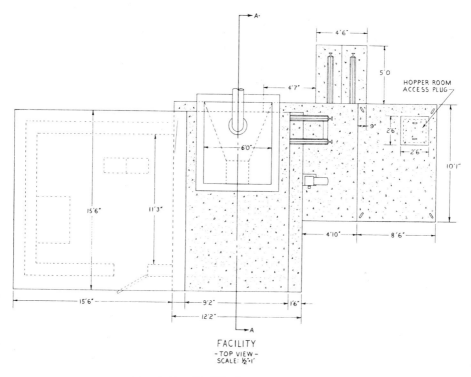

FIG. 6.17c.   Facility Concept B—top view.

room will contain all necessary controls and indicators for normal operating functions.

Material flow in the system will be accomplished by gravity, powered
belt conveyor, and a ribbon conveyor-mixer. Polymer from the input hopper located on top of the shielding structure will flow onto an input belt
conveyor through a gate and will be moved into the irradiation bin. Flow
through the irradiation bin will be accomplished by a ribbon conveyor
equipped with reverse pitch ribbons, thus assuring that homogeneous mixing of the bulk polymer can be attained. This allows the use of a larger irradiation volume than that in Concept A, thereby producing greater irradiation source efficiency. An output belt conveyor will dump the irradiated polymer into a second bin.

A synchronized driving system for the input conveyor, ribbon conveyor-mixer, and output conveyor will result in accurate flow control through
the irradiator.

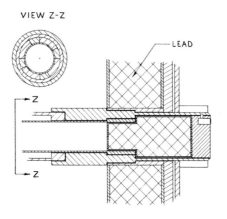

VIEW Z-Z

DETAIL  A-I   LEAD PLUG(REMOVABLE)
SCALE: NONE

FIG. 6.17d.   Facility Concept B—details.

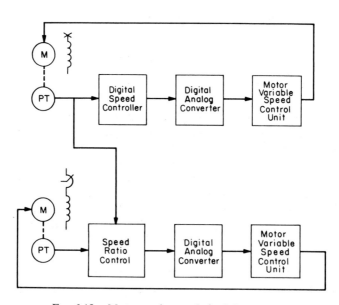

FIG. 6.18.   Motors and controls for belt conveyors.

**3.   Technical Description: Facility Concept A.**   The Facility A concept shown in Fig. 6.16 is for a bulk flow irradiation system where an optimum bin size has been chosen based on processing capacity requirements and source utilization efficiency. The use of gravity feed through the irradiator is a straightforward approach and only the local flow characteristics of Polymer A within the bin and around the source tubes need be investigated before final design is initiated.

a.   PROCESS ENCLOSURE.   The process system will be completely sealed and of stainless steel construction. All interior surfaces will be polished to assure proper product flow. The process enclosures will provide an air tight, dust and moisture proof system that will be free of all materials of a contaminating nature. Air with less than 60% relative humidity will be fed into the process enclosure from the plant air system.

b.   CONVEYOR SYSTEM.   Polymer A will flow through the system by means of gravity and powered belt conveyors. The input hopper positioned on top of the shielding structure will have a 24-hr material capacity for a nominal flow rate of 11.9 ft³/hr of polymer A. The hopper will be of stainless steel construction with the output chute located in one corner to prevent cavitation. The pitch of the tapered section of the output chute will be 60°. Assuming an angle of repose of 45° for Polymer A agglomerates in contact with the polished hopper interior, free flow under operating conditions is assured.

The output chute on the storage hopper will closely match the surface of the stainless steel input conveyor and the chute will have a gate on the front surface operating perpendicular to the direction of belt movement. This gate coupled with belt speed control gives a precise control of volume input. The polymer flows off the belt and enters the irradiation bin.

The output conveyor is identical in construction and operation to the input conveyor with material flowing off the output belt and into the output hopper. Capacity of the output hopper is 24 hr at a nominal product flow rate of 11.9 ft³/hr.

Precise metering of Polymer A through the irradiator is obtained by means of a servo feedback motor control system. The drives on the two belt conveyors are matched through a master-slave motor system to enable precise matching of the input and output conveyor belt speeds. Total drift from predetermined speed settings will be less than 0.5% per year. Figure 6.18 is a schematic representation of the conveyor speed control system.

The stainless steel conveyor belts will have a rough surface and will be wiped clean with reverse rotation stainless steel brushes. All bearings requiring lubrication will be located outside the radiation area and will be sealed.

c. SOURCE CONCEPT ANALYSIS. For a design basis the process rate has been taken to be $2 \times 10^6$ pounds per year with an annual duty cycle of 7,000 hr. With an average bulk density of 24 pounds/ft³ (0.384 g/cm³) the required volume process rate is approximately 11.9 ft³/hr or $3.4 \times 10^5$ cm³/hr.

With the volume process rate as a basic design guide, preliminary source design analyses have been performed to consider alternative concepts and to determine other basic design factors which would be in accordance with the irradiation specifications for Polymer A. Dose rate patterns have been computed on an IBM 7094 Computer using the QAD shielding program. This program computes dose rates from a distributed source by representing the source as a collection of point isotropic sources, performing a point kernel calculation for each source-to-receiver point and summing the results for all sources. For photons, the program does a multigroup calculation using exponential attenuation for materials on the source–receiver point vector to compute uncollided radiation and a fit to moments method data to estimate the scattered portion of the radiation.

The configuration presented is a planar source model, and it is treated in detail since it offers a fairly high efficiency and can be used with single pass flow. The calculational model is illustrated in Fig. 6.19. Source strips (cobalt-60) of about 6 in. active length are arranged in a matrix within the x-y plane, and are housed in threes within 2-in. tubes to form a grating array. The grating is placed and supported within a parallelepiped irradiation chamber. A cross-sectional view of the grating is indicated at the top of Fig. 6.19. Each tube is capped or shaped to enhance the flow of the polymer as it passes through the grating under gravity feed.

Relative strengths of each active source strip are varied to obtain approximate isodose planes as a function of distance above the source plane. Fractional source strengths, normalized to one curie total, are indicated in Fig. 6.19 beside each active stip. Figures 6.20 and 6.21 illustrate dose rates within the polymer for 38 cm by 38 cm receiver point arrays given as a function of distance above the source plane. Since the source array is symmetrically loaded for activity, dose rate patterns are symmetrical and only one quadrant of each receiver point array is shown; that is, the origin of each receiver point array lies on a line that is perpendicular to and through the center of the source plane. All dose rates are in polyethylene rads/hr-Ci and were calculated within the polymer assuming a bulk

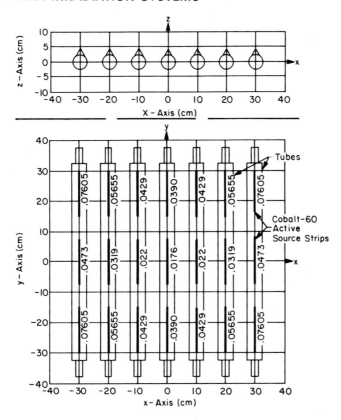

FIG. 6.19.   Plane source calculational model for Facility Concept A.

density of 0.384 g/cm³ and using a mass attenuation coefficient equivalent to that of polyethylene.

A study of the dose rate patterns indicates that a fair degree of uniformity is achieved with the given source loading.

For each plane quadrant, dose rate patterns over a square area of about 35 cm by 35 cm are within or very close to the maximum to minimum dose ratio of 1.4 specified for the polymer irradiation. With the approximate dose rate uniformity over planes above and below the source array, each polymer lamina passing through the irradiation volume under gravity feed and equilibrium conditions will receive an integrated dose that is within the maximum to minimum ratio. The cross sectional area of the source grating, which will allow the polymer to pass is approximately 3350 cm².

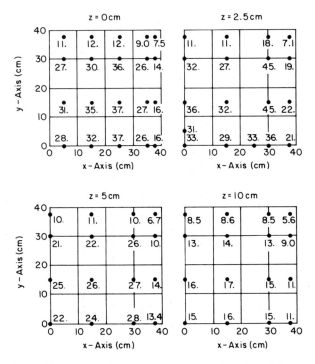

FIG. 6.20.   Plane source dose rate patterns ($z = 0$ to 10 cm) for Facility
Concept A. Dose rates: rads/hr-Ci.

The dose rate distribution for each plane above the source has been
integrated over the plane area using a specially prepared computer program to obtain the area-averaged dose rate. Results of these computations
are plotted as a function of distance above the source plane in Fig. 6.22.
Further integrations over various distances have been performed to obtain the volume-averaged dose rates and other design parameters as a
function of irradiation chamber height. Assuming, as an example, that
the effective irradiation volume is a parallelepiped with a cross-sectional
area of approximately 5770 cm² and height of 115 cm (60 cm above and
below the source with substraction from source space) the irradiation
volume is $6.63 \times 10^5$ cm³ and the volume-averaged dose rate is 8.24 rads/
hr-Ci. With a design volume process rate of $3.4 \times 10^5$ cm³/hr, maximum
dwell time of the polymer within the irradiation volume is 1.95 hr. Since
the required average dose rate is $4 \times 10^5$ rads/hr, the minimum average
dose rate is $2.1 \times 10^5$ rads/hr, and a total source activity of approximately

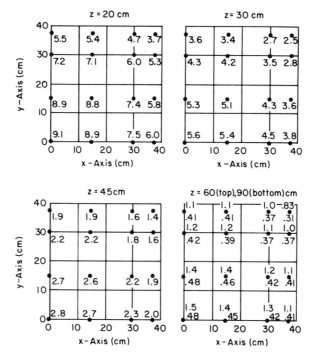

FIG. 6.21.  Plane source dose rate patterns ($z = 20$ to $90$ cm) for Facility Concept A. Dose rates: rads/hr-Ci.

24,900 Ci is obtained by dividing the required average dose rate by the volume-averaged dose rate per curie. Also for a volume of $6.63 \times 10^5$ cm$^3$ and the volume-averaged dose rate of 8.24 rads/hr-Ci the energy absorption rate within the irradiation volume is equal to:

$$8.24 \text{ rads/hr-Ci} \times 100 \text{ ergs/g-rads} \times 1/360 \text{ hr/sec} \times 0.384 \text{ g/cm}^3$$
$$\times 6.63 \times 10^5 \text{ cm}^3 \times 1/1.6 \times 10^{-6} \text{ MeV/ergs}$$
$$= 3.64 \times 10^{10} \text{ MeV/sec-Ci.}$$

Since the energy release of one curie of cobalt-60 is $9.25 \times 10^{10}$ MeV/sec-Ci, the efficiency (ratio of energy absorbed in the irradiation volume to the energy emitted by the source) is about 39%. Other small losses from gamma absorption in the source, source tubes, and source holder are neglected but are estimated to be about 10% or less.

Similar performance calculations have been carried out for other irradiation chamber heights and results are summarized in Table 6.12.

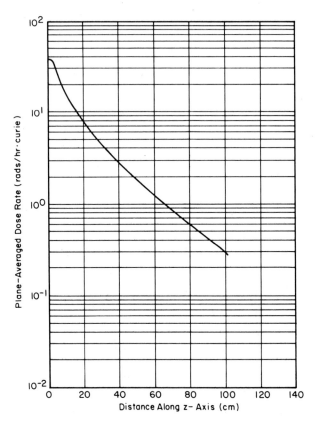

FIG. 6.22.   Dose rates as a function of distance above the plane source model
for Facility Concept A.

Slightly greater efficiency is achieved by increasing the volume height
but a greater sacrifice is made in the volume-averaged dose rate. This will
require a longer irradiation time while the source strength is reduced only
slightly. The practical size of the plane is influenced by other considerations such as structure and shielding cost. For this concept a height of 3
ft (approximately 90 cm) has been chosen as a practical size limitation.
Thus, with 3 ft above and below the source plane, the irradiation volume
is approximately 6 ft × 2.5 ft × 2.5 ft.

The number of sources and approximate specific activities required
are summarized in Table 6.13.

d.   POLYMER HEATING.   Consideration must be given to the temperature rise in the polymer due to gamma heating. Very near the planar

TABLE 6.12

PLANE SOURCE CONFIGURATION PERFORMANCE PARAMETERS

| Height above source plane (cm) | Irradiation volume (cm³) | Maximum irradiation dwelltime (hr) | Required average dose rate (rads/hr) | Volume averaged dose rate (rads/hr Ci) | Required activity (Ci) | Approximate efficiency (%) |
|---|---|---|---|---|---|---|
| 60 | $6.63 \times 10^5$ | 1.95 | $2.1 \times 10^5$ | 8.24 | 24,900 | 39 |
| 70 | $7.79 \times 10^5$ | 2.29 | $1.75 \times 10^5$ | 7.11 | 24,660 | 40 |
| 90 | $1.01 \times 10^6$ | 2.97 | $1.35 \times 10^5$ | 5.67 | 23,900 | 41 |
| 120 | $1.35 \times 10^6$ | 3.97 | $1.01 \times 10^5$ | 4.32 | 23,300 | 42 |

source plaque the dose rate will be on the order of $9.5 \times 10^5$ rads/hr for a 25,000 Ci source. This is equal to a heating rate of 2.3 cal/g hr and with a specific heat of 0.5 cal/g°C (polyethylene) assumed for Polymer A, the temperature rise, without any heat loss, will be 4.6°C/hr. Thus for the polymer temperature to rise from ambient of about 20°C to the maximum allowable of 50°C would require at least 6.5 hr. The exposure time for each lamina of polymer in the peak radiation fields would be far less than this. For a volume-averaged dose rate of 5.67 rads/hr-Ci the time required for the polymer temperature to exceed 50°C would be about 43 hr, far more than the maximum dwell time of 2.97 hr for the polymer in the irradiation volume. In view of these considerations no bulk heating problems will be encountered.

e.  SYSTEM HOUSING.  The structure housing the irradiation facility will be of ordinary concrete construction to the dimensions and design

TABLE 6.13

CALCULATED SOURCE MATERIAL REQUIREMENTS FOR FACILITY CONCEPT A

| Number of strips | Percent of total | Specific activity[a] (Ci/g) | Curies |
|---|---|---|---|
| 4 | 0.314 | 75 | 7800 |
| 4 | 0.226 | 54 | 5620 |
| 4 | 0.172 | 41 | 4260 |
| 2 | 0.095 | 45 | 2290 |
| 2 | 0.078 | 37 | 1890 |
| 2 | 0.064 | 31 | 1580 |
| 2 | 0.044 | 21 | 1070 |
| 1 | 0.0175 | 17 | 455 |
| Totals | | | |
| 21 | 1.0105 | | 24,965 |

[a]Based on strips of 6 in. active length containing 26 g per strip.

shown in Fig. 6.16. All penetrations in the shield will be lined with 0.50 in. thick carbon steel liners painted with Carboline grade radiation resistant paint.

Calculations have been carried out with the QAD program to estimate the required shielding for the planar source concept. The calculational model assumed was that of bulk concrete walls enclosing an irradiation volume of size and form as that shown in Fig. 6.16. Radiation levels within ordinary concrete as determined along the $x$ and $y$ axes of the source configuration are shown in Fig. 6.23. Concrete thicknesses necessary to reduce the radiation leakage to $10^{-2}$ rads/hr were chosen for a design basis, and these estimates of necessary shielding thicknesses taking into account possible streaming paths are indicated in Fig. 6.18.

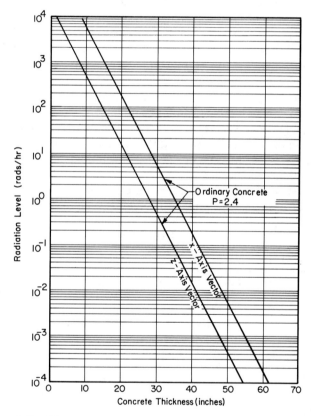

FIG. 6.23.   Plane source concrete shielding for Facility Concept A.

f. MONITORING AND CONTROL INSTRUMENTATION. An operations room will be located adjacent to the system housing which will contain the irradiator operation process control and monitoring panel. The following controls and indicators will be located on the panel: conveyor motor speed control; conveyor speed indicator; polymer flow indicator; source leak check terminals (see Chapter 3); area radiation monitors, access door controls; input and output hopper low and high level indicators; exhaust fan control; and master control power circuit breakers, motor starters, and operation interlock system.

Plant throughput can be adjusted by changing the speed of the input and output conveyors and with no alteration to source strength. All operations at a desired throughput will be completely automatic. Six nuclear density gauging units will be used as level and flow indicators. Three gamma ionization chambers and readout units will monitor the radiation level: (1) inside the system housing adjacent to the irradiation bin, (2) outside the system housing at the input chute, and (3) outside the system housing at the output chute.

Controls for operating the facility access doors will be located on the control panel and will be adequately interlocked to preclude opening until the source is safely secured. A linear recorder will be provided to record polymer throughput on a continuous basis. Gas inlet and outlet lines will be located on the control panel for periodic leak check of the cobalt source. Manual override control for the irradiation bin dust exhaust fan will be located on the control panel.

g. SYSTEM OPERATION AND RELIABILITY. Operation of Facility Concept A will normally be completely automatic. However, allowance will be made for manual override on any phase of operation with the exception of radiation safety interlocks.

The normal sequence of automatic operation will be as shown in Fig. 6.24. All sequencing controls will be of the automatic reset type with the exception of radiation safety interlocks and main power circuit breakers which will be manual reset type. All master controls will be key switch interlocked to preclude inadvertent facility operation by unauthorized personnel.

The belt conveyor drive will be a master–slave motor system as shown in Fig. 6.18. Desired master-motor speed will be dialed into a digital speed controller.

Output from a photo-tachometer will be compared with the dialed-in speed settings. The ratio of the slave motor speed to the master motor

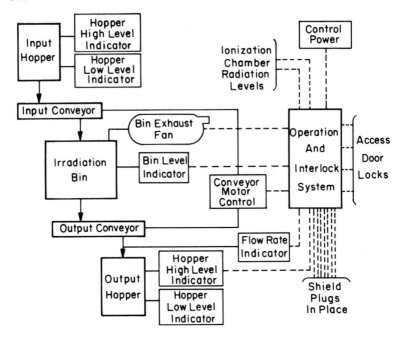

FIG. 6.24.   Operating sequence—Facility Concept A.

Normal Automatic Operating Sequence

| Step | Operating event | Sequence event |
|---|---|---|
| 1 | Access doors closed and locked<br>Radiation levels satisfactory<br>Shield plugs in place and locked | Control power on |
| 2 | Manual start | Input conveyor on<br>Bin exhaust fan on<br>Output conveyor on |
| 3 | Bin level indicator on | Bin exhaust fan off<br>Flow rate permissive energized |
| 4 | Output hopper high level | Input conveyor off |
| 5 | Bin level indicator off | Bin exhaust fan on |
| 6 | Flow rate indicator off | Output conveyor off |
| 7 | Manual reset and restart required | |

Flow rate indicator off after step 3 has been satisfied; de-energizes conveyor motor control

speed will be dialed into the speed ratio control and this ratio control compares the photo-tachometer output of the master and slave motors. An error in either setting will generate digital correction signals which will be fed to the motor's variable speed control unit through the digital–

analog converter. The variable speed control unit will convert ac to dc for motor drive by means of a silicon controlled rectifier circuit on command from the digital speed controller. This control system will provide essentially zero error over a year of continuous operation.

Personnel requirements for operating the facility should be satisfied as follows for normal operation: 1/4 time – 1 technician and 1/4 time – 1 supervisor.

Maintenance requirements for Facility Concept A should be minimal. All enclosures in contact with Polymer A will be of stainless steel construction so as to provide a maintenance-free enclosure.

All conveyors considered in this design concept are designed to provide continuous operation with no maintenance during the duty cycle. All bearings will be sealed and are designed for extended continuous service. All motors and belts are designed so that annual inspection at shutdown will satisfy maintenance requirements. Should unexpected maintenance be required, replacement equipment could be on line in minimum time.

h. SYSTEM SAFETY. The design approach to Facility Concept A presents an inherently safe concept in that maximum assurance is provided against inadvertent personnel entry into the irradiator by electrical and mechanical interlocks. Only after properly satisfying these interlocks, which includes source storage, can access be gained to the conveyors and/ or irradiation room.

Safety of the cobalt source is assured since it is doubly encapsulated in stainless steel, mechanically locked in source carriers, and housed in the sealed source carrier tubes.

Although a dust explosion is highly unlikely in a sealed system a high capacity exhaust fan will be provided and will operate during those periods when there would most likely be dust accumulation in the system. The facility design eliminates potential spark generators and hot surfaces which could cause ignition of an explosive mixture of Polymer A dust in air.

**4. Technical Description: Facility Concept B.** The Facility Concept B shown in Fig. 6.17 is for a bulk mixing irradiation system employing powered belt conveyors, ribbon conveying-mixing, and gravity flow, based on a line source. Selection of this concept for discussion has been made because of the higher source efficiency attainable and reduced shielding requirements.

a. PROCESS ENCLOSURE. The process system will be completely sealed and of stainless steel construction. All interior surfaces will be polished to assure proper product flow. The process enclosures will provide an air-

tight dust and moisture proof system that will be free of all materials of
a contaminating nature. Air with less than 60% relative humidity will be
fed into the process enclosure from the plant air system.

   b. CONVEYOR SYSTEM. Polymer A will flow through the system by
means of gravity powered belt conveyors and a ribbon conveyor-mixer.
The input hopper positioned on top of the shielding structure will have a
24-hr material capacity for a nominal flow rate of 11.9 ft³/hr of Polymer A.
The hopper will be of stainless steel construction with the output chute
located in one corner to prevent cavitation. The pitch of the tapered section of the output chute will be 60°. Assuming on angle of repose of 45°
for Polymer A agglomerates and considering the polished hopper interior,
free flow under operating conditions is assured.

   The output chute on the storage hopper will closely match the surface
of the stainless steel input conveyor and the chute will have a gate on the
front surface operating perpendicular to the direction of belt movement.
This gate coupled with belt speed control gives a precise control of volume
input. The polymer flows off the belt and enters the irradiation bin.

   The ribbon conveyor-mixer is a double ribbon conveyor with opposite-
hand pitch angles on the two ribbons. The shaft of the conveyor-mixer is
hollow and contains the cobalt-60 source. Mixing action by the ribbon
conveyor will provide dose rate uniformity in the polymer as it is convey-
ed through the irradiator. Output from the ribbon conveyor-mixer flows
by gravity on to the output conveyor.

   The output conveyor is identical in construction and operation to the
input conveyor, and material flows off the output belt and into the output
hopper. Capacity of the output hopper is 24 hr at a nominal product flow
rate of 11.9 ft³/hr.

   Precise metering of Polymer A through the irradiator is obtained by
means of a servo feedback motor control system. The drives on the two
belt conveyors are matched through a master–slave motor system to enable precise matching of the input and output conveyor belt speeds. Total
drift from predetermined speed settings will be less than 0.5% per year.
The speed control system is similar to that for Concept A. Figure 6.25 is
a schematic diagram of the conveyor - mixer speed control system.

   The stainless steel conveyor belts will have a rough surface and will be
wiped clean with reverse rotation stainless steel brushes. All bearings requiring lubrication will be located outside the irradiation area and will be
sealed.

   c. SOURCE DESCRIPTION. One of the most efficient irradiation configurations is a line source surrounded by a cylindrical annulus of the poly-

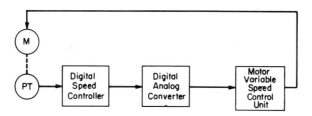

Fig. 6.25.  Motor and controls for double ribbon conveyors, Facility Concept B.

mer. Such a configuration has been examined and the computational model (showing only the lower quadrant) is illustrated in Fig. 6.24. The source is made up of five strips with 12-in. active lengths housed in a thin wall pipe with a diameter of approximately 6 in. Activity of the strip source array is varied to achieve axial dose rate uniformity. The source distribution, normalized to one curie total activity, is given in Table 6.14.

It is assumed that Polymer A fills the volume outside the source housing pipe with a bulk density of 0.384 g/cm³ and with a mass attenuation coefficient equivalent to that of polyethylene. Computed dose rate patterns in rads/hr-Ci are indicated in Fig. 6.26. As seen, the axial uniformity is fair and, except for the extreme ends of the source, is well within the maximum to minimum dose ratio of 1.4. However, radiation intensity decreases rapidly with radial distance and the dose ratio specification cannot be met over a very large volume unless adequate radial mixing of the polymer can be achieved as it passes through the irradiation chamber volume.

The dose rate distribution has been integrated over a fixed volume using a specially prepared computer program to obtain the volume-averaged dose rate and other design parameters. This approach is reasonable since the conveyor will cause mixing of the polymer. Assuming, as an example, that the effective irradiation volume is a cylinder 170 cm high with an inner radius of 7.6 cm and an outer radius of 60 cm, the irradiation volume is $1.89 \times 10^6$ cm³ and the volume-averaged dose rate is 3.8 rads/hr-Ci.

TABLE 6.14

LINE SOURCE DISTRIBUTION

| Source strip | Distance from source bottom (cm) | Curie fraction of cobalt-60 |
|---|---|---|
| 1 | 0 – 33.2 | 0.245 |
| 2 | 33.2 – 66.4 | 0.175 |
| 3 | 66.4 – 99.5 | 0.160 |
| 4 | 99.5 – 132.7 | 0.175 |
| 5 | 132.7 – 165.9 | 0.245 |

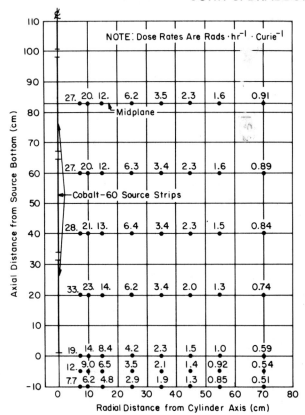

FIG. 6.26.   Line source calculational model with dose rate patterns for Facility Concept B.

With a volume process rate of $3.4 \times 10^5$ cm³/hr the maximum dwell time of the polymer within the irradiation volume is 5.5 hr. Since the required dose is $4 \times 10^5$ rads, the minimum average dose rate is $7.2 \times 10^4$ rads/hr. A minimum total source activity of approximately 19,000 Ci is obtained by dividing the required average dose rate by the volume-averaged dose rate per curie. For a volume of $1.89 \times 10^6$ cm³ and a volume-averaged dose rate 3.8 rads/hr-Ci the energy absorption rate within the irradiation volume is equal to $4.8 \times 10^{10}$ MeV/sec Ci. Since the energy release of one curie of Co-60 is $9.25 \times 10^{10}$ MeV/sec Ci, the efficiency is about 52%. Losses from gamma absorption in the source, source cladding, source holder, and source well pipe are neglected for the conceptual design studies, but are estimated to be about 10%.

TABLE 6.15

LINE SOURCE CONFIGURATION PERFORMANCE PARAMETERS

| Outer radius of cylinder (cm) | Irradiation volume (cm³) | Maximum irradiation dwell time (hr) | Required average dose rate (rads/hr) | Volume averaged dose rate (rads/hr Ci) | Required activity (Ci) | Approximate efficiency (%) |
|---|---|---|---|---|---|---|
| 40 | $8.24 \times 10^5$ | 2.4 | $1.67 \times 10^5$ | 6.46 | 26,000 | 38 |
| 60 | $1.89 \times 10^6$ | 5.5 | $7.21 \times 10^4$ | 3.80 | 19,000 | 52 |
| 70 | $2.58 \times 10^6$ | 7.6 | $5.27 \times 10^4$ | 3.03 | 17,500 | 58 |

The same performance calculations have been conducted for a smaller and larger volume by varying the outer radius of the irradiation volume. Results are summarized in Table 6.15.

Large radius cylinders, of course, give greater efficiency but a lower volume-averaged dose rate as a consequence of the larger radiation intensity range over the volume.

The useful size of the line source irradiation volume is limited primarily by the radius at which adequate radial mixing of the polymer can be maintained to meet the maximum to minimum dose ratio. A radius of 24 in. (approximately 60 cm) has been determined to be feasible for adequate mixing.

The number of strips and approximate specific activities required to assembly the line source are summarized in Table 6.16.

d. POLYMER HEATING. Temperature rise in the polymer due to gamma heating has also been estimated for the line source concept in a manner similar to that for the plane source concept. The volume-averaged dose rate of the recommended line source concept is about 3.8 rads/hr Ci. For a 20,000 Ci source the polymer heating rate is 18 cal/g hr. With a specific heat of 0.5 cal/g°C (polyethylene) assumed for Polymer A the temperature rise neglecting any heat loss is approximately 0.36°C/hr. The time required for the polymer temperature to rise from ambient (assume 20°C) to

TABLE 6.16

CALCULATED SOURCE MATERIAL REQUIREMENTS FOR FACILITY CONCEPT B

| Number of strips | Percent of total | Specific activity[a] (Ci/g) | Curies |
|---|---|---|---|
| 12 | 0.490 | 16 | 9,672 |
| 12 | 0.350 | 11 | 6,864 |
| 6 | 0.160 | 10 | 3,120 |
| Totals | | | |
| 30 | 1.000 | | 19,656 |

[a]Based on strips of 12 in. active length containing 52 g per strip.

50°C would be about 83 hr. This time is far more than the dwell time of 5.5 hr calculated for the line source irradiation volume. Therefore, as for the plane source, temperature rise in the bulk polymer around the line source is not excessive.

e. SYSTEM HOUSING.   The structure housing the irradiation facility will be of ordinary concrete construction to the dimensions and design shown in Fig. 6.17.   All penetrations in the shield will be lined with 0.50-in. thick carbon steel liners painted with Carboline grade radiation resistant paint.

In a manner similar to that for the plane source, calculations were carried out to estimate the required shielding for the line source concept. Radiation levels within ordinary concrete surrounding the line source irradiation volume have been determined as a function of thickness in the axial and radial directions. Results are shown in Fig. 6.27. Concrete thicknesses necessary to reduce the radiation leakage to $10^{-2}$ rads/hr have been chosen as a design basis and the form and amount of shielding required is indicated in Fig. 6.17.

The requirements for monitoring and control instrumentation, system operation and reliability, and system safety will be the same for the B concept as those described for the A concept on pp. 349–352.

**5. Evaluation of Facility Concepts A and B.**   a.   FACILITY CONCEPT A.   Facility Concept A represents a relatively simple approach in materials handling for Polymer A. A minimum amount of piloting work is required to assure that predicated flow characteristics in the system are obtained. The powered conveyors are capable of operating at the desired integrated dose of 2,000,000 pounds/7,000 hr of operation. All operational and interlock control units are off-the-shelf items and the operation of such systems has been proven on many previous applications.

b.   FACILITY CONCEPT B.   Facility Concept B makes use of a unique mixing technique which will result in a significant increase in source efficiency and consequently a reduction in total shielding. Piloting effort would be required to accurately coordinate the driving speed of the multiribbon conveyor-mixer with that of the input–output conveyor systems. Also, the homogeneity of polymer mixing to assure the required dose uniformity must be determined. The powered units will be capable of operating at the desired integrated dose at 2,000,000 lb/7,000 hr of operation. All operational and interlock control units are off-the-shelf items and the operation of such systems has been proven on many previous applications.

c.   EVALUATION SUMMARY.   Although the development problems associated with Facility Concept A are less than those for Facility Concept B, Concept A does represent a less efficient facility with respect to source

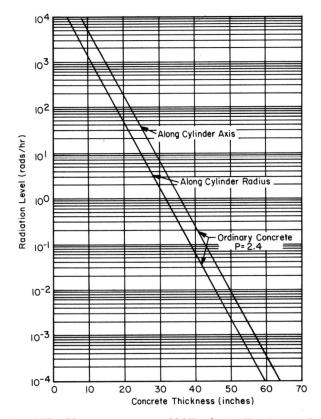

FIG. 6.27. Line source concrete shielding for Facility Concept B.

requirements accompanied by higher shield costs. The specific activity requirements for Concept A are higher, resulting in higher costs per curie for cobalt-60.

Facility Concept B offers a more efficient source design and lower specific activity requirements. Shield costs are subsequently lower because of reduced source strength requirements.

The final economic evaluation can now be made for both facility concepts as in Table 6.17 (10 year write-off is assumed).

### C. Conclusion

The methods of approach to concepting and economically analyzing radioisotope fueled irradiation systems presented in this chapter are not to be used for final design exercises. The accuracies required for large-

TABLE 6.17

COMPARISON OF COST DATA

| Item | Facility Concept A | | Facility Concept B | |
|------|------------------|-----------|------------------|-----------|
| | Total cost per year | Cost/lb-yr | Total cost per year | Cost/lb-yr |
| (1) Cobalt-60 source | $3,260 | $0.00160 | $2,570 | $0.00129 |
| (2) Shield | 6,100 | 0.00328 | 2,860 | 0.00143 |
| (3) Conveyor system | 550 | 0.00030 | 925 | 0.00046 |
| (4) Source plaque conveyor system and storage well | 1,500 | 0.00075 | 1,500 | 0.00075 |
| (5) Miscellaneous equipment | 2,700 | 0.00135 | 2,700 | 0.00135 |
| (6) Annual maintenance costs [a] | 960 | 0.00053 | 960 | 0.00053 |
| (7) Annual operating costs [b] | 17,535 | 0.00877 | 17,535 | 0.00877 |
| (8) Interest on capital investment [c] | 9,870 | 0.00494 | 7,300 | 0.00365 |
| (9) Local taxes and insurance [c] | 2,470 | 0.00123 | 1,825 | 0.00091 |
| (10) Architect and engineering services | 1,235 | 0.00062 | 913 | 0.00046 |
| Total | $46,080 | $0.02337 | $39,088 | $0.01960 |

[a] Based on 160 manhours/yr from service personnel.

[b] Based on 550 manhours/yr from operative personnel and 550 manhours/yr from supervisory personnel.

[c] Includes full initial cost for cobalt-60 source. This analysis is predicated on the basis that the input and output hoppers and their conveyor systems are provided by others.

scale source specification and arrangement can only be gained with exact calculations for each specific application. Cost for shield construction, conveyor systems, operations, etc., will vary with general economic fluctuations and must be compiled based on costs at the time of procurement and construction.

ACKNOWLEDGMENT

(1) Nuclear Analysis Department, Dr. A.O. Burford, Manager, Lockheed–Georgia Company for numerous calculations used in developing this chapter. (2) Division of Isotope Development, U.S. Atomic Energy Commission, Washington, D.C. for numerous figures and data.

REFERENCES

1. C. Jönemalm, *Nomogram for Determining Shield Thickness for Point and Line Sources of Gamma Rays,* Nuclear Structural Engineering **1**, 324-331 (1965).
2. Communication with U.S. AEC Division of Isotopes Development, Washington, D.C.
3. Food Irradiation Check List of Cost Considerations, prepared for delivery by

Harry W. Ketchum, Office of Chemicals and Consumer Products, BDSA, U.S. Department of Commerce at the briefing on Radiation Preservation of Foods, sponsored by the Southern Interstate Nuclear Board, Oak Ridge, Tennessee, Feb. 1, 1967.

4.  Robin P. Gardner and Ralph L. Ely, Jr., *Radioisotope Measurement Applications in Engineering,* Reinhold, New York, 1967.

# 7 RADIOISOTOPES—OR PARTICLE ACCELERATORS?

*E. ALFRED BURRILL*

CONSULTANT, APTOS, CALIFORNIA

Particle accelerators are often considered to be competitive to radio-isotopes in medical and industrial applications. The facts are, however, that many of the engineering-design aspects of the two kinds of radiation facilities cannot readily be compared and that many of the details of applying the various radiations are quite different. A strict economic evaluation is, therefore, difficult to make except in certain selected applications where either type of source (isotopic or accelerator) may optionally be utilized.

Nevertheless, it is of interest to examine typical particle-accelerator systems, their radiation characteristics, and their economics—in practical applications such as radiation therapy, industrial radiography, and radiation processing. From this brief review, the general subject of intense radiation sources and facilities can perhaps be put into better perspective.

## I. CHARACTERISTICS OF ACCELERATOR-PRODUCED RADIATIONS

All of the fundamental nuclear particles and ionizing radiations can be selectively produced by particle acceleration, either as high-velocity primary particles (electrons or ionized atoms), or as penetrating secondary

TABLE 7.1

Commercially Available Particle Accelerators: Range in Rated Particle Energy, Radiations Produced

| Accelerator type[a] | Rated particle energy (MeV) | Electrons | X rays | Ions | Neutrons |
|---|---|---|---|---|---|
| Betatron | 5.0 – 35.0 | x | x | | |
| Cockcroft–Walton | 0.3 – 4.0 | x | x | x | x |
| Cyclotron | 15.0 – 22.0 | | | x | x |
| Cylindrical electrostatic | 0.2 – 1.2 | x | x | x | x |
| Dynamitron | 1.5 – 4.0 | x | x | x | x |
| Electron Linac | 4.0 – 50.0 | x | x | | x |
| Tandem | 8.0 – 20.0 | | | x | x |
| Transformers: | | | | | |
| Insulating-core | 0.3 – 2.5 | x | x | x | x |
| Low-voltage | 0.1 – 0.2 | x | x | x | x |
| Resonant | 1.0 – 2.0 | x | x | | |
| Van de Graaff | 0.4 – 7.0 | x | x | x | x |

[a] Descriptions of these accelerators can be found in Refs. 1, 2, and 3.

radiations (X rays or neutrons) from appropriate targets bombarded by primary-particle beams. Table 7.1 lists the various types of particle accelerators that are commercially available, as well as the species of nuclear particles and radiations that can be produced by them.

*Electrons* are accelerated in well-directed beams that can be electromagnetically deflected and distributed in space. In principle, these charged particles are identical to the beta particles from radioactive decay. In practice, the electron-energy spectra are usually monoenergetic, as contrasted to continuous beta spectra. Electron beams in the 0.2–10 MeV range are in widespread use for industrial radiation processing. Electrons with energies up to 50 MeV are used directly in certain radiation-therapy treatments. For these applications, the electron beams are brought out of the evacuated acceleration region into the atmosphere through a thin electron-permeable window.

*X rays* (bremsstrahlung) are produced by the interaction of electrons and atomic nuclei, usually in heavy metal targets for greater efficiency of X-ray production. These electromagnetic radiations are characterized by a continuous energy spectrum, with a maximum energy corresponding to the impinging electron energy, and a peak in intensity at about one-third the maximum energy. X-ray beams above 1 MeV are generated preferentially in the direction of the accelerated electrons, to an extent that increases markedly with electron energy. In contrast, gamma rays from radioisotopes emanate isotropically and their original spectra consist of one or a few monoenergetic components. The most widespread applications of X rays are in radiation therapy and industrial radiography, where X-ray energies up to 35 MeV are utilized. Radiation processing with X rays has been studied, but no extensive production-line use has yet developed.

*Neutrons* are produced from the interaction of various species of accelerated positive ions with selected atomic nuclei. The most useful accelerator-type neutron-producing reactions, for activation analysis and neutron radiography, are the following:

$^2$H (d, n) $^3$He: 3–6 MeV neutrons (monoenergetic);
$^3$H (d, n) $^4$He: 14 MeV neutrons (monoenergetic);
$^9$Be (d, n) $^{10}$B : 1–6 MeV neutrons (spectrum).

Certain electron accelerators can be used to produce neutrons from photodisintegration ($\gamma$, n) reactions, but the available neutron fluxes are often much lower in magnitude than from the above-listed reactions. The neutron spectra from photodisintegration reactions are continuous, with one or more intensity peaks toward the low-energy end. Through proper choice of nuclear reaction, accelerator-produced neutrons can be obtained with energies ranging from thermal to very high energies. This entire spectrum is of great importance in nuclear and neutron research. Most progress in neutron activation analysis has been made with either thermal or 14-MeV neutrons, although there are certain advantages to the use of moderately fast neutrons in the 2–6 MeV range. The use of thermal neutrons for specialized radiographic purposes has been studied, but results have been somewhat limited by the large apparent source size of thermal neutrons. Neutron therapy is being investigated with very intense neutron beams in the 8–14 MeV range.

Isotopic sources of neutrons are mixtures of selected radioisotopes with beryllium, in which the alpha particles or the gamma rays instigate nuclear or photodisintegration reactions. Certain transplutonium isotopes emit neutrons from the spontaneous fissioning of the isotope. Typical isotopic neutron sources are listed below:

$^{124}$Sb–Be ($\gamma$, n): 0.025-MeV neutrons (spectrum);
$^{210}$Po–Be ($\alpha$, n): 11-MeV (max) neutrons (spectrum);
$^{239}$Pu–Be ($\alpha$, n): 11-MeV (max) neutrons (spectrum);
$^{252}$Cf (fission) : 6-MeV (max) neutrons (spectrum).

*Positive ions* of many species throughout the table of nuclides are accelerated for research purposes, with energies that are more limited by accelerator technology than by their research value. Except for the very high-energy accelerators for fundamental-particle research in the GeV realm, most machines produce ion beams with energies well below 100 MeV. Multiply-charged heavy ions have been accelerated to energies of several hundred MeV in efforts to produce transplutonium isotopes. Singly charged ions, such as $^1$H, $^2$H, $^3$He, $^4$He, are used for the production of quantities of neutron-deficient radioisotopes. Bombarding energies are usually in the 15–30 MeV range for this application.

## II.  ACCELERATOR FACILITIES

For the purpose of the remainder of this chapter, only electron accelerators and supervoltage X-ray generators will be considered in detail, with respect to their applications in radiation therapy, industrial radiography, and radiation processing.

There are about 2,200 particle accelerators now in use throughout the world, about half of which accelerate electrons. Scores of different models, involving several different principles of operation, are now commercially available from about 30 manufacturers (4). Each of these models has its own specific installation requirements and facility design, depending on the particle energy (or the energies of the secondary radiations), the accelerated-beam power, and the particular application. Consequently, it is difficult to provide more than a few generalizations about these facilities, in this chapter.

Most accelerators are rated in terms of their electrical parameters, such as accelerating voltage (millions of volts, MV), or corresponding particle energy (millions of electron-volts, MeV) and beam current (milliamperes, mA). Quite often, beam power (kilowatts, kW = MeV × mA) is used for purposes of comparison, especially when beam energy is not an important parameter. Figure 7.1 illustrates the broad choice in beam current and energy, for several types of accelerators, with an indication of the beam powers that can be attained.

A few figures of merit may be useful, in relating accelerated-beam power to the strength of radioisotope sources, as follows:

One kilowatt of electron-beam power is equivalent *in ionizing energy* to 67 kCi of $^{60}$Co. The electrons are of course much less penetrating than the cobalt gamma rays.
One kilowatt of 2-MeV electron-beam power, impinging on a thick X-ray-producing target, produces a radiation output in the forward di-

rection roughly equivalent in intensity and attenuation characteristics to 8 kCi of $^{60}$Co in a teletherapy configuration. At 10 MeV, one kilowatt of electron-beam power would produce an X-ray output in the forward direction about 16 times more intense.

One kilowatt of deuteron-beam power at 1 MeV, or 1 kW of electron-beam power at 10 MeV, can produce a neutron output of the order of $10^{11}$ n/sec, approximately equivalent to the output from 60 kCi of an Sb–Be isotopic neutron source.

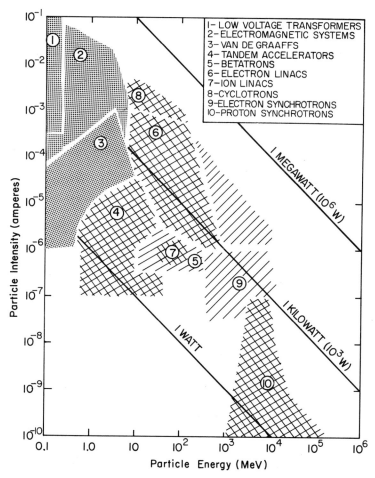

FIG. 7.1. Particle-beam intensity versus particle energy, for several types of accelerators. (Dark-toned areas relate to accelerators of both electrons and ions; middle tones relate to ion accelerators only; light tones relate to electron accelerators only.)

The inference can certainly be made from the above comparisons that accelerator facilities require more radiation shielding as compared with most massive radioisotope facilities, because of the relatively high radiation intensities and great penetrating powers. Where both species of radiation are produced from small source diameters or from target dimensions that are small in comparison with room dimensions, this inference is a valid one.

On the other hand, the radiation-shielding design for radiation-processing gamma-ray facilities can be quite elaborate, to accommodate extensive arrays of rods or plaques of radioactivity for the large-scale irradiation of materials, with a minimum of radiation attenuation in the source itself. The facility design must also include provisions for withdrawing the radioactive arrays from the production line, during servicing of the materials-handling apparatus or during replenishment of the source.

The shielding design for an "equivalent" electron accelerator or X-ray generator tends to be less complex for two major reasons: the radiation is produced from a relatively small area (1 in. × 18–72 in., depending on the width of the scanned-beam width); and there is no necessity for withdrawing the accelerator during servicing because the radiation can be electrically turned off at any time. At electron energies below 10 MeV, there is no radiation hazard from possible induced radioactivity in the vicinity of the accelerator.

In radiation-therapy installations, teletherapy units generally require less space than supervoltage X-ray generators having the same radiation output and radiation-positioning features. A similar amount of shielding and collimation is required about each source or target. In addition, however, the accelerator that generates the X rays must be accommodated, either in the same room or in adjacent space. This bulk often requires a higher ceiling and, occasionally, a larger room area than the corresponding teletherapy unit. However, accelerator designers are becoming more ingenious in producing compact, powerful machines. For example, electron linacs are now available for radiation therapy with configurations that can be accommodated in rooms designed for cobalt sources.

## III.  BASIS FOR COMPARING ECONOMICS OF RADIATION FACILITIES

The relative economics of radiation facilities, whether accelerator or radioisotope, must be studied on a case-by-case basis. A simple comparison of equipment costs is usually misleading, unless the radiation parameters, equipment sizes, applications, and servicing requirements are closely similar. Even hourly costs or annual outlays for an entire facility provide only part of the story, unless they can be related to the productivity of the facility.

In the next three sections, that are concerned with facilities for radiation therapy, industrial radiography, and radiation processing, the following components of cost will be tabulated or discussed:

A. *Fixed costs* (based on capital investment):
   (1)  radiation-producing equipment;
   (2)  building to house the equipment, including the necessary radiation-protective features;
   (3)  materials-handling equipment;
   (4)  necessary instrumentation associated with the application or radiation-protection procedures.

*Note:* The total fixed costs are amortized over 5–10 years, on a straight-line basis, with no consideration of "pay-back time" or return on investment, since these would vary depending on the specific application and accounting methods; 5 years is sometimes chosen as the amortization period, to protect against equipment (or process) obsolescence; 2,000–6,000 operating hours per year are assumed, depending on the usage of the facility.

B. *Operating costs* (based on use of the facility):
   (1)  Direct labor for operation and maintenance of the equipment and its facility;
   (2)  Servicing costs, including replacement parts or source replenishment;
   (3)  Electric power, cooling water, insulating gas, special coolants; these are usually negligible in comparison with other components of cost.

*Note:* Accelerator manufacturers are often prepared to offer terms for leasing their equipment, and for guaranteed-service contracts; in general, the use of these options would result in similar or slightly greater costs than presented in this chapter because of necessary risk factors and shorter amortization periods.

In the tables and graphs to follow, total hourly costs (amortized fixed costs plus operating costs) are compared mainly to illustrate the spread in cost among various types of accelerators. Wherever possible, these costs are related to the radiation parameters or the productivity of the accelerator. The costs of accelerators and their radiation characteristics should be considered only as approximations, for whatever rough comparisons with corresponding radioisotopes may be deemed advisable. Accelerator technology is continually changing, so that details of a particular design may be rapidly obsoleted by new models and kinds of equipment.

The subject of accelerator operating costs has been discussed over the years, mainly because of the unreliability of prototype machines that were technologically inadequate to perform a continuing function in a hospital or industrial environment. The situation has changed markedly during the past few years, and it is now possible to put forth realistic estimates of accelerator operating costs, based on performance in the field. An amount equivalent to 5–10% of the accelerator cost should be budgeted for a shift-year. This amount varies from one type of accelerator to another, but in general there is a decreasing trend in the percentage as the equipment becomes more powerful. This percentage can be compared with the 14% radioactive decay of $^{60}$Co per year.

## IV. RADIATION THERAPY

There are about 300 supervoltage X-ray generators in clinical use today throughout the world, including betatrons, electron linacs, resonant transformers, and Van de Graaffs (4, 6). This population can be compared with perhaps 2,500 $^{60}$Co and 200 $^{137}$Cs units. The prices of the X-ray generators range from $75,000 to $300,000, with some specialized machines that are priced even higher. Table 7.2 lists typical machines and their fixed and operating costs.

The accelerators are best used in clinics with a high patient load, and 50 treatments per day are not unusual for the larger units. Reliability of operation is continually improving, especially with scheduled service and preventive maintenance programs.

The choice of a supervoltage X-ray generator for a radiation-therapy facility is dependent to a great extent on the judgment of the individual radiologist. There is much to be said concerning the relative therapeutic benefits from X rays throughout the spectrum from 1 to 50 MeV. Consequently, there is a broad selection of accelerator types and ratings from which the radiologist can choose—in addition to the many models of cobalt and cesium teletherapy units. In fact, some of the larger medical centers have several different types of radiation facilities to accommodate the patient load.

TABLE 7.2

SUPERVOLTAGE X-RAY EQUIPMENT FOR RADIATION THERAPY

| Type: | Van de Graaff | Linac | Linac | Betatron | Betatron | $^{60}$Co | $^{60}$Co | Notes |
|---|---|---|---|---|---|---|---|---|
| MeV: | 2.0 | 4.0 | 8.0 | 25.0 | 35.0 | 75 | 150 | |
| Rad/min (100 cm): | 85 | 350 | 250 | 55 | 100 | | | |
| | (flat) | (flat) | (flat) | (flat) | (flat) | | | |
| | * | * | ** ‡ | * ‡ | * ‡ | ** | ** | |
| *Fixed cost* | | | | | | | | |
| Accelerator | $75,000 | $150,000 | $300,000 | $170,000 | $300,000 | $25,000 | $40,000 | mt. |
| Facility $^a$ | 25,000 | 40,000 | 25,000 | 30,000 | 35,000 | 30,000 | 60,000 | source |
| | | | | | | 20,000 | 20,000 | — |
| Total | 100,000 | 190,000 | 325,000 | 200,000 | 335,000 | 75,000 | 100,000 | — |
| Cost/hour $^b$ | 5.00 | 9.50 | 16.25 | 10.00 | 16.75 | 6.00 | 10.50 | source 4-yr. |
| *Operating cost* | | | | | | | | |
| Service/year $^c$ | 7,000 | 7,000 | 15,000 | 9,000 | 15,000 | 1,000 | 1,500 | |
| Service/hour $^b$ | 3.50 | 3.50 | 7.50 | 4.50 | 7.50 | 0.50 | 0.75 | |
| Total costs/hour | 8.50 | 13.00 | 23.75 | 14.50 | 24.50 | 6.50 | 11.25 | |
| Number treatment/hour $^d$ | 4.5 | 4.5 | 5.0 | 4.0 | 4.5 | 4.5 | 5.0 | |
| Cost/treatment | $1.90 | $2.90 | $4.75 | $3.60 | $5.40 | $1.60 | $2.25 | |

$^a$Therapy room, auxiliary apparatus.
$^b$10-year amortization, 2,000 hr/yr = 20,000 hr total.
$^c$Includes parts, labor, utilities, etc. (source replenish).
$^d$10-min. setup, 200-rad treatment at 100 cm (also includes run-up time).
  * Vertical travel, target angulation.
 ** Isocentric rotation of target axis.
 ‡ Also direct electrons for therapy.

The variation in accelerator price for radiation therapy arises from the relative complexity of the mounting, the desired X-ray energy, and the radiation output. In addition, there are special features offered in some accelerators, e.g., facilities for treating patients with direct electron beams, for producing radioactive isotopes, for conducting research programs in medicine and biology, and for sterilization of hospital supplies.

Accelerators can readily be designed to provide intense radiation outputs, but there is little point in increasing presently available performance much beyond 400 rads per minute at one meter distance. Average radiation doses per treatment are in the 200–400 rad range. It is usually not practical to reduce treatment time to less than a minute because the treatment cycle may take a longer period. In some specialized treatment techniques, however, whole-body irradiation is prescribed, in which case the irradiation distance must be considerably greater than a meter for uniformity of dose distribution. Thus, very high radiation outputs are sometimes desired to shorten these treatment times.

Despite the broad range of supervoltage X-ray generator prices, the costs per treatment are in the $2–$5 range. The lower costs are comparable to those for $^{60}$Co facilities (see Table 7.2), and the higher costs are attributable to more complex and versatile machines.

The radiation-shielding walls surrounding a therapy room are usually not as thick as those required for other types of accelerator applications. Hence, the facility costs tend to be a smaller fraction of the total fixed costs. The justification for these relatively thin, yet protective, walls, lies in the fact that most therapy X-ray generators are designed with extensive local shielding around the X-ray target and the envelope of the machine to protect patients from excessive spurious radiation. Some isocentric-mounted X-ray generators are counterweighted with an X-ray beam shield that rotates in opposition to the target, thereby preventing the direct X-ray beam from impinging on the walls of the treatment room.

The competition between accelerator manufacturers and radioisotope suppliers of radiation-therapy equipment is intense, judging from the great numbers of teletherapy units that are in use as compared with the numbers of supervoltage X-ray generators. In no other field of radiation application is the competition so obviously keen. Perhaps it is because the competitive edge is so slim, on either side of the controversy. The effects of the ionizing radiations and the economics of the respective facilities are closely similar. There are those radiologists who will continue to rely on "maintenance-free" teletherapy units, just as there are those who will wish to avail themselves of the fringe benefits to be derived from the use of accelerators. The ratio of popularity between these markedly different sources of radiation will probably not change appreciably over the next few years.

## V.  INDUSTRIAL RADIOGRAPHY

Over 250 supervoltage X-ray generators are in use throughout the world for industrial radiography, with X rays in the 1–35 McV range (4). Most of these machines produce useful X-ray outputs greater than 50 roentgens per minute at a meter (Rmm). There are also countless radioisotopic sources for radiography, mainly $^{60}$Co and $^{192}$Ir, with strengths ranging from a few curies to a few hundred curies.

The gamut of radiographic X-ray machines is extremely broad, ranging from 50-kVp units for inspecting thin spot welds to powerful supervoltage electron accelerators for the radiographic inspection of steel sections up to 24 in. in thickness. The prices of these machines are similarly spread, from a few thousand dollars for a small X-ray machine, to several hundred thousand dollars for the more sophisticated radiographic linear accelerators (see Fig. 7.2). Gamma-ray sources, by contrast, are generally priced in the range of a few hundred to a few thousand dollars (with a few expensive exceptions), but they are relatively weak in radiation output.

Radiographic inspection is considered by many organizations to be expensive, time-consuming, and a general deterrent to productivity. On the other hand, radiography is more often than not a *required* inspection method to assure that the inspected material meets certain minimum standards or specifications. As a consequence, radiography is usually performed with equipment of the lowest practical cost, in the fastest possible time, with marginally acceptable results—to ameliorate the overall costs of production, and yet to satisfy the minimum inspection requirements.

For the inspection of steel sections below 2 in. in thickness, the field is adequately served by conventional X-ray machines in the 50–250 kVp range and by isotopic sources such as $^{192}$Ir and (to a lesser extent) $^{137}$Cs. Exposure times of 10 min or less, using moderate-speed film at 36-in. distance, are preferred for radiographs of these relatively thin steel sections. A large fraction of the work done by these machines and sources requires equipment mobility in the field. Some machines are indeed portable, i.e., they can be carried and positioned by one man. Isotopic sources

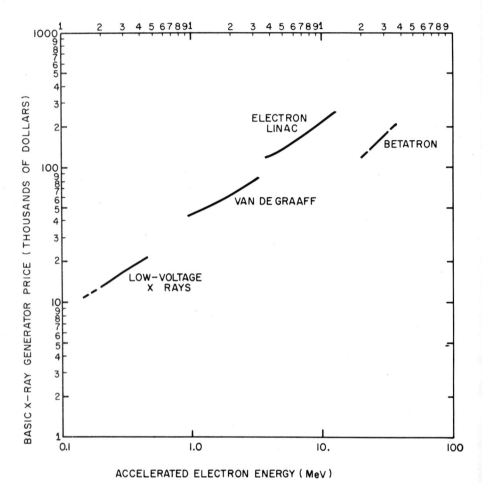

FIG. 7.2.   Radiographic X-ray generator price versus electron energy producing the X-rays.

or "cameras" are not only portable, but also self-contained, i.e., they require no external power source.

Very thick steel sections (above 5 in.) are inspected either through long exposures using mobile $^{60}$Co isotopic sources, or through relatively short exposures using expensive and complex supervoltage X-ray generators, such as Van de Graaffs, betatrons, or electron linacs. With very few exceptions, these machines are permanently housed in radiation-protective facilities.

The 2- to 5-in. steel-thickness range is usually inspected either by mobile gamma-ray equipment or (somewhat inadequately) by low-voltage X-ray equipment in the field, or by supervoltage X-ray equipment at permanent locations. The latter method is expensive, not only because of the inherent costs of radiography with such machines, but also because of the cost of transporting the material or fabrications to the inspection site. This latter method is, of course, impractical in the case of field-erected fabrications, such as nuclear-reactor containment vessels. Recently, electron-linac designs have been offered that feature equipment compactness and mobility for use in the field.

The gamma rays from $^{60}$Co have limited usefulness in the radiographic inspection of 2-8 in. steel sections. The practical strength limit is about 100 Ci; beyond this the source size becomes too large for radiographs with reasonable definition. In radiography, it is important to cast a sharp "shadow" onto a film from the preferential attenuation of the radiation. A small-diameter source, a few millimeters in diameter, is to be preferred, to permit radiographic examination at relatively short distances or under cramped conditions. It is possible to consider high specific $^{60}$Co activity, to reduce source size. However, a second limitation becomes important, namely the weight and bulk of the necessary radiation shielding.

The fixed and operating costs of a few typical supervoltage X-ray generators are summarized in Table 7.3. The accelerator cost includes the basic X-ray generator only. The facility cost includes radiation shielding, typical mounting arrangements for the X-ray generator, associated radiographic darkroom, jigs and fixtures for positioning the objects to be inspected. Because the dimensions and bulk of materials and fabrications tend to increase with the thickness of the sections to be inspected, facility costs tend toward the same magnitude as the accelerator cost. One-shift operation is assumed in Table 7.3, although several facilities now in operation function on a three-shift basis. Service costs have been assumed to be comparable to those for X-ray generators used in radiation therapy.

The total costs per hour are not dissimilar from the labor costs that are directly associated with the radiographic effort. The larger X-ray machines are usually needed for the inspection of very bulky fabrications or castings; hence a number of technicians would be required to maneuver them into position for radiography.

Which X-ray generator should be used depends strongly on the rapidity with which the inspection should be made, to minimize hold-up time in production. A figure of merit is the thickness of steel that can be

TABLE 7.3

SUPERVOLTAGE X-RAY EQUIPMENT FOR INDUSTRIAL RADIOGRAPHY

| Type:<br>MeV:<br>Rad/min (100 cm) | Van de Graaff<br>1.0<br>8 | Van de Graaff<br>2.5<br>170 | Linac<br>4.0<br>500 | Linac<br>7.5<br>1,500 | Linac<br>12.<br>6,000 | Betatron<br>25.<br>140 | $^{60}$Co<br><br>(100 Ci) |
|---|---|---|---|---|---|---|---|
| *Fixed costs* | | | | | | | |
| Accelerator | $50,000 | $75,000 | $120,000 | $170,000 | $250,000 | $150,000 | |
| Facility[a] | 30,000 | 65,000 | 85,000 | 120,000 | 200,000 | 100,000 | |
| Total | 80,000 | 140,000 | 205,000 | 290,000 | 450,000 | 250,000 | |
| Cost/hour[b] | 4.00 | 7.00 | 10.25 | 14.50 | 22.50 | 12.50 | |
| *Operating costs* | | | | | | | |
| Service/year[c] | 5,000 | 7,000 | 9,000 | 10,000 | 15,000 | 9,000 | |
| Service/hour[b] | 2.50 | 3.50 | 4.50 | 5.00 | 7.50 | 4.50 | |
| Total costs/hr | $6.50 | $10.50 | $14.75 | $19.50 | $30.00 | $17.00 | |
| Steel thickness (in.) radio-<br>graphed with 10-min.<br>exposure | 4.5 | 8.9 | 9.0 | 12.6 | 15.0 | 10.4 | 4.0 |

[a]Building shielding, accelerator mounting, auxiliary facilities and equipment.
[b]10-yr amortization, 2,000 hr/yr = 20,000 hr total.
[c]Includes parts, labor, utilities, etc.

radiographed in 10 min, at a distance sufficient to cover the diagonal of a 14 × 17-in. radiographic film with reasonable uniformity of X-ray intensity. Figure 7.3 shows a family of radiographic exposure-steel thickness curves for typical X-ray machines and isotopic sources, from which were derived the steel thicknesses listed in Table 7.3.

## VI. RADIATION PROCESSING

At present (1969) there is a total of about 1,028 kW of installed radiation-processing power throughout the world, the majority of which is being used on a multiple-shift basis. About two-thirds of this available power (700 kW) is installed in the U.S.A. Electron accelerators and isotopic sources are both being applied, with the following contributions to the total:

> *Electron accelerators:*
>     91 units, averaging 9 kW each      818 kW
> *Cobalt-irradiation facilities:*
>     30 units, averaging 7 kW each*      210 kW
>   Total installed power      1,028 kW

The term "radiation processing" is a general expression that covers a number of techniques of utilizing various kinds of ionizing radiation to change the characteristics of materials in an industrially practical sense. Among the many radiation processes that have been accepted and exploited by industry are the following:

(a) Cross-linking of polyethylene film, sheet, tubing, and miscellaneous shapes—to improve their temperature resistance, to provide heat-shrinkable properties, to stabilize their dimensions.

(b) Graft-polymerization of textiles, e.g., to impart a durable press and easy soil release to clothing.

(c) Curing of surface coatings by radiation-induced polymerization, e.g., prefinished plywood.

(d) Sterilization of medical supplies, e.g., surgical sutures, disposable hypodermic syringes, blood-donor kits, bandages.

(e) Polymerization of monomers impregnated in wood, to enhance the strength, appearance, and surface properties of wood.

---

* 1 kW electron power is roughly equivalent *in ionizing power* to 67 kCi $^{60}$Co. Thus, there is a total of 15 MCi $^{60}$Co, installed in 30 facilities.

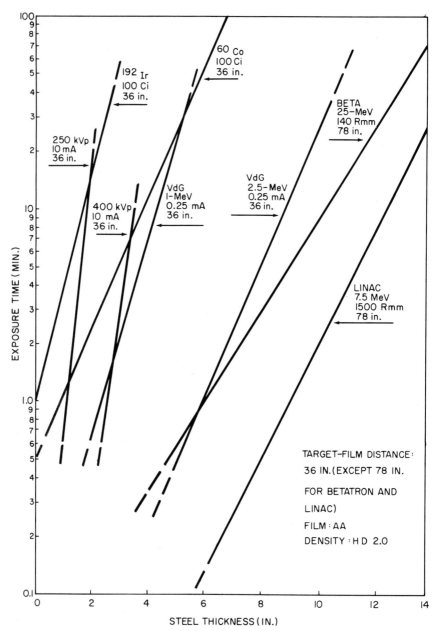

Fig. 7.3. Radiographic exposure time as a function of steel thickness, for several types of X-ray generators and radioisotope sources.

(f)  Synthesis of chemicals, e.g. ethyl bromide, polyethylene oxide, biodegradable detergents.

Sterilization or pasteurization of food is being studied extensively, but as yet this general process is not considered to be economically or politically acceptable, either by industry or by the U.S. Food and Drug Administration. The general subject of radiation processing has been extensively described in the literature. Four recent articles are referenced because of their comparisons in the relative usage of accelerators and isotopes (2, 6, 7, 8) (see also Section 1.5).

Accelerators are utilized mainly for the irradiation of surfaces or thin films, as exemplified by categories (a), (b), and (c) above. Radioisotopes are being used for (d), (e), and (f), although some productive work has also been done with accelerators in these categories. Food-irradiation techniques are being developed with both accelerators and isotopes. A detailed comparison of the economics of electron linacs and $^{60}$Co for food irradiation has been made by the U. S. Army Quartermaster Corps (8).

In certain radiation-chemical processes, accelerator-produced radiation is somewhat at a disadvantage because of the dose-rate dependency of the particular reaction, in which the efficiency of the process typically decreases with the square-root of the dose rate. This tendency inhibits the use of accelerators for producing some materials in (e) and (f). The electron linac is at a further disadvantage because its electron output is in the form of very intense, short bursts rather than a continous flow (dc), which is characteristic of lower-energy machines. The decrease in reaction-rate efficiency can sometimes be offset, however, by the relatively economical power that is available from most commercial accelerators.

The low dose rate produced by presently economic radioisotopes (as compared with accelerators) can be both an advantage and a disadvantage. Where high-volume throughput is required in a process, thin plaques or arrays of rods of radioactivity are needed to irradiate progressively the material for a prolonged time. The reason for these arrays is that the self-absorption in the Source would otherwise greatly reduce the efficiency of utilizing the radioisotope and would, in the larger installations, create a heating problem. It is important to concede, however, that this extensive array also provides a very uniform dose, with proper materials-conveying techniques.

There is a broad spectrum of electron accelerators that are adaptable to practical radiation processing. A selection of electron energy and beam power is needed to provide an appropriate match between the capability of the machine, the throughput of the plant, and the thickness of the irradiated product. To show the wide range of available electron energies

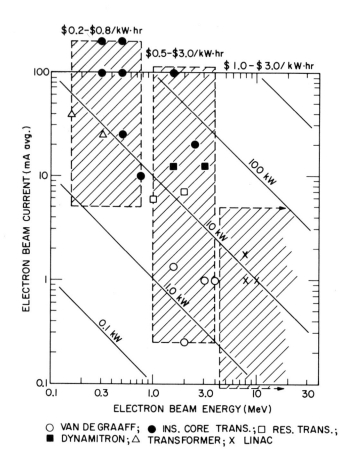

Fig. 7.4. Electron-beam current versus electron-beam energy, for several accelerators designed for radiation processing.

and powers, Fig. 7.4 summarizes the characteristics of typical electron accelerators. This graph is divided into three sections:

Low-voltage            (0.2 – 0.75 MeV)
Direct accelerators    (1.0 – 4.0  MeV)
Electron linacs        (above 4.0* MeV)

*Probably 4–10 MeV, to minimize the possibility of inducing radioactivity in either the product or in the accelerating apparatus.

Electron beams are brought out of the evacuated acceleration region through an electron-permeable window. These beams are usually scanned or spread, by electromagnetic techniques, to provide a uniformity of electron-intensity distribution across wide swaths (from a few inches to at least 72 in.), and to distribute the powerful beam over a large area of the window, thereby minimizing window failure.

Technical feasibility of accelerating electrons is not a sufficient criterion of judging the industrial practicality of a particular machine. Economic and reliable operation is of utmost importance. Table 7.4 summarizes the fixed and operating costs of several commercially available accelerators. The ultimate cost-per-kilowatt-hour is a figure of merit that can readily be applied to a process to determine the overall costs per processed unit of material.

Sheer power is a crude basis for evaluating accelerator systems and it is of little value if the particular process cannot utilize all the available power from a radiation-producing machine. At a matched power level, economics can better be judged by the efficiency with which the radiation is applied to the product. Ingenuity of the accelerator designer, in cooperation with the process company, can result in more pounds of processed material per kilowatt-hour than could have been predicted by considering ordinary irradiation techniques.

It is difficult to compare the economics of cobalt facilities with accelerator facilities for radiation processing, but the following commentary may be helpful.

The installed cost of a 500-kCi $^{60}$Co irradiation facility is in the neighborhood of $350,000. In ionizing power, such a facility would be equivalent to a 7-kW electron-accelerator processing installation. Applying the same use factors as in Table 7.4, the total "costs per kilowatt-hour" amount to about $2.70. Thus, $^{60}$Co is relatively expensive for radiation processing, *if* a process can as readily be carried out with electrons as with gamma rays.

If electrons cannot be used in a particular process because of their inadequate penetration into material, some consideration can be given to the use of X rays. The conversion of electron power to X-ray power is not, however, very efficient (2). For example, at 3 MeV the practical efficiency of power conversion is about 6%. Hence, a 3-MeV electron accelerator, whose total costs per kW-hr are in the vicinity of $0.60 *as an electron source,* could be adapted to X-ray production with economics of $10.00 per *X-ray* kW-hr. The efficiency of X-ray production is better at 10 MeV (about 20%), but the cost per kW-hr is also greater. A 10-MeV

TABLE 7.4

ELECTRON ACCELERATORS FOR RADIATION PROCESSING

| Type:<br>MeV:<br>Power (kW): | Low Volt.<br>0.3<br>7.5 | Res. Trans<br>1.0<br>7.0 | ICT<br>0.5<br>12.5 | ICT<br>0.5<br>100. | ICT<br>2.5<br>50. | Van de<br>Graaff<br>1.5<br>2.5 | Dyn.<br>3.0<br>2.5 | Linac<br>10.<br>10. | $^{60}$Co<br>500 kCi<br>(7 kW) |
|---|---|---|---|---|---|---|---|---|---|
| *Fixed costs* | | | | | | | | | |
| Accelerator | $50,000 | $130,000 | $115,000 | $250,000 | $440,000 | $ 65,000 | $225,000 | $300,000 | $350,000 |
| Facility[a] | 30,000 | 60,000 | 40,000 | 70,000 | 160,000 | 60,000 | 150,000 | 150,000 | |
| Total | 80,000 | 190,000 | 155,000 | 320,000 | 600,000 | 125,000 | 375,000 | 450,000 | 350,000 |
| Cost/hour[b] | 2.67 | 6.33 | 5.17 | 10.67 | 20.00 | 4.17 | 12.50 | 15.00 | 11.67 |
| *Operating costs* | | | | | | | | | |
| Service/year[c] | 10,000 | 19,000 | 12,000 | 45,000 | 60,000 | 18,000 | 60,000 | 50,000 | 42,000[d] |
| Service/hour[b] | 1.67 | 3.33 | 2.00 | 7.50 | 10.00 | 3.00 | 10.00 | 8.33 | 7.00 |
| Total costs/hr | 4.34 | 9.66 | 7.17 | 18.17 | 30.00 | 7.17 | 22.50 | 23.33 | 18.67 |
| Costs/kW-hr | $0.72 | $1.39 | $0.57 | $0.18 | $0.60 | $2.87 | $0.63 | $2.33 | $2.67 |

[a] Building, shielding, materials handling, instruments, etc.
[b] 5-yr amortization, 6000=hr/yr (3-shift) = 30,000 hr.
[c] Parts, labor, utilities, 6000 hr.
[d] Replenish 14% $^{60}$Co, plus miscellaneous servicing.

electron linac has a cost of about \$2.30 per kW-hr, at the 10-kW level. The cost per *X-ray* kW-hr would be about \$11.50. If, on the other hand, that same linac could be made to operate at 20 kW reliably, the costs per kW-hr would be reduced to \$5.75.

There is obviously a cross-over in costs per kW-hr, but the cross-over point will continue to move, as cobalt becomes less expensive and as machine designers provide a more economical package.

## VII.   CONCLUSION

Electron accelerators and massive radioisotope sources are both important—in radiation therapy, industrial radiography, and radiation processing. The characteristics of the two basic kinds of radiation sources are sufficiently different that their usage is correspondingly different, with only a few exceptions at present.

Radiation therapy is undoubtedly an application in which there will continue to be well-matched competition, springing from the relative resources of accelerator manufacturers and isotope suppliers.

Industrial radiography will continue to be served by the compact and portable isotope cameras, as well as the specialized supervoltage X-ray generators. Machines may start to move out into the field, despite the radiation-protection problem. If higher specific-activity cobalt becomes more available at reasonable prices, the strength of cobalt cameras in radiography may well increase, thus giving the accelerator manufacturers a run for their money. Machine technology exists, however, to provide portable and low-cost equipment in the very realm that now is served by cobalt.

Radiation processing has always been a tantalizing application, for both accelerator and isotope champions. The obvious reason for continuing enthusiasm by both parties is that a mass market for irradiation facilities can be envisaged—the only mass market for radiation that has yet appeared. This "will-o'-the-wisp" market will continue to goad accelerator manufacturers and isotope suppliers, to bring the economics of their respective irradiation facilities closer to the point where low-margin industries can afford to take another look.

### REFERENCES

*1.*  A. Charlesby (ed.), *Radiation Sources,* Pergamon Press, London and New York, 1964.
*2.*  H. W. Koch and E. H. Eisenhower, *Radiation Preservation of Foods,* Publication

1273, National Academy of Science, National Research Council, Washington, D.C. (1965).

3. R. G. Jaeger (ed.), *Engineering Compendium on Radiation Shielding, Vol. I,* Springer-Verlag, New York, 1968.

4. E. A. Burrill, *The World-Wide Usefulness of Particle Accelerators,* NUCLEX-66 International Nuclear Exposition, Basel, Switzerland, Sept. 1966.

5. *Planning of Radiotherapy Facilities,* World Health Organization Technical Report Series, No. 328, Geneva, Switzerland, 1966.

6. R. H. Lafferty, Jr., *Isotopes Radiation Technol.* **6,** 227 (1969).

7. E. A. Burrill, *Isotopes Radiation Technol.* **3,** 297 (1966).

8. E. S. Josephson, A. Brynjolfsson, and E. Wierbick, *Trans. N.Y. Acad. Sci.* **30,** 600 (1968).

# APPENDIX A

## USEFUL PHYSICAL CONSTANTS AND CONVERSION FACTORS

| | |
|---|---|
| Avogadro's number | $N_A = 6.0226 \times 10^{23}$ mol$^{-1}$ |
| Planck's constant | $h = 6.6255 \times 10^{-27}$ erg-sec |
| Boltzmann constant | $k = 1.3805 \times 10^{-16}$ erg °K$^{-1}$ |
| Velocity of light in vacuum | $c = 2.9979 \times 10^{10}$ cm-sec$^{-1}$ |
| Electron rest mass | $m_e = 9.1090 \times 10^{-28}$ g |
| Elementary charge | $e = 1.6021 \times 10^{-19}$ C |
| | $= 1.6021 \times 10^{-20}$ emu |
| | $= 4.8030 \times 10^{-10}$ esu |
| Energy equivalent of electron mass | $m_e c^2 = 0.51101$ MeV |
| Energy equivalent of proton mass | $m_p c^2 = 938.25$ MeV |
| Quantum energy × wavelength | $hv \times \lambda = 12.398$ keV-Å |
| Density of dry air at 0°C, 760 Torr | 0.001293 g/cm$^3$ |
| Specific $\gamma$-ray constant ($\Gamma$) of radium in 0.5 mm Pt shield | 0.825 R m$^2$ hr$^{-1}$ g$^{-1}$ |
| Specific $\gamma$-ray constant ($\Gamma$) of $^{60}$Co | 1.30 R m$^2$ hr$^{-1}$Ci$^{-1}$ |
| Specific $\gamma$-ray constant ($\Gamma$) of $^{137}$Cs | 0.31 R m$^2$ hr$^{-1}$Ci$^{-1}$ |

In general, the $\gamma$-ray exposure rate in R/hr at 1 meter from an unshielded point source is approximately

$$\triangle X/\triangle t \approx 0.5 \times \text{(activity in Ci)} \times \text{(average } \gamma\text{-ray energy in MeV)}$$
$$\times \text{(number of } \gamma \text{ rays emitted per disintegration)}$$

| | |
|---|---|
| 1 curie (Ci) | $3.700 \times 10^{10}$ disintegrations/second |
| Half-life ($\tau_{1/2}$) of $^{60}$Co | 5.26 years |
| Half-life ($\tau_{1/2}$) of $^{137}$Cs | 29.7 years |

In general the activity $A$ at time t is related to the initial activity $A_0$ by the formula

TABLE 8.1

CONVERSION FACTORS

| Multiply | By | To obtain |
|----------|-----|-----------|
| MeV | $1.517 \times 10^{-16}$ | Btu |
| MeV | $4.44 \ \times 10^{-20}$ | kW-hr |
| MeV | $3.83 \ \times 10^{-14}$ | g-cal |
| MeV | $1.602 \times 10^{-6}$ | erg |
| erg | $6.24 \ \times 10^{5}$ | MeV |
| erg | $9.49 \ \times 10^{-11}$ | Btu |
| erg | $2.78 \ \times 10^{-14}$ | kW-hr |
| erg | $2.39 \ \times 10^{-8}$ | g-cal |
| g-cal | $2.61 \ \times 10^{13}$ | MeV |
| g-cal | $3.97 \ \times 10^{-3}$ | Btu |
| g-cal | $1.163 \times 10^{-6}$ | kW-hr |
| g-cal | $4.18 \ \times 10^{7}$ | erg |
| kW-hr | $2.25 \ \times 10^{19}$ | MeV |
| kW-hr | $3.41 \ \times 10^{3}$ | Btu |
| kW-hr | $8.60 \ \times 10^{5}$ | g-cal |
| kW-hr | $3.60 \ \times 10^{13}$ | erg |
| Btu | $6.59 \ \times 10^{15}$ | MeV |
| Btu | $2.93 \ \times 10^{-4}$ | kW-hr |
| Btu | 252 | g-cal |
| Btu | $1.055 \times 10^{10}$ | erg |
| watt | $6.24 \ \times 10^{12}$ | MeV/sec |
| MeV/sec | $1.602 \times 10^{-13}$ | watt |
| Btu/sec | $1.055 \times 10^{3}$ | watt |
| MeV/(cm²) (sec) | $1.485 \times 10^{-10}$ | watt/ft² |
| MeV/(cm²) (sec) | $1.409 \times 10^{-13}$ | Btu/(ft²) (sec) |
| kW/ft² | $3.42 \ \times 10^{3}$ | Btu/(ft²) (hr) |
| watt/cm² | $3.18 \ \times 10^{3}$ | Btu/(ft²) (hr) |
| MeV/(cm³) (sec) | $4.54 \ \times 10^{-9}$ | watt/ft³ |
| MeV/(cm³) (sec) | $4.30 \ \times 10^{-12}$ | Btu/(ft³) (hr) |
| kW/liter | $9.7 \ \times 10^{-4}$ | Btu/(ft³) (hr) |

$$A/A_0 = e^{-0.693t/\tau_{1/2}},$$

where $\tau_{1/2}$ is the half-life, at which time $A = A_0/2$

| | |
|---|---|
| 1 ampere | 1 coulomb/second $= 2.9979 \times 10^9$ esu/second |
| | $= 6.2418 \times 10^{18}$ electrons/second |
| 1 g-calorie (mean) | $4.1860 \times 10^7$ erg |
| 1 MeV | $1.6021 \times 10^{-6}$ erg |
| 1 erg | $6.2418 \times 10^{11}$ eV |
| 1 rad | 100 erg/g |

One roentgen (R) of X- or $\gamma$-radiation produces in dry air under charged particle equilibrium conditions:

> 1 esu of charge of either sign per 0.001293 g
> $2.580 \times 10^{-7}$ coulombs of either sign per gram
> 1 esu of charge of either sign per $cm^3$ (0 °C, 760 Torr)
> $3.336 \times 10^{-10}$ coulombs of either sign per $cm^3$ (0 °C, 760 Torr)
> $1.610 \times 10^{12}$ ion pairs/g
> $2.082 \times 10^9$ ion pairs/$cm^3$ (0 °C, 760 Torr)
> 86.9 erg/g or 0.869 rad ($W_{air} = 33.7$ eV/ion pair)

One roentgen (R) of X- or $\gamma$-radiation produces in soft tissue (muscle) under charged particle equilibrium conditions:

> 95.1 erg/g at 0.1 MeV ($W_{air} = 33.7$ eV/ion pair)
> 96.0 erg/g at 0.3 MeV ($W_{air} = 33.7$ eV/ion pair)
> 95.6 erg/g at 1.0 MeV ($W_{air} = 33.7$ eV/ion pair)
> 95.3 erg/g at 3.0 MeV ($W_{air} = 33.7$ eV/ion pair)

## I. NUCLIDE DESIGNATION (SUBSCRIPTS AND SUPERSCRIPTS)

In accordance with recommendations of the International Union of Pure and Applied Chemistry, the following designations are used for nuclides:

The *MASS NUMBER* of a nuclide is placed as a *superscript* to the left of the symbol for the chemical element of the nuclide, rather than to its right, as formerly; for example, $^{14}N$, rather than $N^{14}$ for nitrogen-14.

The *ATOMIC NUMBER* is placed as a left *subscript;* for example, $^{14}_6C$ for carbon-14, or $^{235}_{92}U$ for uranium-235.

The state of *IONIZATION* is shown as a *right superscript;* for example, $Ca^{++}$ or $SO_4^{--}$.

The number of NEUTRONS in the nucleus is shown as a *right subscript;* for example, $^{40}_{20}Ca_{20}$ for the isotope of calcium-40 containing 20 protons (its atomic number) (left subscript), and 20 neutrons (right subscript) in its nucleus.

Excited states are shown either as part of the *left superscript,* or sometimes the *right superscript;* for example: $^{110m}Ag$ or $^{110}Ag^m$ indicates an excited state of a silver-110 nucleus; $He^*$ indicates an excited state of a helium atom.

| 1<br>H | | | | | | | | | | | | | | | | | | 2<br>He |
|---|---|---|---|---|---|---|---|---|---|---|---|---|---|---|---|---|---|---|
| 3<br>Li | 4<br>Be | | | | | | | | | | | 5<br>B | 6<br>C | 7<br>N | 8<br>O | 9<br>F | 10<br>Ne |
| 11<br>Na | 12<br>Mg | | | | | | | | | | | 13<br>Al | 14<br>Si | 15<br>P | 16<br>S | 17<br>Cl | 18<br>Ar |
| 19<br>K | 20<br>Ca | 21<br>Sc | 22<br>Ti | 23<br>V | 24<br>Cr | 25<br>Mn | 26<br>Fe | 27<br>Co | 28<br>Ni | 29<br>Cu | 30<br>Zn | 31<br>Ga | 32<br>Ge | 33<br>As | 34<br>Se | 35<br>Br | 36<br>Kr |
| 37<br>Rb | 38<br>Sr | 39<br>Y | 40<br>Zr | 41<br>Nb | 42<br>Mo | 43<br>Tc | 44<br>Ru | 45<br>Rh | 46<br>Pd | 47<br>Ag | 48<br>Cd | 49<br>In | 50<br>Sn | 51<br>Sb | 52<br>Te | 53<br>I | 54<br>Xe |
| 55<br>Cs | 56<br>Ba | 57-71<br>La*<br>Series | 72<br>Hf | 73<br>Ta | 74<br>W | 75<br>Re | 76<br>Os | 77<br>Ir | 78<br>Pt | 79<br>Au | 80<br>Hg | 81<br>Tl | 82<br>Pb | 83<br>Bi | 84<br>Po | 85<br>At | 86<br>Rn |
| 87<br>Fr | 88<br>Ra | 89-103<br>Act<br>Series | | | | | | | | | | | | | | | |

*Lanthanide Series

| 57<br>La | 58<br>Ce | 59<br>Pr | 60<br>Nd | 61<br>Pm | 62<br>Sm | 63<br>Eu | 64<br>Gd | 65<br>Tb | 66<br>Dy | 67<br>Ho | 68<br>Er | 69<br>Tm | 70<br>Yb | 71<br>Lu |
|---|---|---|---|---|---|---|---|---|---|---|---|---|---|---|

†Actinide Series

| 89<br>Ac | 90<br>Th | 91<br>Pa | 92<br>U | 93<br>Np | 94<br>Pu | 95<br>Am | 96<br>Cm | 97<br>Bk | 98<br>Cf | 99<br>Es | 100<br>Fm | 101<br>Md | 102<br>No | 71<br>Lu<br>(103)<br>Lr |
|---|---|---|---|---|---|---|---|---|---|---|---|---|---|---|

FIG. 8.1. Periodic table of the elements. Transuranium elements are shown in shaded squares. The actinide series of elements as a group occupies a single square in the main figure. The lanthanide series of elements also occupies a single square in the larger chart.

## II.  LEGAL DEFINITIONS (EXTRACTED FROM 10 U.S. CFR PART 20)

Units of measurement of dose (rad, rem) defined in § 20.4;
Units of measurement of radioactivity defined in § 20.5.

§ 20.4  Units of radiation dose.

(a)  *Dose*, as used in this part, is the quantity of radiation absorbed, per unit of mass, by the body or by any portion of the body. When the regulations in this part specify a dose during a period of time, the dose means the total quantity of radiation absorbed, per unit of mass, by the body or by any portion of the body during such period of time. Several different units of dose are in current use. Definitions of units as used in this part are set forth in paragraphs (b) and (c) of this section.

(b)  The *rad,* as used in this part, is a measure of the dose of any ionizing radiation to body tissues in terms of the energy absorbed per unit mass of the tissue. One rad is the dose corresponding to the absorption of 100 ergs per gram of tissue. (One millirad (mrad) = 0.001 rad.)

(c)  The *rem,* as used in this part, is a measure of the dose of any ionizing radiation to body tissue in terms of its estimated biological effect relative to a dose of one roentgen (R) of X-rays. (One millirem (mrem) = 0.001 rem.) The relation of the rem to other dose units depends upon the biological effect under consideration and upon the conditions of irradiation. For the purpose of the regulations in this part, any of the following is considered to be equivalent to a dose of one rem:

(1)  A dose of 1 R due to X- or gamma radiation;
(2)  A dose of 1 rad due to X-, gamma, or beta radiation;
(3)  A dose of 0.1 rad due to neutrons or high energy protons;
(4)  A dose of 0.05 rad due to particles heavier than protons and with sufficient energy to reach the lens of the eye.

If it is more convenient to measure the neutron flux, or equivalent, than to determine the neutron dose in rads, as provided in subparagraph (3) of this paragraph, one rem of neutron radiation may, for purposes of the regulations in this part, be assumed to be equivalent to 14 million neutrons per square centimeter incident upon the body, or, if there exists sufficient information to estimate with reasonable accuracy the approximate distribution in energy of the neutrons, the incident number of neutrons per square centimeter equivalent to one rem may be estimated from the following table:

TABLE 8.2

NEUTRON FLUX DOSE EQUIVALENTS

| Neutron energy (MeV) | Number of neutrons per square centimeter equivalent to a dose of 1 rem (neutrons/cm²) | Average flux to deliver 100 millirem in 40 hours (neutrons/cm² per sec) |
|---|---|---|
| Thermal | $970 \times 10^6$ | 670 |
| 0.0001 | $720 \times 10^6$ | 500 |
| 0.005 | $820 \times 10^6$ | 570 |
| 0.02 | $400 \times 10^6$ | 280 |
| 0.1 | $120 \times 10^6$ | 80 |
| 0.5 | $43 \times 10^6$ | 30 |
| 1.0 | $29 \times 10^6$ | 18 |
| 2.5 | $26 \times 10^6$ | 20 |
| 5.0 | $26 \times 10^6$ | 18 |
| 7.5 | $24 \times 10^6$ | 17 |
| 10 | $24 \times 10^6$ | 17 |
| 10 to 30 | $14 \times 10^6$ | 10 |

(d)   For determining exposures to X or gamma rays up to 3 MeV, the dose limits specified in § § 20.101 to 20.104, inclusive, may be assumed to be equivalent to the "air dose." For the purpose of this part "air dose" means that the dose is measured by a properly calibrated appropriate instrument in air at or near the body surface in the region of highest dosage rate.

§ 20.5   Units of radioactivity.

(a)   Radioactivity is commonly, and for purposes of the regulations in this part shall be, measured in terms of disintegrations per unit time or in curies. One curie (Ci) $= 3.7 \times 10^{10}$ disintegrations per second (dps) $= 2.2 \times 10^{12}$ disintegrations per minute (dpm). A commonly used sub-multiple of the curie is the microcurie (μCi). One μCi $= 0.000001$ Ci $= 3.7 \times 10^4$ dps $= 2.2 \times 10^6$ dpm.

§ 20.101   Exposure of individuals to radiation in restricted areas.

(a)   Except as    ovided in paragraph (b) of this section, no licensee shall possess, u    r transfer licensed material in such a manner as to cause any indiv    l in a restricted area to receive in any period of one calendar quarte    om radioactive material and other sources of radiation in the licensee's possession a dose in excess of the limits specified in the following table:

*Rems per calendar quarter*

1. Whole body; head and trunk; active blood-forming organs; lens of eyes; or gonads ........................................................ $1\frac{1}{4}$
2. Hands and forearms; feet and ankles ............................ $18\frac{3}{4}$
3. Skin of whole body ..................................................... $7\frac{1}{2}$

(b)  A licensee may permit an individual in a restricted area to receive a dose to the whole body greater than that permitted under paragraph (a) of this section, provided:

(1)  During any calendar quarter the dose to the whole body from radioactive material and other sources of radiation in the licensee's possession shall not exceed 3 rems; and

(2)  The dose to the whole body, when added to the accumulated occupational dose to the whole body, shall not exceed $5(N-18)$ rems, where "N" equals the individual's age in years at his last birthday.

TABLE 8.3

| Name | Symbol | Dimensions[a] | Units mksa | Units cgs | Units Special |
|------|--------|---------------|------|-----|---------|
| Energy imparted (integral absorbed dose) | — | $E$ | J | erg | g rad |
| Absorbed dose | $D$ | $EM^{-1}$ | J kg$^{-1}$ | erg g$^{-1}$ | rad |
| Absorbed dose rate | — | $EM^{-1}T^{-1}$ | J kg$^{-1}$ s$^{-1}$ | erg g$^{-1}$ s$^{-1}$ | rad s$^{-1}$, etc. |
| Particle fluence or fluence | $\Phi$ | $L^{-2}$ | m$^{-2}$ | cm$^{-2}$ | — |
| Particle flux density | $\varphi$ | $L^{-2}T^{-1}$ | m$^{-2}$ s$^{-1}$ | cm$^{-2}$ s$^{-1}$ | — |
| Energy fluence | $F$ | $EL^{-2}$ | J m$^{-2}$ | erg cm$^{-2}$ | — |
| Energy flux density or intensity | $I$ | $EL^{-2}T^{-1}$ | J m$^{-2}$ s$^{-1}$ | erg cm$^{-2}$ s$^{-1}$ | — |
| Kerma | $K$ | $EM^{-1}$ | J kg$^{-1}$ | erg g$^{-1}$ | — |
| Kerma rate | — | $EM^{-1}T^{-1}$ | J kg$^{-1}$ s$^{-1}$ | erg g$^{-1}$ s$^{-1}$ | — |
| Exposure | $X$ | $QM^{-1}$ | C kg$^{-1}$ | esu g$^{-1}$ | R (roentgen) |
| Exposure rate | — | $QM^{-1}T^{-1}$ | C kg$^{-1}$ s$^{-1}$ | esu g$^{-1}$ s$^{-1}$ | R s$^{-1}$, etc. |
| Mass attenuation coefficient | $\mu/\rho$ | $L^2M^{-1}$ | m$^2$ kg$^{-1}$ | cm$^2$ g$^{-1}$ | — |
| Mass energy-transfer coefficient | $\mu_k/\rho$ | $L^2M^{-1}$ | m$^2$ kg$^{-1}$ | cm$^2$ g$^{-1}$ | — |
| Mass energy-absorption coefficient | $\mu_{en}/\rho$ | $L^2M^{-1}$ | m$^2$ kg$^{-1}$ | cm$^2$ g$^{-1}$ | — |
| Mass stopping power | $S/\rho$ | $EL^2M^{-1}$ | J m$^2$ kg$^{-1}$ | erg cm$^2$ g$^{-1}$ | — |
| Linear energy transfer | $L$ | $EL^{-1}$ | J m$^{-1}$ | erg cm$^{-1}$ | keV $(\mu m)^{-1}$ |
| Average energy per ion pair | $W$ | $E$ | J | erg | eV |
| Activity | $A$ | $T^{-1}$ | s$^{-1}$ | s$^{-1}$ | Ci (curie) |
| Specific $\gamma$-ray constant | $\Gamma$ | $QL^2M^{-1}$ | C m$^2$kg$^{-1}$ | esu cm$^2$ g$^{-1}$ | R m$^2$ h$^{-1}$ Ci$^{-1}$, etc. |
| Dose equivalent | $DE$ | — | — | — | rem |

[a] It was desired to present only one set of dimensions for each quantity, a set that would be suitable in both the mksa and electrostatic-cgs systems. To do this it was necessary to use a dimension Q, for the electrical charge, that is not a fundamental dimension in either system. In the mksa system (fundamental dimensions $M, L, T, I$) $Q$ represents the product $IT$; in the electrostatic-cgs system $(M, L, T)$ it represents $M^{1/2}L^{3/2}T^{-1}$.

# APPENDIX B

## CONDENSED GLOSSARY OF NUCLEAR TERMS*

| | |
|---|---|
| *A* | Symbol for mass number. |
| absorbed dose | When ionizing radiation passes through matter, some of its energy is imparted to the matter. The amount absorbed per unit mass of irradiated material is called the absorbed dose, and is measured in rems and rads. |
| absorber | Any material that absorbs or diminishes the intensity of ionizing radiation. Neutron absorbers, like boron, hafnium, and cadmium, are used in control rods for reactors. Concrete and steel absorb gamma rays and neutrons in reactor shields. A thin sheet of paper or metal will absorb or attenuate alpha particles and all except the most energetic beta particles. |
| absorption | The process by which the number of particles or photons entering a body of matter is reduced by interaction of the particles or radiation with the matter; similarly, the reduction of the energy of a particle while traversing a body of matter. This term is sometimes erroneously used for capture. |
| accelerator | A device for increasing the velocity and energy of charged elementary particles, for example, electrons or protons, through application of electrical and/or magnetic forces. Accelerators have made particles move at velocities approaching the speed of light. Types of accelerators include betatrons, Cockcroft–Walton accelerators, cyclotrons, linear accelerators, |

---

* Adapted from "Nuclear Terms–A Brief Glossary," U.S. AEC., Div. of Technical Information, 1967.

synchrocyclotrons, synchrotrons, and Van de Graaff generators.

actinide series
The series of elements beginning with actinium, Element No. 89, and continuing through lawrencium, Element No. 103, which together occupy one position in the Periodic Table. The series includes uranium, Element No. 92, and all the man-made transuranic elements. The group is also referred to as the "actinides."

activation
The process of making a material radioactive by bombardment with neutrons, protons, or other nuclear particles. Also called radioactivation.

alpha particle
[Symbol $\alpha$] A positively charged particle emitted by certain radioactive materials. It is made up of two neutrons and two protons bound together, hence is identical with the nucleus of a helium atom. It is the least penetrating of the three common types of radiation (alpha, beta, gamma) emitted by radioactive material, being stopped by a sheet of paper. It is not dangerous to plants, animals, or man unless the alpha-emitting substance has entered the body.

alpha ray
A stream of alpha particles. Loosely, a synonym for alpha particle.

atom
A particle of matter indivisible by chemical means. It is the fundamental building block of the chemical elements. The elements, such as iron, lead, and sulfur, differ from each other because they contain different kinds of atoms. There are about six sextillion $(6 \times 10^{21})$ atoms in an ordinary drop of water. According to present-day theory, an atom contains a dense inner core (the nucleus) and a much less dense outer domain consisting of electrons in motion around the nucleus. Atoms are electrically neutral.

atomic mass unit
[Symbol $amu$] One-twelfth the mass of a neutral atom of the most abundant isotope of carbon, $^{12}C$.

atomic number
[Symbol $Z$] The number of protons in the nucleus of an atom, and also its positive charge. Each chemical element has its characteristic atomic number, and the atomic numbers of the known elements form a complete series from 1 (hydrogen) to 103 (lawrencium).

atomic reactor    A nuclear reactor.

atomic weight     The mass of an atom relative to other atoms. The present-day basis of the scale of atomic weights is carbon; the commonest isotope of this element has arbitrarily been assigned an atomic weight of 12. The unit of the scale is 1/12 the weight of the carbon-12 atom, or roughly the mass of one proton or one neutron. The atomic weight of any element is approximately equal to the total number of protons and neutrons in its nucleus.

background        The radiation in man's natural environment, including cosmic rays and radiation from the naturally radioactive elements, both outside and inside the bodies of men and animals. It is also called natural radiation. The term may also mean radiation that is unrelated to a specific experiment.
radiation

backscatter       When radiation of any kind strikes matter (gas, liquid, or solid), some of it may be reflected or scattered back in the general direction of the source. An understanding or exact measurement of the amount of backscatter is important when beta particles are being counted in an ionization chamber, in medical treatment with radiation, or in use of industrial radioisotopic thickness gauges.

barn              [Symbol b] A unit area used in expressing the cross sections of atoms, nuclei, electrons, and other particles. One barn is equal to $10^{-24}$ square centimeters.

beam              A stream of particles or electromagnetic radiation, going in a single direction.

beta particle     [Symbol $\beta$] An elementary particle emitted from a nucleus during radioactive decay, with a single electrical charge and a mass equal to 1/1837 that of a proton. A negatively charged beta particle is identical to an electron. A positively charged beta particle is called a *positron*.

binding energy    The binding energy of a nucleus is the minimum energy required to dissociate it into its component neutrons and protons. Neutron or proton binding energies are those required to remove a neutron or a proton, respectively, from a nucleus. Electron binding energy is that required to remove an electron from an atom or a molecule.

biological dose — The radiation dose absorbed in biological material. Measured in *rems*.

biological half-life — The time required for a biological system, such as a man or an animal, to eliminate, by natural processes, half the amount of a substance (such as a radioactive material) that has entered it.

breeder reactor — A reactor that produces fissionable fuel as well as consuming it, especially one that creates more than it consumes. The new fissionable material is created by capture in fertile materials of neutrons from fission. The process by which this occurs is known as breeding.

breeding ratio — The ratio of the number of fissionable atoms produced in a breeder reactor to the number of fissionable atoms consumed in the reactor. Breeding gain is the breeding ratio minus one.

bremsstrahlung — Electromagnetic radiation emitted (as photons) when a fast-moving charged particle (usually an electron) loses energy upon being accelerated and deflected by the electric field surrounding a positively charged atomic nucleus. X rays produced in ordinary X-ray machines are bremsstrahlung. (In German, the term means "braking radiation.")

cladding — The outer jacket of nuclear fuel elements. It prevents corrosion of the fuel and the release of fission products into the coolant. Aluminum or its alloys, stainless steel, and zirconium alloys are common cladding materials.

coffin — A heavily shielded shipping cask for spent (used) fuel elements. Some coffins weigh as much as 75 tons.

collimator — A device for focusing or confining a beam of particles or radiation, such as X rays.

collision — A close approach of two or more particles, photons, atoms, or nuclei, during which such quantities as energy, momentum, and charge may be exchanged.

Compton effect — Elastic scattering of photons (X rays or gamma rays) by electrons. In each such process the electron gains energy and recoils, and the photon loses energy. This

is one of three ways photons lose energy upon inter-
acting with matter, and is the usual method with photons of intermediate energy and materials of low
atomic number. It is named for A. H. Compton,
American physicist, who discovered it in 1923.

counter
A general designation applied to radiation detection
instruments or survey meters that detect and measure
radiation in terms of individual ionizations, display-
ing them either as the accumulated total or their rate
of occurrence.

cross section
[Symbol $\sigma$] A measure of the probability that a
nuclear reaction will occur. Usually measured in
barns, it is the apparent (or effective) area presented
by a target nucleus (or particle) to an oncoming particle or other nuclear radiation, such as a photon of
gamma radiation.

curie
[Symbol Ci] The basic unit to describe the intensity
of radioactivity in a sample of material. The curie is
equal to 37 billion disintegrations per second, which
is approximately the rate of decay of 1 gram of radium. A curie is also a quantity of any nuclide having
1 curie of radioactivity. Named for Marie and Pierre
Curie, who discovered radium in 1898.

cyclotron
A particle accelerator in which charged particles receive repeated synchronized accelerations by electrical fields as the particles spiral outward from their
source. The particles are kept in the spiral by a powerful magnetic field.

daughter
A nuclide formed by the radioactive decay of another
nuclide, which in this context is called the parent.

decay chain
A radioactive series.

decay heat
The heat produced by the decay of radioactive nuclides.

decay, radio-
active
The spontaneous transformation of one nuclide into
a different nuclide or into a different energy state of
the same nuclide. The process results in a decrease,
with time, of the number of the original radioactive
atoms in a sample. It involves the emission from the
nucleus of alpha particles, beta particles (or electrons), or gamma rays; or the nuclear capture or

ejection of orbital electrons; or fission. Also called radioactive disintegration.

decontamination   The removal of radioactive contaminants from surfaces or equipment, as by cleaning and washing with chemicals.

delayed neutrons   Neutrons emitted by radioactive fission products in a reactor over a period of seconds or minutes after a fission takes place. Fewer than 1 % of the neutrons are delayed, the majority being prompt neutrons. Delayed neutrons are important considerations in reactor design and control.

detector   Material or a device that is sensitive to radiation and can produce a response signal suitable for measurement or analysis. A radiation detection instrument.

deuterium   [Symbol $^2$H or D] An isotope of hydrogen whose nucleus contains one neutron and one proton and is therefore about twice as heavy as the nucleus of normal hydrogen, which is only a single proton. Deuterium is often referred to as heavy hydrogen; it occurs in nature as 1 atom to 6500 atoms of normal hydrogen. It is nonradioactive.

deuteron   The nucleus of deuterium. It contains one proton and one neutron.

dose rate   The radiation dose delivered per unit time and measured, for instance, in *rems per hour*.

dosimeter   A device that measures radiation dose, such as a film badge or ionization chamber.

doubling time   The time required for a breeder reactor to produce as much fissionable material as the amount usually contained in its core plus the amount tied up in its fuel cycle (fabrication, reprocessing, etc.). It is estimated as 10 to 20 years in typical reactors.

electron   [Symbol $e^-$] An elementary particle with a unit negative electrical charge and a mass 1/1837 that of the proton. Electrons surround the positively charged nucleus and determine the chemical properties of the atom. Positive electrons, or *positrons*, also exist.

electron capture   [Abbreviation EC] A mode of radioactive decay of a nuclide in which an orbital electron is captured by and merges with the nucleus, thus forming a new nuclide with the mass number unchanged but the atomic number decreased by one.

electron volt
[Abbreviation eV] The amount of kinetic energy gained by an electron when it is accelerated through an electric potential difference of 1 volt. It is equivalent to $1.602 \times 10^{-12}$ erg. It is a unit of energy, or work, not of voltage.

element
One of the 103 known chemical substances that cannot be divided into simpler substances by chemical means. A substance whose atoms all have the same atomic number. Examples: hydrogen, lead, uranium. (Not to be confused with fuel element.)

enriched material
Material in which the percentage of a given isotope present in a material has been artificially increased, so that it is higher than the percentage of that isotope naturally found in the material. Enriched uranium contains more of the fissionable isotope uranium-235 than the naturally occurring percentage (0.7 %).

fast breeder reactor
A reactor that operates with fast neutrons and produces more fissionable material than it consumes.

fast neutron
A neutron with energy greater than approximately 100,000 electron volts.

fast reactor
A reactor in which the fission chain reaction is maintained primarily by fast neutrons rather than by thermal or intermediate neutrons. Fast reactors contain little or no moderator to slow down the neutrons from the speeds at which they are ejected from fissioning nuclei.

film badge
A light-tight package of photographic film worn like a badge by workers in nuclear industry or research, used to measure possible exposure to ionizing radiation. The absorbed dose can be calculated by the degree of film darkening caused by the irradiation.

fission
The splitting of a heavy nucleus into two approximately equal parts (which are nuclei of lighter elements), accompanied by the release of a relatively large amount of energy and generally one or more neutrons. Fission can occur spontaneously, but usually is caused by nuclear absorption of gamma rays, neutrons, or other particles.

fission fragments   The two nuclei which are formed by the fission of a nucleus. Also referred to as primary fission products. They are of medium atomic weight, and are radioactive.

fission products    The nuclei (fission fragments) formed by the fission of heavy elements, plus the nuclides formed by the fission fragments' radioactive decay.

fission yield        The amount of energy released by fission in a thermonuclear (fusion) explosion as distinct from that released by fusion. Also the amount (percentage) of a given nuclide produced by fission.

flux (neutron)       A measure of the intensity of neutron radiaton. It is the number of neutrons passing through 1 square centimeter of a given target in 1 second. Expressed as $nv$, where $n$ = the number of neutrons per cubic centimeter and $v$ = their velocity in centimeters per second.

fuel                 Fissionable material used or usable to produce energy in a reactor. Also applied to a mixture, such as natural uranium, in which only part of the atoms are readily fissionable, if the mixture can be made to sustain a chain reaction.

fuel cycle           The series of steps involved in supplying fuel for nuclear power reactors. It includes mining, refining, the original fabrication of fuel elements, their use in a reactor, chemical processing to recover the fissionable material remaining in the spent fuel, re-enrichment of the fuel material, and refabrication into new fuel elements.

fuel element         A rod, tube, plate, or other mechanical shape or form into which nuclear fuel is fabricated for use in a reactor. (Not to be confused with element.)

fuel reprocessing    The processing of reactor fuel to recover the unused fissionable material.

fundamental
  particles          Elementary particles.

gamma rays           [Symbol $\gamma$] High-energy, short-wavelength electromagnetic radiation. Gamma radiation frequently accompanies alpha and beta emissions and always accompanies fission. Gamma rays are very penetrating and are best stopped or shielded against by dense materials, such as lead or depleted uranium. Gamma rays are essentially similar to X rays, but are usually more energetic, and are nuclear in origin.

gauging
The measurement of the thickness, density, or quantity of material by the amount of radiation it absorbs. This is the most common use of radioactive isotopes in industry.

genetic effects of radiation
Radiation effects that can be transferred from parent to offspring. Any radiation-caused changes in the genetic material of sex cells.

geometry
The spatial configuration, pattern, or relationship of components in an experiment or apparatus. In nuclear physics, it refers to the arrangement of source and detecting equipment. In counting and scanning, the term commonly indicates the percentage of the radiation leaving a sample which reaches the sensitive volume of a counter.

half-life
The time in which half the atoms of a particular radioactive substance disintegrate to another nuclear form. Measured half-lives vary from millionths of a second to billions of years.

half-life,effective
The time required for a radionuclide contained in a biological system, such as a man or an animal, to reduce its activity by half as a combined result of radioactive decay and biological elimination.

half-thickness
The thickness of any given absorber that will reduce the intensity of a beam of radiation to one-half its initial value.

half-value layer
The thickness of any particular material necessary to reduce the dose rate of an X-ray beam to one-half its original value.

health physics
The science concerned with recognition, evaluation, and control of health hazards from ionizing radiation.

hydrogen
[Symbol H] The lightest element, No. 1 in the atomic series. It has two natural isotopes of atomic weights 1 and 2. The first is ordinary hydrogen, or light hydrogen; the second is deuterium, or heavy hydrogen. A third isotope, tritium, atomic weight 3, is a radioactive form produced in reactors by bombarding lithium-6 with neutrons.

| | |
|---|---|
| induced radio-activity | Radioactivity that is created when substances are bombarded with neutrons, as from a nuclear explosion or in a reactor, or with charged particles produced by accelerators. |
| integrated neutron flux | Flux multiplied by time, usually expressed as *nvt,* when $n =$ the number of neutrons per cubic centimeter, $v =$ their velocity in centimeters per second, and $t =$ time in seconds. |
| intensity | The energy or the number of photons or particles of any radiation incident upon a unit area or flowing through a unit of solid material per unit of time. In connection with radioactivity, the number of atoms disintegrating per unit of time. |
| intermediate (epithermal) neutron | A neutron having energy greater than that of a thermal neutron but less than that of a fast neutron. The range is generally considered to be between about 0.5 and 100,000 electron volts. |
| ion exchange | A chemical process involving the reversible interchange of various ions between a solution and a solid material usually a plastic or a resin. It is used to separate and purify chemicals, such as fission products, rare earths, etc., in solutions. |
| ion pair | A closely associated positive ion and negative ion (usually an electron) having charges of the same magnitude and formed from a neutral atom or molecule by radiation. |
| ionization | The process of adding one or more electrons to, or removing one or more electrons from, atoms or molecules, thereby creating ions. High temperatures, electrical discharges, or nuclear radiations can cause ionization. |
| ionization chamber | An instrument that detects and measures ionizing radiation by measuring the electrical current that flows when radiation ionizes gas in a chamber, making the gas a conductor of the electricity. |
| ionizing event | Any occurrence in which an ion or group of ions is produced; for example, by passage of a charged particle through matter. |
| ionizing radiation | Any radiation displacing electrons from atoms or molecules, thereby producing ions. Examples, alpha, |

|  |  |
|---|---|
| | beta, gamma radiation, short-wave ultraviolet light. Ionizing radiation may produce severe skin or tissue damage. |
| irradiation | Exposure to radiation, as in a nuclear reactor. |
| isobar | One of two or more nuclides having about the same atomic mass but different atomic numbers, hence different chemical properties. Example: $^{14}_6C$, $^{14}_7N$, and $^{14}_8O$ are isobars. |
| isodose curves | Curves or lines drawn to connect points where identical amounts of radiant energy reach a certain depth in tissue. |
| isointensity contours | Imaginary lines on the surface of the ground or water, or lines drawn on a map, joining points in a radiation field which have the same radiation intensity at a given time. |
| isomer | One of two or more nuclides with the same numbers of neutrons and protons in their nuclei, but with different energies; a nuclide in the excited state and a similar nuclide in the ground state are isomers. |
| isotone | One of several nuclides having the same number of neutrons but a different number of protons in their nuclei. Example: potassium-39 ($^{39}_{19}K_{20}$) and calcium-40 ($^{40}_{20}Ca_{20}$) are isotones. |
| isotope | One of two or more atoms with the same atomic number (the same chemical element) but with different atomic weights. An equivalent statement is that the nuclei of isotopes have the same number of protons but different numbers of neutrons. Thus $^{12}_6C$, $^{13}_6C$, and $^{14}_6C$ are isotopes of the element carbon, the subscripts denoting their common atomic numbers, the superscripts denoting the differing mass numbers, or approximate atomic weights. Isotopes usually have very nearly the same chemical properties, but somewhat different physical properties. |
| isotope separation | The process of separating isotopes from one another, or changing their relative abundances, as by gaseous diffusion or electromagnetic separation. All systems are based on the mass differences of the isotopes. Isotope separation is a step in the isotopic enrichment process. |

isotope enrich-
ment

A process by which the relative abundances of the isotopes of a given element are altered, thus producing a form of the element which has been enriched in one particular isotope. Example: enriching natural uranium in the uranium-235 isotope.

K-capture

The capture by an atomic nucleus of an orbital electron from the first (innermost) orbit or shell, or K-shell, surrounding the nucleus.

mass number

[Symbol $A$] The sum of the neutrons and protons in a nucleus. It is the nearest whole number to an atom's atomic weight. For instance, the mass number of uranium-235 is 235.

maximum cred-
ible accident

The most serious reactor accident that can reasonably be imagined from any adverse combination of equipment malfunction, operating errors, and other foreseeable causes. The term is used to analyze the safety characteristics of a reactor. Reactors are designed to be safe even if a maximum credible accident should occur.

maximum per-
missible con-
centration
(MPC)

The amount of radioactive material in air, water, or food which might be expected to result in a maximum permissible dose to persons consuming them at a standard rate of intake.

maximum per-
missible dose
(MPD) (max-
imum permis-
sible exposure)

That dose of ionizing radiation established by competent authorities as an amount below which there is no reasonable expectation of risk to human health, and which at the same time is somewhat below the lowest level at which a definite hazard is believed to exist.

mean free path

The average distance traveled by a particle, atom, or molecule between collisions or interactions.

mean life

The average time during which an atom, an excited nucleus, a radionuclide, or a particle exists in a particular form.

megawatt-day
per ton

A unit used for expressing the burnup of fuel in a reactor; specifically, the number of megawatt-days of heat output per metric ton of fuel in the reactor.

quality factor

The factor by which absorbed dose is to be multiplied to obtain a quantity that expresses on a common scale, for all ionizing radiations, the irradiation incurred by exposed persons.

| | |
|---|---|
| quantum | Unit quantity of energy according to the quantum theory. It is equal to the product of the frequency of radiation of the energy and $6.6256 \times 10^{-27}$ erg- sec. The photon carries a quantum of electromagnetic energy. |
| rad | (Acronym for *r*adiation *a*bsorbed *d*ose.) The basic unit of absorbed dose of ionizing radiation. A dose of one rad means the absorption of 100 ergs of radiation energy per gram of absorbing material. |
| radiation | The emission and propagation of energy through matter or space by means of electromagnetic disturbances which display both wave-like and particle-like behavior; in this context the "particles" are known as photons. Also, the energy so propagated. The term has been extended to include streams of fast-moving particles (alpha and beta particles, free neutrons, cosmic radiation, etc.). Nuclear radiation is that emitted from atomic nuclei in various nuclear reactions, including alpha, beta, and gamma radiation and neutrons. |
| radiation accidents | Accidents resulting in the spread of radioactive material or in the exposure of individuals to radiation. |
| radiation area | Any accessible area in which the level of radiation is such that a major portion of an individual's body could receive in any one hour a dose in excess of 5 millirem, or in any 5 consecutive days a dose in excess of 150 millirem. |
| radiation biology | (See radiobiology.) |
| radiation burn | Radiation damage to the skin. Beta burns result from skin contact with or exposure to emitters of beta particles. Flash burns result from sudden thermal radiation. |
| radiation chemistry | The branch of chemistry that is concerned with the chemical effects, including decomposition, of energetic radiation or particles on matter. |
| radiation damage | A general term for the harmful effects of radiation on matter. |
| radiation detection instruments | Devices that detect and record the characteristics of ionizing radiation. |
| radiation dosimetry | The measurement of the amount of radiation delivered to a specific place or the amount of radiation that was absorbed there. |

radiation illness    An acute organic disorder that follows exposure to relatively severe doses of ionizing radiation. It is characterized by nausea, vomiting, diarrhea, blood cell changes, and in later stages by hemorrhage and loss of hair.

radioactive series    A succession of nuclides, each of which transforms by radioactive disintegration into the next until a stable nuclide results. The first member is called the parent, the intermediate members are called daughters, and the final stable member is called the end product.

radioactive source    A radiation source.

radioactive standard    A sample of radioactive material, usually with a long half-life, in which the number and type of radioactive atoms at a definite reference time is known. These are used in calibrating radiation measuring equipment or for comparing measurements in different laboratories.

radioactive tracer    A small quantity of radioactive isotope (either with carrier or carrier-free) used to follow biological, chemical, or other processes, by detection, determination, or localization of the radioactivity.

radioactivity    The spontaneous decay or disintegration of an unstable atomic nucleus, usually accompanied by the emission of ionizing radiation. (Often shortened to "activity.")

radiobiology    The body of knowledge and the study of the principles, mechanisms, and effects of ionizing radiation on living matter.

radiochemistry    The body of knowledge and the study of the chemical properties and reactions of radioactive materials.

radioelement    An element containing one or more radioactive isotopes; a radioactive element.

radiogenic    Of radioactive origin; produced by radioactive transformation.

radiography    The use of ionizing radiation for the production of shadow images on a photographic emulsion. Some of the rays (gamma rays or X rays) pass through the subject, while others are partially or completely absorbed by the more opaque parts of the subject and thus cast a shadow on the photographic film.

| | |
|---|---|
| radioisotope | A radioactive isotope. An unstable isotope of an element that decays or disintegrates spontaneously, emitting radiation. More than 1300 natural and artificial radioisotopes have been identified. |
| radionuclide | A radioactive nuclide. |
| radioresistance | A relative resistance of cells, tissues, organs, or organisms to the injurious action of radiation. |
| radiosensitivity | A relative susceptibility of cells, tissues, organs or organisms to the injurious action of radiation. |
| recycling | The reuse of fissionable material, after it has been recovered by chemical processing from spent or depleted reactor fuel, re-enriched, and then refabricated into new fuel elements. |
| reflector | A layer of material immediately surrounding a reactor core which scatters back or reflects into the core many neutrons that would otherwise escape. The returned neutrons can then cause more fissions and improve the neutron economy of the reactor. Common reflector materials are graphite, beryllium, and natural uranium. |
| relative biological effectiveness (RBE) | A factor used to compare the biological effectiveness of different types of ionizing radiation. It is the inverse ratio of the amount of absorbed radiation, required to produce a given effect, to a standard (or reference) radiation required to produce the same effect. |
| rem | (Acronym for *r*oentgen *e*quivalent *m*an.) The unit of dose of any ionizing radiation which produces the same biological effect as a unit of absorbed dose of ordinary X rays. The RBE dose (in rems) = RBE × absorbed dose (in rads). |
| rep | (Acronym for *r*oentgen *e*quivalent *p*hysical.) An obsolete unit of absorbed dose of any ionizing radiation, with a magnitude of 93 ergs per gram. It has been superseded by the rad. |
| reprocessing | Fuel reprocessing. |
| roentgen | [Abbreviation R] A unit of exposure to ionizing radiation. It is that amount of gamma or X rays required to produce ions carrying 1 electrostatic unit of electrical charge (either positive or negative) in 1 |

cubic centimeter of dry air under standard conditions. Named after Wilhelm Roentgen, German scientist who discovered X rays in 1895.

scanning radioisotope  A method of determining the location and amount of radioactive isotopes within the body by measurements taken with instruments outside the body; usually the instrument, called a *scanner,* moves in a regular pattern over the area to be studied, or over the whole body, and makes a visual record.

scattering  A process that changes a particle's trajectory. Scattering is caused by particle collisions with atoms, nuclei, and other particles or by interactions with fields of magnetic force. If the scattered particle's internal energy (as contrasted with its kinetic energy) is unchanged by the collision, elastic scattering prevails; if there is a change in the internal energy, the process is called inelastic scattering.

scavenging  In chemistry, the use of a nonspecific precipitate to remove one or more undesirable radionuclides from solution by absorption or coprecipitation. In atmospheric physics, the removal of radionuclides from the atmosphere by the action of rain, snow, or dew.

shield (shielding)  A body of material used to reduce the passage of radiation.

slow neutron  A thermal neutron.

SNAP  (Acronym for *s*ystems for *n*uclear *a*uxiliary *p*ower.) An Atomic Energy Commission program to develop small auxiliary nuclear power sources for specialized space, land, and sea uses. Two approaches are employed; the first uses heat from radioisotope decay to produce electricity directly by thermoelectric or thermionic methods; the second uses heat from small reactors to produce electricity by thermoelectric or thermionic methods or by turning a small turbine and electric generator.

somatic effects of radiation  Effects of radiation limited to the exposed individual, as distinguished from genetic effects (which also affect subsequent, unexposed generations). Large radiation doses can be fatal. Smaller doses may make the individual noticeably ill, may merely produce temporary changes in blood cell levels detectable only in the laboratory, or may produce no detectable effects whatever. Also called physiological effects of radiation.

source            (See radiation source.)

source material    In atomic energy law any material, except special nuclear material, which contains 0.05 % or more of uranium, thorium, or any combination of the two.

special nuclear material    In U.S. atomic energy law, this term refers to plutonium-239, uranium-233, uranium containing more than the natural abundance of uranium-235, or any artificially enriched material in any of these substances.

species    A particular kind of atomic nucleus, atom, molecule, or ion; a nuclide.

specific activity    The radioactivity of a radioisotope of an element per unit weight of the element in a sample. The activity per unit mass of a pure radionuclide. The activity per unit weight of any sample of radioactive material.

specific ionization    The number of ion pairs formed per unit of distance along the track of an ion passing through matter.

specific power    The power generated in a nuclear reactor per unit mass of fuel. It is expressed in kilowatts of heat per kilogram of fuel.

spontaneous fission    Fission that occurs without an external stimulus. Several heavy isotopes decay mainly in this manner; examples: californium-252 and californium-254. The process occurs occasionally in all fissionable materials, including uranium-235.

stable    Incapable of spontaneous change. Not radioactive.

stable isotope    An isotope that does not undergo radioactive decay.

stopping power    A measure of the effect of a substance upon the kinetic energy of a charged particle passing through it.

thermal efficiency    The ratio of the electric power produced by a power plant to the amount of heat produced by the fuel; a measure of the efficiency with which the plant converts thermal to electrical energy.

thermal (slow) neutron    A neutron in thermal equilibrium with its surrounding medium. Thermal neutrons are those that have been slowed down by a moderator to an average

|                          | speed of about 2200 meters per second (at room temperature) from the much higher initial speeds they had when expelled by fission. This velocity is similar to that of gas molecules at ordinary temperatures. |
| --- | --- |
| thermal reactor | A reactor in which the fission chain reaction is sustained primarily by thermal neutrons. Most reactors are thermal reactors. |
| thermal shield | A layer or layers of high density material located within a reactor pressure vessel or between the vessel and the biological shield to reduce radiation heating in the vessel and the biological shield. |
| thermionic conversion | The conversion of heat into electricity by evaporating electrons from a hot metal surface and condensing them on a cooler surface. No moving parts are required. |
| thermocouple | A device consisting essentially of two conductors made of different metals, joined at both ends, producing a loop in which an electric current will flow when there is a difference in temperature between the two junctions. |
| thermoelectric conversion | The conversion of heat into electricity by the use of thermocouples. |
| waste, radioactive | Equipment and materials (from nuclear operations) which are radioactive and for which there is no further use. Wastes are generally classified as high-level (having radioactivity concentrations of hundreds to thousands of curies per gallon or cubic foot), low-level (in the range of 1 microcurie per gallon or cubic foot), or intermediate (between these extremes). |
| X ray | A penetrating form of electromagnetic radiation emitted either when the inner orbital electrons of an excited atom return to their normal state (these are characteristic X rays), or when a metal target is bombarded with high-speed electrons (these are bremsstrahlung). X rays are always nonnuclear in origin. |
| yield | The total energy released in a nuclear explosion. It is usually expressed in equivalent tons of TNT (the quantity of TNT required to produce a corresponding amount of energy). Low yield is generally considered |

to be less than 20 kilotons; low intermediate yield from 20 to 200 kilotons; intermediate yield from 200 kilotons to 1 megaton. There is no standardized term to cover yields from 1 megaton upward.

$Z$     The symbol for atomic number.

# INDEX

411